USERS' GUIDES TO THE MEDICAL LITERATURE

Essentials of
Evidence-Based
Clinical Practice

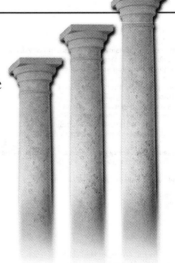

The Evidence-Based
Medicine Working Group

Edited by
Gordon Guyatt, MD
Drummond Rennie, MD

JAMA
&
ARCHIVES
JOURNALS
American Medical Association

AMA Press

Vice President, Business Products: Anthony J. Frankos
Editorial Director: Mary Lou White
Director, Production and Manufacturing: Jean Roberts
Senior Acquisitions Editor: Barry Bowlus
Developmental Editor: Susan Moss
Director, Marketing: JD Kinney
Marketing Manager: Amy Roberts
Senior Production Coordinator: Rosalyn Carlton
Senior Print Coordinator: Ronnie Summers
Project Manager: Katharine Dvorak

McMaster University and University of Alberta Staff:
Christina Lacchetti and Tanya Voth

JAMA **Book Liaison:** Annette Flanagin

ISBN 1-57947-191-9
BP92:0129-00:07/01

CONTENTS

Part 1

The Basics: Using the Medical Literature

Part 2

Beyond the Basics: Using and Teaching the Principles of Evidence-Based Medicine

FOREWORD

When I was attending school in wartime Britain, staples of
the curriculum, along with cold baths, mathematics, boiled
cabbage, and long cross-country runs, were Latin and
French. It was obvious that Latin was a theoretical exercise—
the Romans were dead, after all. However, while France was
clearly visible just across the Channel, for years it was either
occupied or inaccessible, so learning the French language
seemed just as impractical and theoretical an exercise.
It was unthinkable to me and my teachers that I would
ever put it to practical use—that French was a language to
be spoken.

This is the relationship too many practitioners have with
the medical literature—clearly visible but utterly inaccessible. We recognize that practice should be based on discover-
ies announced in the medical journals. But we also recognize
that every few years the literature doubles in size, and every
year we seem to have less time to weigh it,[1] so every day the
task of taming the literature becomes more hopeless. The
translation of those hundreds of thousands of articles into
everyday practice appears to be an obscure task left to others.
And as the literature becomes more inaccessible, so does the
idea that the literature has any utility for a particular patient
become more fanciful.

This book is designed to change all that. It's designed to
make the clinician fluent in the language of the medical literature in all its forms. To free the clinician from practicing
medicine by rote, by guesswork, and by their variably inte-
grated experience. To put a stop to clinicians being ambushed
by drug company representatives, or by their patients, telling
them of new therapies the clinicians are unable to evaluate.
To end their dependence on out-of-date authority. To enable
the practitioner to work with the patient and use the literature as a tool to solve the patient's problems. To provide the

clinician access to what is relevant and the ability to assess its validity and whether it applies to a specific patient. In other words, to put the clinician in charge of the single most powerful resource in medicine.

The Users' Guides Series in *JAMA*

I have left it to Gordon Guyatt, the moving force, principal editor, and most prolific coauthor of the *Users' Guides to the Medical Literature* series in *JAMA,* to describe the history of this series and of this book in the accompanying Preface. But where did *JAMA* come into this story?

In the late 1980s, at the invitation of my friend David Sackett, I visited his department at McMaster University to discuss another Sackett/*JAMA* venture—a series examining the evidence behind the clinical history and examination. Following these discussions, a series of articles and systematic reviews was developed and, with the enthusiastic support of then *JAMA* editor-in-chief, George Lundberg, *JAMA* began publishing the *Rational Clinical Examination* series in 1992.[1] By that time, I had formed an excellent working relationship with the brilliant group at McMaster. Like Sackett, their leader, they tended to be iconoclastic, expert at working together and forming alliances with new and talented workers, and intellectually exacting. Like their leader, they delivered on their promises.

So, when I heard that they were thinking of updating the wonderful series of "Readers' Guides" published in 1981 in the *Canadian Medical Association Journal*, I took advantage of this working relationship to urge that they update and expand the series for *JAMA*. Together with Sackett, and first with Andy Oxman, and then with Gordon Guyatt taking the lead (when Oxman left to take his present position in Oslo), the *Users' Guides* series was born. We began publishing articles in the series in *JAMA* in 1993.[2,3]

At the start, we thought we might have eight or 10 articles, but the response from readers was so enthusiastic, and the variety of types of article in the literature so great, that 7 years later I still found myself receiving, sending for review, and editing new articles for the series. In the end, Gordon Guyatt and I closed this series at 25, appearing as 33 separate journal articles.

The passage of 8 years during the preparation of the series had a particularly useful result. Some subjects that in 1992-1993 were scarcely discussed in the major medical journals, but that have burgeoned recently, could receive the attention that had become their due. For instance, in 2000, *JAMA* published two Users' Guides on how readers should approach reports of qualitative research in health care.[4,5] To take another example, systematic reviews and meta-analyses, given a huge boost by the activities of the Cochrane Collaboration, have become prominent features of the literature. An article in the series discusses how to use such studies.[6] Another example would be the guide on electronic health information resources.[7]

The Book

From the start, readers kept urging us to put the series together as a book. That had been our intention right from the start, but each new article delayed its implementation. How fortunate! When the original *Readers' Guides* appeared in the *CMAJ* in 1981, Gordon Guyatt's phrase "evidence-based medicine" had never been coined, and only a tiny proportion of health care workers possessed computers. The Internet did not exist and electronic publication was only a dream. In 1992, the Web—for practical purposes—had scarcely been invented, the dot.com bubble hadn't appeared, let alone burst, and the health professions were only beginning to become computer-literate. But at the end of the 1990s, when Guyatt and I approached AMA Press with the idea of publishing not merely the standard printed book, but also Web-based and CD-ROM formats of the book, they were immediately receptive. Putting the latter part into practice has been the notable achievement of Dr Rob Hayward, of the University of Alberta.

In addition, the science and art of evidence-based medicine, which this series does so much to reinforce, has developed remarkably during the past 8 years, and this is reflected in every page of the book.

The requirements for individual articles in a journal series are different from those of separate chapters in a book. To make it possible to understand each article by itself, a good deal of redundancy had to be built in, and one of Guyatt's tasks when editing the book was to remove this extra material. In addition, the Evidence-Based Medicine Working Group has updated the articles in the series so that they all reflect the latest practice.

First, I must thank Gordon Guyatt, who has become a good friend over the years, for making my own task, first as editor of the *JAMA* series and then as co-editor of the book, extraordinarily easy and pleasant, as well as educational. I know personally and greatly admire a good number of his colleagues, but it would be invidious to name them, given the huge collective effort this 9-year effort has entailed. On the *JAMA* side, I must thank Annette Flanagin, a wonderfully efficient, creative, and diplomatic colleague at *JAMA*. The book would not exist without the vision of Tony Frankos and the hard work, enthusiasm, and dedication of Barry Bowlus, both of AMA Press. Susan Moss has been an exemplary book editor, meticulous, thoughtful, and long-suffering. Between her and Gordon, I was left little to do. I also wish to thank Jean Roberts, Katharine Dvorak, and Amy Roberts of AMA Press. Finally, I thank my wonderful new boss, Cathy DeAngelis, Editor-in-Chief of *JAMA*, for her strong backing of me, my colleagues, and this project; for her tolerance; and for keeping up everyone's spirits with her dreadful jokes.

Drummond Rennie, MD

University of California, San Francisco
Deputy Editor, JAMA

References

1. Durack DT. The weight of medical knowledge. *N Engl J Med*. 1978;298:773-775.

2. Sackett DL, Rennie D. The science of the art of the clinical examination. *JAMA*. 1992;267:2650-2652.

3. Guyatt GH, Rennie D. Users' guides to the medical literature. *JAMA*. 1993;270:2096-2097.

4. Giacomini MK, Cook DJ. Users' guides to the medical literature, XXIII: qualitative research in health care. A. Are the results of the study valid? Evidence-Based Medicine Working Group. *JAMA*. 2000;284:357-362.

5. Giacomini MK, Cook DJ. Users' guides to the medical literature, XXIII: qualitative research in health care. B. What are the results and how do they help me care for my patients? Evidence-Based Medicine Working Group. *JAMA*. 2000;284:478-482.

6. Oxman AD, Cook DJ, Guyatt GH. Users' guides to the medical literature, VI: how to use an overview. Evidence-Based Medicine Working Group. *JAMA*. 1994;272:1367-1371.

7. Hunt DL, Jaeschke R, McKibbon KA. Users' guides to the medical literature, XXI: using electronic health information resources in evidence-based practice. Evidence-Based Medicine Working Group. *JAMA*. 2000;283:1875-1879.

Users' Guides to Medical Literature Series in *JAMA*

VIII. Wilson MC, Hayward RS, Tunis SR, Bass EB, Guyatt G. How to use clinical practice guidelines. B. What are the recommendations and will they help you in caring for your patients? The Evidence-Based Medicine Working Group. *JAMA*. 1995;274:1630-1632.

IX. Guyatt GH, Sackett DL, Sinclair JC, Hayward R, Cook DJ, Cook RJ. A method for grading health care recommendations. Evidence-Based Medicine Working Group. *JAMA*. 1995;274:1800-1804.

X. Naylor GH, Guyatt GH. How to use an article reporting variations in the outcomes of health services. The Evidence-Based Medicine Working Group. *JAMA*. 1996;275:554-558.

XI. Naylor CD, Guyatt GH. How to use an article about a clinical utilization review. The Evidence-Based Medicine Working Group. *JAMA*. 1996;275:1435-1439.

XII. Guyatt G, Naylor CD, Juniper E, Heyland DK, Jaeschke R, Cook DJ. How to use articles about health-related quality of life measurements. The Evidence-Based Medicine Working Group. *JAMA*. 1997;277:1232-1237.

XIII. Drummond MF, Richardson WS, O'Brien BJ, Levine M, Heyland D. How to use an article on economic analysis of clinical practice. A. Are the results of the study valid? *JAMA*. 1997;277:1552-1557.

XIII. O'Brien BJ, Heyland D, Richardson WS, Levine M, Drummond MF. How to use an article on economic analysis of clinical practice. B. What are the results and will they help me in caring for my patients? The Evidence-Based Medicine Working Group. *JAMA*. 1997;277:1802-1806.

XIV. Dans AL, Dans LF, Guyatt GH, Richardson S. How to decide on the applicability of clinical trials results to your patient. *JAMA*. 1998;279:545-549.

XV. Richardson WS, Wilson MC, Guyatt GH, Nishikawa J. How to use an article about disease probability for differential diagnosis. The Evidence-Based Medicine Working Group. *JAMA*. 1999;281:1214-1219.

XVI. Guyatt GH, Sinclair J, Cook DJ, Glasziou P. How to use a treatment recommendation. The Evidence-Based Medicine Working Group and the Cochrane Applicability Methods Working Group. *JAMA*. 1999;281:1836-1843.

XVII. Barratt A, Irwig L, Glasziou P, Cumming RG, Raffle A, Hicks N, Gray JA, Guyatt GH. How to use guidelines and recommendations about screening. The Evidence-Based Medicine Working Group. *JAMA*. 1999;281:2029-2034.

PREFACE

This book grew out of a series of 25 articles published in
JAMA between 1993 and 2000, the original Users' Guides to
the Medical Literature. Clinicians and medical educators
have found this series, which includes contributions by
approximately 50 clinicians expert in evidence-based medicine, to be invaluable.

*The Users' Guides to the Medical Literature: Essentials for
Evidence-Based Clinical Practice* goes beyond the Users'
Guides in a number of ways. First, it incorporates the
advances in clinical research that have taken place during the
past 7 years relevant to understanding sources of bias in
research studies, quantifying the magnitude of benefits and
risks, and incorporating patient values. Second, it incorporates what we have learned about how to better teach evidence-based medicine (EBM) concepts and approaches to
clinicians. Third, it clearly distinguishes what we believe
every clinician should know about EBM (Part 1 of this
book) from what those who wish to delve farther might like
to know (Part 2 of the written book), and from those who
wish to role-model and teach EBM should know (the larger
Part 2 on the CD-ROM). Fourth, we have eliminated redun-
dancies, linked different sections, and ensured consistency of
style and conceptual presentation. Fifth, the focus on clinical
decision making, already prominent in the Users' Guides, has
been further strengthened through the addition of clinical
examples* and through highlighting of the role of patient
values in choosing optimal therapy.

Finally, this book is available in both paper and electronic
formats. Robert Hayward has taken primary responsibility

---

* Most clinical scenarios and their resolutions were finalized at the end of
  August 2000; they do not include evidence that has appeared since that time.

for translation of the material into both CD-ROM and Web-based formats, the latter of which includes a large number of additional aids for the practice of EBM. Rob has done a magnificent job as coeditor of the electronic versions, and his contribution, representing an enormous expenditure of both time and energy, has been vital.

How It All Began

During the late 1970s, a group of clinical epidemiologists at McMaster University, led by David Sackett and including Brian Haynes, Peter Tugwell, and Victor Neufeld, were planning a series of articles advising clinicians on how to read clinical journals. The series appeared in the *Canadian Medical Association Journal* beginning in 1981. The group proposed the term *critical appraisal* to describe the application of the basic rules of evidence presented in that series. After teaching critical appraisal for a number of years, members of the group became increasingly aware of both the necessity and the challenges of motivating clinicians to go beyond merely browsing the literature and, rather, to actually use the information in solving patient problems. David Sackett suggested the term *bringing critical appraisal to the bedside* to describe the process of the practical application of evidence from the medical literature to patient care.

In 1990, I assumed the position of Residency Director of the internal medicine program at McMaster. Through Dave Sackett's leadership, the concept of bringing critical appraisal to the bedside had evolved into a philosophy of medical practice based on knowledge and understanding of the medical literature supporting each clinical decision. We believed this represented a fundamentally different style of practice warranting a formal term that would capture this difference.

In the spring of 1990, with the mission to train physicians who would practice this new brand of medicine, I presented our plans for changing the program to the members of the Department of Medicine, many of whom were not sympathetic. The term I suggested to describe the new approach was *scientific medicine*. Those already hostile to the challenge to the traditional sources of medical authority were incensed by the term; specifically, they were disturbed at the implication that they had previously been unscientific. My second try at a name for our philosophy of medical practice, *evidence-based medicine*, proved felicitous.

The term *evidence-based medicine* first appeared in the autumn of 1990 in an informational document intended for residents entering or considering application to our residency program. An excerpt follows:

> Residents are taught to develop an attitude of "enlightened scepticism" toward the application of diagnostic, therapeutic, and prognostic technologies in their day-to-day management of patients. This approach, which has been called "evidence-based medicine," is based on principles outlined in the text "Clinical Epidemiology." The goal is to be aware of the evidence on which one's practice is based, the soundness of the evidence, and the strength of inference the evidence permits. The strategy employed requires a clear delineation of the relevant question(s); a thorough search of the literature relating to the questions; a critical appraisal of the evidence, and its applicability to the clinical situation; and a balanced application of the conclusions to the clinical problem.

The term subsequently appeared in print in the *ACP Journal Club* in 1991.[1] Meanwhile, our group of enthusiastic evidence-based medical educators at McMaster, led by Deborah Cook, Roman Jaeschke, Jim Nishikawa, Pat Brill-Edwards, and Akbar Panju, in addition to the four original innovators, were refining our practice and teaching of EBM. Because the process proved exciting and productive, we concluded that the concept of a new approach to medical practice would prove useful for the larger community of medical educators.

Consequently, we linked up with a larger group of academic physicians, primarily from the United States, to form the first international Evidence-based Medicine Working Group, and we published an article that expanded greatly on the existing description of evidence-based medicine, labeling it a paradigm shift.[2]

The Evidence-based Medicine Working Group then addressed the task of producing a new set of articles, the successor to the *Canadian Medical Association Journal* "Readers' Guides" series, to present a much more practical approach to applying the medical literature to clinical practice. Although many people made important contributions, the non-McMaster faculty who provided the greatest input to the intensive development of educational strategies included Scott Richardson, Mark Wilson, Robert Hayward, and Virginia Moyer. With the unflagging support and wise counsel of *JAMA* editor Drummond Rennie, the Evidence-based Medicine Working Group created a 25-part series called *The Users' Guides to the Medical Literature.* This series was published in *JAMA* between 1993 and 2000,[3] and the book you are now reading is the direct descendent of those Users' Guides.

It did not take long for health care practitioners to realize that the principles of EBM were equally applicable to such allied health care workers as nurses, dentists, orthodontists, physical therapists, occupational therapists, chiropractors, podiatrists, and others. Thus, terms such as *evidence-based health care* or *evidence-based practice* are appropriate to cover the full range of clinical applications of the evidence-based approach to patient care. However, since this book is directed primarily to physicians, we have stayed with the term *evidence-based medicine* (EBM).

Who Should Read This Book?

Any clinician who wishes to understand the medical literature, and to use it more effectively in solving patient problems, will benefit from this book. The written book, focusing
on the essentials, is designed for those who wish to develop a
core knowledge of basic. Most medical students, residents,
and community practitioners will likely be satisfied with this
level of understanding. They will find Part 1 filled with case
scenarios and clinical examples that facilitate their understanding, and they will also uncover tips for finding the best
information and applying it to their practice.

A Note About Authorship

Among the innovative aspects of this book is the way we have
dealt with authorship, which is shared by all 50 members of
the EBM Working Group. For most sections of the book, we
began with the relevant Users' Guides as they appeared in
JAMA; in most cases, the authors of those guides participated
in their revision and retain authorship. In addition to the
input of the primary authors, other members of the EBM
Working Group have reviewed each section in detail. In certain instances, the magnitude of their input has warranted a
coauthorship role. In other cases, we have acknowledged their
valuable suggestions by means of prominent placement of
their names immediately below the author byline. On page
xvii we acknowledge the members of the EBM Working
Group who participated in the creation of this book.

Producing this book has proved to be an enormously
stimulating collaborative adventure. We hope the results
provide a sense of how exciting it is to practice evidence-
based medicine.

Gordon Guyatt, MD
McMaster University

References

1. Guyatt GH. Evidence-based medicine. *ACP Journal Club*. 1991;114:A-16.

2. Evidence-based medicine working group. Evidence-based medicine: a new approach to the teaching of medicine. *JAMA*. 1992;268:2420-2425.

3. Guyatt GH, Rennie D. Users' Guides to the Medical Literature [editorial]. *JAMA*. 1993;270:2096-2097.

CONTRIBUTORS

John Attia, MD, MSc, PhD
Centre for Clinical Epidemiology
  and Biostatistics
Royal Newcastle Hospital
Newcastle, NSW, Australia

**Alexandra Barratt, MBBS, MPH,
  PhD**
Public Health and Community
  Medicine
University of Sydney
Sydney, NSW, Australia

Eric Bass, MD, MPH
Division of Internal Medicine
Johns Hopkins University School
  of Medicine
Baltimore, Maryland, USA

Patrick Bossuyt, PhD
Clinical Epidemiology and
  Biostatistics
University of Amsterdam
Amsterdam, the Netherlands

Heiner Bucher, MD
Department of Internal Medicine
University Hospital Basel
Basel, Switzerland

Deborah Cook, MD, MSc
Department of Medicine
Faculty of Health Sciences
McMaster University
Hamilton, Ontario, Canada

Jonathan Craig, FRACP, PhD
Department of Public Health
  and Community Medicine
Faculty of Medicine
University of Sydney
Sydney, NSW, Australia

**Robert Cumming, MB BS, MPH,
  PhD, FAFPHM**
Department of Public Health
  and Community Medicine
University of Sydney
Sydney, NSW, Australia

Antonio Dans, MD
Clinical Epidemiological Unit
University of the Philippines
Manila, Philippines

Leonila Dans, MD
Clinical Epidemiological Unit
University of the Philippines
Manila, Philippines

Alan Detsky, MD, PhD
Department of Clinical
  Epidemiology and Biostatistics
McMaster University
Hamilton, Ontario, Canada

P J Devereaux, BSc, MD
Department of Medicine
McMaster University
Hamilton, Ontario, Canada

Michael Drummond, BSc, MCom, DPhil
Centre for Health Economics
University of York
York, England, UK

Mita Giacomini, PhD
Centre for Health Economics
and Policy Analysis
McMaster University
Hamilton, Ontario, Canada

Paul Glasziou, MBBS, PhD
Department of Social and
Preventative Medicine
University of Queensland Medical
School
Herston, QLD, Australia

Lee Green, MD, MPH
Department of Family Medicine
University of Michigan Medical
Centre
Ann Arbor, Michigan, USA

Trisha Greenhalgh, MA, MD, FRCP, FRCGP
Unit for Evidence-Based Practice
and Policy
Royal Free and University College
Medical School
London, England, UK

Gordon Guyatt, MD, MSc
Chair, Evidence-Based Medicine
Working Group
Clinical Epidemiology and
Biostatistics and Medicine
McMaster University
Hamilton, Ontario, Canada

Ted Haines, MD, MSc
Departments of Clinical
Epidemiology and Biostatistics,
and Occupational Health
Program
McMaster University
Hamilton, Ontario, Canada

David Haslam, MD, FRCPC
North Bay Psychiatric Hospital
North Bay, Ontario, Canada

Rose Hatala, MD, MSc, FRCPC
Department of Medicine
McMaster University
Hamilton, Ontario, Canada

Brian Haynes, MD, MSc, PhD
Department of Clinical
Epidemiology and Biostatistics
McMaster University
Hamilton, Ontario, Canada

Robert Hayward, MD, MPH, FRCPC
Centres for Health Evidence
University of Alberta
Edmonton, Alberta, Canada

Daren Heyland, MD, FRCPC, MSc
Medicine and Community Health
and Epidemiology
Queen's University
Kingston, Ontario, Canada

Anne Holbrook, MD, PharmD, MSc
Centre for Evaluation
 of Medicines
Faculty of Sciences
McMaster University
Hamilton, Ontario, Canada

Dereck Hunt, MD
Health Information Research Unit
Faculty of Health Sciences
McMaster University
Hamilton, Ontario, Canada

Les Irwig, MBBCh, PhD, FFPHM
Department of Public Health
 and Community Medicine
University of Sydney
Sydney, NSW, Australia

Roman Jaeschke, MD, MSc
Department of Medicine
McMaster University
Hamilton, Ontario, Canada

Elizabeth Juniper, MCSP, MSc
Department of Clinical
 Epidemiology and Biostatistics
McMaster University
Hamilton, Ontario, Canada

Regina Kunz, MD, MSc
Department of Nephrology
Charite Humboldt-University
Berlin, Germany

Christina Lacchetti, MHSc
Departments of Clinical
 Epidemiology and Biostatistics
 and Medicine
McMaster University
Hamilton, Ontario, Canada

Andreas Laupacis, MD, MSc
Departments of Medicine and
 Epidemiology and Community
 Medicine
University of Ottawa
Ottawa, Ontario, Canada

Hui Lee, MD, MSc, FRCPC
Department of Medicine
McMaster University
Hamilton, Ontario, Canada

Luz Letelier, MD
General Internal Medicine
Servicio de Medicina
Hospital Dr. Sotero del Rio
U.D.A. Universidad Catolica
 de Chile
Santiago, Chile

Raymond Leung, MDCM
Centres for Health Evidence
 Department of Cardiology
University of Alberta
Edmonton, Alberta, Canada

Mitchell Levine, MD, MSc
Centre for Evaluation
 of Medicines
St. Joseph's Hospital
Hamilton, Ontario, Canada

Jeroen Lijmer, MD
Clinical Epidemiology
    and Biostatistics
University of Amsterdam
Amsterdam, the Netherlands

**Finlay McAlister, MD, MSc,
    FRCPC**
Department of Medicine
University of Alberta
Edmonton, Alberta, Canada

Thomas McGinn, MD
Primary Care Medicine
Mount Sinai Medical Center
New York, New York, USA

Ann McKibbon, MLS
Department of Clinical
    Epidemiology and Biostatistics
Health Information Research Unit
McMaster University
Hamilton, Ontario, Canada

**Maureen Meade, MD, FRCPC,
    MSc**
Department of Medicine
McMaster University
Hamilton, Ontario, Canada

Victor Montori, MD
Department of Medicine
Mayo Clinic and Foundation
Rochester, Minnesota, USA

Virginia Moyer, MD, MPH
Department of Pediatrics
University of Texas
Houston, Texas, USA

David Naylor, MD DPhil
Faculty of Medicine
University of Toronto
Toronto, Ontario, Canada

Thomas Newman, MD, MPH
Departments of Epidemiology
    and Biostatistics, Pediatrics
    and Laboratory Medicine
University of California,
    San Francisco
San Francisco, California, USA

Jim Nishikawa, MD, FRCPC
Departments of Clinical
    Epidemiology and Biostatistics
    and Medicine
McMaster University
Hamilton, Ontario, Canada

Bernie O'Brien, PhD
Centre for Evaluation
    of Medicines
St. Joseph's Hospital
Hamilton, Ontario, Canada

Andrew Oxman, MD, MSc
Health Services Research Unit
National Institute of Public Health
Oslo, Norway

Peter Pronovost, MD, PhD
Anesthesiology and Critical
    Care Medicine
Johns Hopkins University
Baltimore, Maryland, USA

Adrienne Randolph, MD, MSc
The Children's Hospital
Boston, Massachusetts, USA

Drummond Rennie, MD
Institute for Health Policy Studies
University of California,
    San Francisco
San Francisco, California, USA

Scott Richardson, MD
Audie L. Murphy Memorial
    Veterans Hospital
San Antonio, Texas, USA

Holger Schünemann, MD
Departments of Medicine
    and Social and
    Preventative Medicine
University at Buffalo
Buffalo, New York, USA

Jack Sinclair, MD
Departments of Clinical
    Epidemiology and Biostatistics
    and Pediatrics
McMaster University
Hamilton, Ontario, Canada

**Martin Stockler, MBBS, MSc,
    FRACP**
Department of Medicine
University of Sydney
Sydney, NSW, Australia

Sharon Straus, MD
Department of Medicine
    University of Toronto
and Mount Sinai Hospital
Toronto, Ontario, Canada

Peter Tugwell, MD, MSc
Clinical Epidemiology Unit
    and Departments of Medicine
    and Epidemiology
University of Ottawa
Ottawa, Ontario, Canada

Stephen Walter, PhD
Department of Clinical
    Epidemiology and Biostatistics
McMaster University
Hamilton, Ontario, Canada

George Wells, MSc, PhD
Clinical Epidemiology Unit and
    Departments of Medicine and
    Epidemiology
University of Ottawa
Ottawa, Ontario, Canada

Mark Wilson, MD, MPH
Department of Medicine
Wake Forest University School
    of Medicine
Winston-Salem, North Carolina,
    USA

Jeremy Wyatt, MD
Knowledge Management Centre
University College London
London, England, UK

Peter Wyer, MD
Department of Medicine
Columbia University College
    of Physicians and Surgeons
Pelham, New York, USA

How to Use This Book

Gordon Guyatt

The following EBM Working Group members also made substantive contributions to this section: John Attia, Roman Jaeschke, Maureen Meade, Andrew Oxman, Trisha Greenhalgh, Jack Sinclair, Anne McKibbon, Deborah Cook, and Eric Bass

Like evidence-based medicine (EBM), this book is about clinical decision making. In particular, our objective is to make efficient use of the published literature to help with patient care. What does the published literature comprise? Our definition is broad. Evidence may be published in a wide variety of sources, including original journal articles, reviews and synopses of primary studies, practice guidelines, and traditional and innovative medical textbooks. Increasingly, clinicians can most easily access many of these sources through the World Wide Web. In the future, the Internet may be the only route of access for some resources.

PART 1: THE BASICS: USING THE MEDICAL LITERATURE

Part 1 of our clinicians' guide covers the basics: what every medical student, every intern and resident, and every practicing physician should know about reading the medical literature. We have kept this section as simple and succinct as possible. From an instructor's point of view, Part 1 constitutes a curriculum for a short course in using the literature for medical students or house staff; it is also appropriate for a continuing education program for practicing physicians.

Part 1 of this book teaches a systematic approach that involves three steps to using an article from the medical literature. The clinician should ask whether new information is likely to be true, what the information says about patient care, and how the information can be used. In the first step, the clinician considers the validity or likelihood of bias. In the second and third steps, the clinician comes to understand the results and to apply those results to the care of individual patients. These three steps provided the inspiration for the three pillars that you see on the cover of this book. To help demonstrate the clinical relevance of this approach, we begin each section with a clinical scenario, demonstrate a search for relevant literature, and present a table that summarizes criteria for using the three steps.

Although Part 1 of this book is concise, after you have mastered its concepts you will be able to ensure that your practice is evidence-based. You will have learned:

- To distinguish stronger evidence from weaker evidence;

- To become familiar with the full process of detailed critical appraisal, summarization of evidence, and balancing of benefits and risks that should precede management decisions;

- To identify, locate, and understand preappraised evidence summaries and evidence-based recommendations; and

- To understand the issues involved in applying evidence from the literature to your clinical practice and, in particular, to individualizing the application to each unique patient.

A wide array of preappraised evidence-based resources already exist and most are easily accessed by computer. The number and quality of these resources are certain to increase dramatically during the next few years. Part 1A1, "Finding the Evidence," will teach you how to identify the right databases—ones providing evidence that is both valid and applicable to your practice—and to find the information you want within them. Sections B through F of Part 1 will teach you how to make optimal use of what you find to address patient management problems.

In fact, you need not read all of Part 1. The book is designed so that each section is largely self-contained. If all you need is guidance on formulating and carrying out searches, read only Part 1A1. If the only original articles you are interested in are primary studies concerning therapy and systematic reviews of those studies, read only the Therapy and Harm section of Parts 1B, 1B1, and 1B2 and the systematic reviews section in Part 1E. We have avoided excessive redundancy, so there are times when we do not repeat a concept common to two sections. You will find such instances clearly denoted.

PART 2: BEYOND THE BASICS: USING AND TEACHING THE PRINCIPLES OF EVIDENCE-BASED MEDICINE

Part 2 of this book is directed to clinicians who want to practice EBM at a more sophisticated level. In Part 2 of the written book, we included what those who wish to delve farther might like to know. In the larger Part 2 on the CD-ROM, we included all of the information those who wish to role-model and teach EBM should know.

Reading Part 2 will deepen your understanding of study methodology, of statistical issues, and of how to use the numbers that emerge from medical research in helping each patient make the best health care choices. We wrote Part 2 mindful of an additional audience: those who teach evidence-based practice. You will find that many entries in Part 2 read like a guideline for an interactive discussion with a group of learners in tutorial, or on the ward. That is natural enough, as the material originated in just such small-group settings.

How should you use Part 2? Note first that the organization of Part 2 roughly parallels that of Part 1. Each major section includes more detailed discussion of concepts introduced in the corresponding section of Part 1. For instance, in the Therapy and Harm section of Part 2 you will find discussions concerning standards for appraising studies that address cost issues, studies evaluating screening programs, and studies evaluating computer decision support systems. We judged each of these as being outside the core knowledge needed for a basic application of EBM in your practice.

Each expansion in Part 2 has a corresponding cross-reference in Part 1. For instance, you will find an expanded version of our introductory discussion of the philosophy of EBM in Part 2A on the CD-ROM. In most cases, the expansion in Part 2 will be directly linked to core knowledge presented in Part 1. For instance, Part 1 tells you that when using an article about therapy, you need to ask whether the investigators have measured all important outcomes of treatment, both good and bad. It mentions that health-related quality of life is often an important outcome, and it includes some brief remarks about how it should be measured. Part 2, by contrast, includes a major expansion of this topic, with a full discussion of quality-of-life measurement.

Some may find the CD-ROM version, in which a mouse-click moves you from Part 1 to the relevant section of Part 2, easier to use than the written text. Either way, many will find the glossary of terms a useful reminder of formal definition of terms used in the book. We hope that this organization is well suited to the needs of any clinician who is eager to achieve an evidence-based practice.

Please look for future tools and EBM information at the *Users' Guides* Web site at www.usersguides.org.

Part 1

The Basics: Using The Medical Literature

Clinicians are primarily interested in making accurate diagnoses and selecting optimal treatments for patients in their practice. They must also avoid harmful exposures and offer patients prognostic information. Part 1 of this book provides clinicians with the essential skills they need to use the medical literature for these four aspects of patient care.

Before clinicians can incorporate the best evidence, they must find it. Part 1 begins with an approach to formulating clinical questions and locating the best studies that address those questions. Opportunities for efficient searching have grown enormously during in recent years, and our section concerning "Finding the Evidence" (see Section 1A1) incorporates the latest developments.

Primary Studies

One can distinguish between individual studies presenting original data—which we shall call primary studies—and reports that summarize a number of primary studies. After we have offered instruction on how to find the best evidence, we provide an approach to critically appraising primary studies and applying the results to patient care. The principles of assessing articles on therapy and harm are closely linked, as are the principles of assessing diagnostic and prognostic studies. Throughout, our discussion highlights these links.

Systematic Reviews

When someone has gone to the trouble of systematically summarizing primary studies addressing a specific clinical question, clinicians should take advantage of that summary. Indeed, efficient evidence-based practice dictates bypassing the critical assessment of primary studies and moving straight to the evaluation of rigorous systematic literature reviews. Thus, clinicians must be aware of how to recognize a systematic review, appraise its methodologic quality, and apply its results to patients in their practice. After discussing primary studies, Part 1 provides clinicians with the skills needed to use a systematic review.

Treatment Recommendations

Even more efficient than using a systematic review is moving directly to a treatment recommendation. Ideally, treatment recommendations—which are summarized in practice guidelines or decision analyses—will rigorously incorporate the best evidence and make explicit the value judgments used in moving from evidence to recommendations for action. Once again, there are methodologically weak practice guidelines and decision analyses that clinicians should ignore—and methodologically rigorous recommendations to which they should attend. Our section on "Moving From Evidence to Action" (see Section 1F) provides instruction in how to differentiate weak practice guidelines and decision analyses from strong ones, to understand their limitations, and to judiciously use these recommendations in clinical practice.

INTRODUCTION: THE PHILOSOPHY OF EVIDENCE-BASED MEDICINE

Gordon Guyatt, Brian Haynes, Roman Jaeschke,
Deborah Cook, Trisha Greenhalgh, Maureen Meade,
Lee Green, C. David Naylor, Mark Wilson,
Finlay McAlister, and W. Scott Richardson

The following EBM Working Group members also made
substantive contributions to this section: Victor Montori
and Heiner Bucher

IN THIS SECTION

CLINICAL SCENARIO

Who's Right?

A senior resident, a junior attending physician, a senior attending physician, and an emeritus professor were discussing evidence-based medicine over lunch in a hospital cafeteria. "EBM," announced the resident with some passion, "is a revolutionary development in medical practice." She went on to describe EBM's fundamental innovations in solving patient problems. "A compelling exposition," remarked the emeritus professor. "Wait a minute," the junior attending exclaimed with some heat, and then proceeded to present an alternative position: that EBM has merely provided a set of additional tools for traditional approaches to patient care. "You make a strong and convincing case," the emeritus professor commented. "Something's wrong here," the senior attending exclaimed to her older colleague, "their positions are diametrically opposed. They can't both be right." The emeritus professor looked thoughtfully at the puzzled doctor and, with the barest hint of a smile, replied, "Come to think of it, you're right too."

Evidence-based medicine (EBM) is about solving clinical problems.[1] In 1992, we described EBM as a shift in medical paradigms.[2] In contrast to the traditional paradigm of medical practice, EBM acknowledges that intuition, unsystematic clinical experience, and pathophysiologic rationale are insufficient grounds for clinical decision making; and it stresses the examination of evidence from clinical research. In addition, EBM suggests that a formal set of rules must complement medical training and common sense for clinicians to interpret the results of clinical research effectively. Finally, EBM places a lower value on authority than the traditional medical paradigm does.

We continue to find this paradigm shift a valid way of conceptualizing EBM. As our opening vignette about the lunchtime conversation suggests, the world is often complex enough to invite more than one useful way of thinking about an idea or a phenomenon. In this section, we describe the way of thinking about EBM that currently appeals to us most. We explain two key principles of EBM relating to the value-laden nature of clinical decisions, along with a hierarchy of evidence. We note the additional skills necessary for optimal clinical practice, and we conclude with a discussion of the challenges facing EBM in the new millennium.

TWO FUNDAMENTAL PRINCIPLES OF EBM

As a distinctive approach to patient care, EBM involves two fundamental principles. First, evidence alone is never sufficient to make a clinical decision. Decision makers must always trade the benefits and risks, inconvenience, and costs associated with alternative management strategies, and in doing so consider the patient's values.[1] Second, EBM posits a hierarchy of evidence to guide clinical decision making.

1. Clinical Decision Making: Evidence Is Never Enough

Picture a patient with chronic pain resulting from terminal cancer. She has come to terms with her condition, has resolved her affairs and said her goodbyes, and she wishes to receive only palliative therapy. The patient develops pneumococcal pneumonia. Now, evidence that antibiotic therapy reduces morbidity and mortality from pneumococcal pneumonia is strong. Almost all clinicians would agree, however, that even evidence this convincing does not dictate that this particular patient should receive antibiotics. Despite the fact that antibiotics might reduce symptoms and prolong the patient's life, her values are such that she would prefer a rapid and natural death.

Now envision a second patient—an 85-year-old man with severe dementia, who is incontinent, contracted, and mute, without family or friends, who spends his days in apparent discomfort. This man develops pneumococcal pneumonia. Although many clinicians would argue that those responsible for this patient's care should not administer antibiotic therapy because of his circumstances, others, by contrast, would suggest that they should do so. Again, evidence of treatment effectiveness does not automatically imply that treatment should be administered. The management decision requires a judgment about the tradeoff between risks and benefits; and because values or preferences differ, the best course of action will vary from patient to patient and among clinicians.

Finally, picture a third patient—a healthy, 30-year-old mother of two children who develops pneumococcal pneumonia. No clinician would doubt the wisdom of administering antibiotic therapy to this patient. However, this does not mean that an underlying value judgment has been unnecessary. Rather, our values are sufficiently concordant, and the benefits so overwhelm the risks, that the underlying value judgment is unapparent.

In current health care practice, judgments often reflect clinicial or societal values concerning whether intervention benefits are worth the cost.[2] Consider the decisions regarding administration of tissue plasminogen activator (tPA) versus streptokinase to patients with acute myocardial infarction, or administration of clopidogrel versus aspirin to patients with transient ischemic attack. In both cases, evidence from large randomized trials suggests that the more expensive agents are more effective. In both cases, many authorities recommend first-line treatment with the less expensive, less effective drug, presumably because they believe society's resources would be better used in other ways. Implicitly, they are making a value or preference judgment about the tradeoff between deaths and strokes prevented, and resources spent.

By *values* and preferences, we mean the underlying processes we bring to bear in weighing what our patients and our society will gain—or lose—when we make a management decision. The explicit enumeration and balancing of benefits and risks that is central to EBM brings the underlying value judgments involved in making management decisions into bold relief.

Acknowledging that values play a role in every important patient care decision highlights our limited understanding of eliciting and incorporating societal and individual values. Health economists have played a major role in developing a science of measuring patient preferences.[3,4] Some decision aids incorporate patient values indirectly: If patients truly understand the potential risks and benefits, their decisions will likely reflect their preferences.[5] These developments constitute a promising start. Nevertheless, many unanswered questions remain concerning how to elicit preferences and how to incorporate them in clinical encounters already subject to crushing time pressures. Addressing these issues constitutes an enormously challenging frontier for EBM.

2. A Hierarchy of Evidence

What is the nature of the "evidence" in EBM? We suggest a broad definition: any empirical observation about the apparent relation between events constitutes potential evidence. Thus, the unsystematic observations of the individual clinician constitute one source of evidence, and physiologic experiments constitute another source. Unsystematic observations can lead to profound insight, and experienced clinicians develop a healthy respect for the insights of their senior colleagues in issues of clinical observation, diagnosis, and relations with patients and colleagues. Some of these insights can be taught, yet rarely appear in the medical literature.

At the same time, unsystematic clinical observations are limited by small sample size and, more importantly, by deficiencies in human processes of making inferences.[6] Predictions about intervention effects on clinically important outcomes based on physiologic experiments usually are right, but occasionally are disastrously wrong.

Given the limitations of unsystematic clinical observations and physiologic rationale, EBM suggests a hierarchy of evidence. Table 1A-1 presents a hierarchy of study designs for treatment issues; very different hierarchies are necessary for issues of diagnosis or prognosis. Clinical research goes beyond unsystematic clinical observation in providing strategies that avoid or attenuate spurious results. Because few—if any—interventions are effective in all patients, we would ideally test a treatment in a patient to whom we would like to apply that treatment. Numerous factors can lead clinicians astray as they try to interpret the results of conventional open trials of therapy. These include natural history, placebo effects, patient and health worker expectations, and the patient's desire to please.

TABLE 1A-1

A Hierarchy of Strength of Evidence for Treatment Decisions

- N of 1 randomized controlled trial
- Systematic reviews of randomized trials
- Single randomized trial
- Systematic review of observational studies addressing patient-important outcomes
- Single observational study addressing patient-important outcomes
- Physiologic studies (studies of blood pressure, cardiac output, exercise capacity, bone density, and so forth)
- Unsystematic clinical observations

The same strategies that minimize bias in conventional therapeutic trials involving multiple patients can guard against misleading results in studies involving single patients.[7] In the N of 1 randomized controlled trial (RCT), patients undertake pairs of treatment periods in which they receive a target treatment during one period of each pair, and a placebo or alternative during the other. Patients and clinicians are blind to allocation, the order of the target and control is randomized, and patients make quantitative ratings of their symptoms during each period. The N of 1 RCT continues until both the patient and clinician conclude that the patient is, or is not, obtaining benefit from the target intervention. N of 1 RCTs are often feasible,[8,9] can provide definitive evidence of treatment effectiveness in individual patients, and may lead to long-term differences in treatment administration.[10]

When considering any other source of evidence about treatment, clinicians are generalizing from results in other people to their patients, inevitably weakening inferences about treatment impact and introducing complex issues of how trial results apply to individual patients. Inferences may nevertheless be very strong if results come from a systematic review of methodologically strong RCTs with consistent results. However, inferences generally will be somewhat weaker if only a single RCT is being considered, unless it is very large and investigators have enrolled a diverse patient population (see Table 1A-1). Because observational studies may under-estimate treatment effects in an unpredictable fashion,[11,12] their results are far less trustworthy than those of randomized trials. Physiologic studies and unsystematic clinical observations provide the weakest inferences about treatment effects.

This hierarchy is not absolute. If treatment effects are sufficiently large and consistent, for instance, observational studies may provide more compelling evidence than most RCTs. By way of example, observational studies have allowed extremely strong inferences about the efficacy of insulin in diabetic ketoacidosis or that of hip replacement in patients with debilitating hip osteoarthritis. At the same time, instances in which RCT results contradict consistent results from observational studies reinforce the need for caution. Defining the extent to which clinicians should temper the strength of their inferences when only observational studies are available remains one of the important challenges for EBM. The challenge is particularly important given that much of the evidence regarding the harmful effects of therapies comes from observational studies.

The hierarchy implies a clear course of action for physicians addressing patient problems: they should look for the highest available evidence from the hierarchy. The hierarchy makes clear that any statement to the effect that there is no evidence addressing the effect of a particular treatment is a non sequitur. The evidence may be extremely weak—it may be the unsystematic observation of a single clinician or a generalization from physiologic studies that are related only indirectly—but there is always evidence.

Next we will briefly comment on additional skills that clinicians must master for optimal patient care and the relation of those skills to EBM.

CLINICAL SKILLS, HUMANISM, SOCIAL RESPONSIBILITY, AND EBM

The evidence-based process of resolving a clinical question will be fruitful only if the problem is formulated appropriately. One of us, a secondary care internist, developed a lesion on his lip shortly before an important presentation. He was quite concerned and, wondering if he should take acyclovir, proceeded to spend the next 2 hours searching for the highest quality evidence and reviewing the available RCTs. When he began to discuss his remaining uncertainty with his partner, an experienced dentist, she quickly cut short the discussion by exclaiming, "But, my dear, that isn't herpes!"

This story illustrates the necessity of obtaining the correct diagnosis before seeking and applying research evidence in practice, the value of extensive clinical experience, and the fallibility of clinical judgment. The essential skills of obtaining a history and conducting a physical examination and the astute formulation of the clinical problem come only with thorough background training and extensive clinical experience. The clinician makes use of evidence-based reasoning—applying the likelihood ratios associated with positive or negative physical findings, for instance—to interpret the results of the history and physical examination. Clinical expertise is further required to define the relevant treatment options before examining the evidence regarding the expected benefits and risks of those options.

Finally, clinicians rely on their expertise to define features that have an impact on the generalizability of the results to the individual patient. We have noted that, except when clinicians have conducted N of 1 RCTs, they are attempting to generalize (or, one might say, particularize) results obtained in other patients to the individual patient before them. The clinician must judge the extent to which differences in treatment (local surgical expertise or the possibility of patient noncompliance, for instance), the availability of monitoring, or patient characteristics (such as age, comorbidity, or concomitant treatment) may impact estimates of benefit and risk that come from the published literature.

Thus, knowing the tools of evidence-based practice is necessary but not sufficient for delivering the highest quality of patient care. In addition to clinical expertise, the clinician requires compassion, sensitive listening skills, and broad perspectives from the humanities and social sciences. These attributes allow understanding of patients' illnesses in the context of their experience, personalities, and cultures. The sensitive understanding of the patient links to evidence-based practice in a number of ways. For some patients, incorporation of patient values for major decisions will mean a full enumeration of the possible benefits, risks, and inconvenience associated with alternative management strategies that are relevant to the particular patient. For some of these patients and problems, this discussion should involve the patients' family. For other problems— the discussion of screening with prostate-specific antigen with older male patients, for instance—attempts to involve other family members might violate strong cultural norms.

Many patients are uncomfortable with an explicit discussion of benefits and risks, and they object to having what they perceive as excessive responsibility for decision making being placed on their shoulders.[13] In such patients, who would tell us they want the physician to make the decision on their behalf, the physician's responsibility is to develop insight to ensure that choices will be consistent with patients' values and preferences. Understanding and implementing the sort of decision-making process patients desire and effectively communicating the information they need requires skills in understanding the patient's narrative and the person behind that narrative.[14,15] A continuing challenge for EBM—and for medicine in general—will be to better integrate the new science of clinical medicine with the time-honored craft of caring for the sick.

Ideally, evidence-based technical skills and humane perspective will lead physicians to become effective advocates for their patients both in the direct context of the health system in which they work and in broader health policy issues. Most physicians see their role as focusing on health care interventions for their patients. Even when they consider preventive therapy, they focus on individual patient behavior. However, we consider this focus to be too narrow.

Observational studies have documented the strong and consistent association between socioeconomic status and health. Societal health is associated more strongly with income gradients than with the total wealth of the society. In other words, the overall health of the populace tends to be higher in poorer countries with a relatively equitable distribution of wealth than in richer countries with larger disparities between rich and poor. These considerations suggest that physicians concerned about the health of their patients as a group, or about the health of the community, should consider how they might contribute to reducing poverty.

Observational studies have shown a strong and consistent association between pollution levels and respiratory and cardiovascular health. Physicians seeing patients with chronic obstructive pulmonary disease will suggest that they stop smoking. But should physicians also be concerned with the polluted air that patients are breathing? We believe they should.

ADDITIONAL CHALLENGES FOR EBM

In 1992, we identified skills necessary for evidence-based practice. These included the ability to precisely define a patient problem and to ascertain what information is required to resolve the problem, conduct an efficient search of the literature, select the best of the relevant studies, apply rules of evidence to determine their validity, extract the clinical message, and apply it to the patient problem as the skills necessary for evidence-based practice.[1] To these skills we would now add an understanding of how the patient's values impact the balance between advantages and disadvantages of the available management options and the ability to appropriately involve the patient in the decision.

A further decade of experience with EBM has not changed the biggest challenge to evidence-based practice: time limitation. Fortunately, new resources to assist clinicians are available and the pace of innovation is rapid. One can consider a classification of information sources that comes with a mnemonic device, 4S: the individual study or studies, the systematic review of all the available studies on a given problem, a synopsis of individual studies or systematic reviews or both, and systems of information. By systems we mean summaries that link a number of synopses related to the care of a particular patient problem (for example, acute upper gastrointestinal bleeding) or type of patient (for example, an outpatient with diabetes) (Table 1A-2). Evidence-based selection and summarization is becoming increasingly available at each level (see Part 1A1, "Finding the Evidence").

TABLE 1A-2

A Hierarchy of Preprocessed Evidence

Studies	Preprocessing involves selecting only those studies that are both highly relevant and characterized by study designs that minimize bias and thus permit a high strength of inference.
Systematic Reviews	Systematic reviews provide clinicians with an overview of all of the evidence addressing a focused clinical question.
Synopses	Synopses of individual studies or of systematic reviews encapsulate the key methodologic details and results required to apply the evidence to individual patient care.
Systems	Practice guidelines, clinical pathways, or evidence-based textbook summaries of a clinical area provide the clinician with much of the information needed to guide the care of individual patients.

This book deals primarily with decision making at the level of the individual patient. Evidence-based approaches can also inform health policy making,[16] day-to-day decisions in public health, and systems-level decisions such as those facing hospital managers. In each of these arenas, EBM can support the appropriate goal of gaining the greatest health benefit from limited resources. On the other hand, evidence—as an ideology, rather than a focus for reasoned debate—has been used as a justification for many agendas in health care, ranging from crude cost cutting to the promotion of extremely expensive technologies with minimal marginal returns.

In the policy arena, dealing with differing values poses even more challenges than in the arena of individual patient care. Should we restrict ourselves to alternative resource allocation within a fixed pool of health care resources, or should we be trading off health care services against, for instance, lower tax rates for individuals or lower health care costs for corporations? How should we deal with the large body of observational studies suggesting that social and economic factors may have a larger impact on the health of populations than health care delivery? How should we deal with the tension between what may be best for a person and what may be optimal for the society of which that person is a member? The debate about such issues is at the heart of evidence-based health policy making, but, inevitably, it has implications for decision making at the individual patient level.

References

1. Haynes RB, Sackett RB, Gray JMA, Cook DC, Guyatt GH. Transferring evidence from research into practice, 1: the role of clinical care research evidence in clinical decisions. *ACP Journal Club*. Nov-Dec 1996 ;125:A-14-15.

2. Napodano RJ. *Values in Medical Practice*. New York, NY: Human Sciences Press; 1986.

3. Drummond MF, Richardson WS, O'Brien B, Levine M, Heyland DK, for the Evidence-Based Medicine Working Group. Users' Guides to the Medical Literature XIII. How to use an article on economic analysis of clinical practice. A. Are the results of the study valid? *JAMA*. 1997;277:1552-1557.

4. Feeny DH, Furlong W, Boyle M, Torrance GW. Multi-attribute health status classification systems: health utilities index. *Pharmacoeconomics*. 1995;7:490-502.

5. O'Connor AM, Rostom A, Fiset V, et al. Decision aids for patients facing health treatment or screening decisions: systematic review. *BMJ*. 1999;319:731-734.

6. Nisbett R, Ross L. *Human Inference*. Englewood Cliffs, NJ: Prentice-Hall; 1980.

7. Guyatt GH, Sackett DL, Taylor DW, et al. Determining optimal therapy: randomized trials in individual patients. *N Engl J Med*. 1986;314:889-892.

8. Guyatt GH, Keller JL, Jaeschke R, Rosenbloom D, Adachi JD, Newhouse MT. The n-of-1 randomized controlled trial: clinical usefulness. Our three-year experience. *Ann Intern Med*. 1990;112:293-299.

9. Larson EB, Ellsworth AJ, Oas J. Randomized clinical trials in single patients during a 2-year period. *JAMA*. 1993;270:2708-2712.

10. Mahon J, Laupacis A, Donner A, Wood T. Randomised study of n of 1 trials versus standard practice. *BMJ*. 1996;312:1069-1074.

11. Guyatt GH, DiCenso A, Farewell V, Willan A, Griffith L. Randomized trials versus observational studies in adolescent pregnancy prevention. *J Clin Epidemiol*. 2000;53:167-174.

12. Kunz R, Oxman AD. The unpredictability paradox: review of empirical comparisons of randomised and non-randomised clinical trials. *BMJ*. 1998;317:1185-1190.

13. Sutherland HJ, Llewellyn-Thomas HA, Lockwood GA, Tritchler DL, Till JE. Cancer patients: their desire for information and participation in treatment decisions. *J R Soc Med*. 1989;82:260-263.

14. Greenhalgh T. Narrative based medicine: narrative based medicine in an evidence based world. *BMJ*. 1999;318:323-325.

15. Greenhalgh T, Hurwitz B. Narrative based medicine: why study narrative? *BMJ*. 1999;318:48-50.

16. Muir Gray FA, Haynes RB, Sackett DL, Cook DJ, Guyatt GH. Transferring evidence from research into practice, III: developing evidence-based clinical policy. *ACP Journal Club*. 1997;A14.

FINDING THE EVIDENCE

Ann McKibbon, Dereck Hunt, W. Scott Richardson,
Robert Hayward, Mark Wilson, Roman Jaeschke,
Brian Haynes, Peter Wyer, Jonathan Craig,
and Gordon Guyatt

The following EBM Working Group members also made
substantive contributions to this section: Patrick Bossuyt,
Trisha Greenhalgh, Sharon Straus, and Deborah Cook

IN THIS SECTION

WAYS OF USING THE MEDICAL LITERATURE

This book is about using the medical literature. But not, as we describe in the following section, in the ways medical students most typically use it.

Background and Foreground Questions

There are several reasons that medical students, early in their training, seldom consult the original medical literature. First, they are not usually responsible for managing patients and solving specific patient problems. Even if they attend a school that uses problem-oriented learning as an educational strategy, their interest is primarily in understanding normal human physiology and the pathophysiology associated with a patient's condition or problem. Once they have grasped these basic concepts, they will turn to the prognosis, available diagnostic tests, and possible management options. Finally, when students are presented with a patient-related problem, their questions are likely to include, for example, what is diabetes, why did this patient present with polyuria, and how might we manage the problem.

By contrast, experienced clinicians responsible for managing a patient's problem ask very different sorts of questions. They are interested less in the diagnostic approach to a presenting problem and are more interested in how to interpret a specific diagnostic test; less in the general prognosis of a chronic disease and more in a particular patient's prognosis; less in the management strategies that might be applied to a patient's problems and more in the risks and benefits of a particular treatment in relation to an alternative management strategy.

Think of the first set of questions, those of the medical student, as background questions; think of the second set as foreground questions. In most situations, you need to understand the background thoroughly before it makes sense to address issues in the foreground.

On her first day on the ward, a medical student will still have a great deal of background knowledge to acquire. However, in deciding how to manage the first patient she sees, she may well need to address a foreground issue. A senior clinician, while well versed in all issues that represent the background of her clinical practice, may nevertheless also occasionally require background information. This is most likely when a new condition or medical syndrome appears (consider the fact that as recently as 20 years ago, experienced clinicians were asking, "What is the acquired immunodeficiency syndrome?") or when a new diagnostic test ("How does PCR work?") or treatment modality ("What are COX-2 inhibitors?") is introduced into the clinical arena. At every stage of training and experience, clinicians' grasp of the relevant background issues of disease inform their ability to identify and formulate the most pertinent foreground questions for an individual patient.

Figure 1A-1 represents the evolution of the questions we ask as we progress from being novices (who pose almost exclusively background questions) to being experts (who pose almost exclusively foreground questions). This book is devoted to how clinicians can use the medical literature to solve their foreground questions.

FIGURE 1A-1

Asking Questions

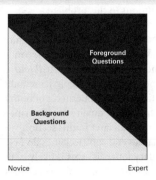

Browsing and Problem Solving

Traditionally, clinicians subscribed to a number—sometimes a large number—of target medical journals in which articles relevant to their practice were likely to appear. They would keep up to date by skimming the table of contents and reading articles relevant to their practice. One might label this the browsing mode of using the medical literature.

Traditional approaches to browsing have major limitations of inefficiency and resulting frustration. Picture a clinician with a number of subscriptions placing journals in a pile on her desk awaiting browsing review. She may even be aware that less than 10% of articles that are published in the core medical journals are both high quality and clinically useful. Unable to spend sufficient time to browse, she finds the pile growing until it becomes intimidating. At this point, she tosses the whole pile and starts the process again.

Although it is somewhat of a parody, most experienced clinicians can relate easily to this scenario. Physicians at every stage of training often feel overwhelmed by the magnitude of the medical literature. Evidence-based medicine offers some solutions to this problem.

Browse Secondary Journals. Perhaps the most efficient strategy is to restrict your browsing to secondary journals. For internal and general medicine, *ACP Journal Club* (www.acponline.org/journals/acpjc/jcmenu.htm) publishes synopses of articles that meet criteria of both clinical relevance and methodologic quality. We describe such secondary journals in more detail later in this section.

Many specialties and subspecialties do not yet have devoted secondary journals. This is likely to be a temporary phenomenon, at least for the major specialties. In the meantime, you can apply your own relevance and methodologic screen to articles in your target journals. Most clinical publications serve a dual purpose: as a forum for both investigator-to-investigator communication and investigator-to-clinician communication.[1] However, only the latter articles will be directly relevant to your practice. Part 1 of this book is devoted to providing the tools that will allow you to screen journals for high-quality, relevant evidence. When you have learned the skills, you will be surprised both at the small proportion of studies to which you need to attend—and at the efficiency with which you can identify them.

Operate in a Problem-Solving Mode. Another part of the solution to the overwhelming-amount-of-literature problem is for clinicians to spend more of the time they have available for consulting the literature in what we call a problem-solving mode. Here, questions raised in caring for patients are defined and then the literature is consulted to resolve these questions. Whether you are operating in the browsing mode or problem-solving mode, this book can help you to judge the validity of the information in the articles you are examining, gain a clear understanding of their results, and apply them to patients.

The remainder of this section focuses on skills you will need to use the literature effectively when you are in the problem-solving mode.

FRAMING THE QUESTION

Clinical questions often spring to practitioners' minds in a form that makes finding answers in the medical literature a challenge. Dissecting the question into its component parts to facilitate finding the best evidence is a fundamental EBM skill.[2,3] Most questions can be divided into three parts.

1. **The population**. Who are the relevant patients?

2. **The interventions or exposures** (diagnostic tests, foods, drugs, surgical procedures, etc). What are the management strategies we are interested in comparing, or the potentially harmful exposure about which we are concerned? For issues of therapy or harm, there will always be two or more parts to this: the intervention or exposure and a control or alternative intervention(s) or exposure(s).

3. **The outcome**. What are the patient-relevant consequences of the exposure in which we are interested?

We will now provide examples of the transformation of unstructured clinical questions into the structured questions that facilitate use of the medical literature.

Example 1: Diabetes and Target Blood Pressure

A 55-year-old white woman presents with type 2 diabetes mellitus and hypertension. Her glycemic control is excellent on metformin and she has no history of complications. To manage her hypertension, she takes a small daily dose of a thiazide diuretic. Over a 6-month period, her blood pressure hovers around a value of 155/88 mm Hg.

Initial Question: When treating hypertension, at what target blood pressure should we aim?

Digging Deeper: One limitation of this formulation of the question is that it fails to specify the population in adequate detail. The benefits of tight control of blood pressure may differ in diabetic patients vs nondiabetic patients, in type 1 vs type 2 diabetes mellitus, as well as in those with and without diabetic complications. We may wish to specify that we are interested in the addition of a specific antihypertensive agent. Alternatively, the intervention of interest may be any antihypertensive treatment. Furthermore, a key part of the intervention will be the target for blood pressure control. For instance, we might be interested in knowing whether it makes any difference if our target diastolic blood pressure is < 80 mm Hg vs < 90 mm Hg. The major limitation of the initial question formulation is that it fails to specify the criteria by which we will judge the appropriate target for our hypertensive treatment. The target outcomes of interest would include stroke, myocardial infarction, cardiovascular death, and total mortality.

Improved (Searchable) Question: A searchable question would specify the relevant patient population, the management strategy and exposure, and the patient-relevant consequences of that exposure as follows:

- *Patients:* Hypertensive type 2 diabetic patients without diabetic complications

- *Intervention:* Any antihypertensive agent aiming at a target diastolic blood pressure of 90 mm Hg vs a target of 80 mm Hg

- *Outcomes:* Stroke, myocardial infarction, cardiovascular death, total mortality

Example 2: Suspected Unstable Angina

A 39-year-old man without previous chest discomfort presented to the emergency department at the end of his working day. Early that day he had felt unwell and nauseated; he had had a vague sensation of chest discomfort and had begun to sweat profusely. The unpleasant experience lasted for about 2 hours, after which the patient felt tired but otherwise normal. At the end of his work day, feeling rather nervous about the episode, he came to the emergency department. The patient has no family history of coronary artery disease. He has had hypertension for 5 years that is controlled with a thiazide, has a 15-pack-year smoking history, and has a normal lipid profile. His physical examination, electrocardiogram (ECG), creatine kinase level, and troponin I level are all normal.

Initial Question: Can I send this man home or should I admit him to a monitored hospital bed?

Digging Deeper: The initial question gives us little idea of where to look in the literature for an answer. We can break down the issue by noting that the patient has suspected unstable angina. However, a number of distinguishing features differentiate him from other patients with possible unstable angina. He is relatively young, he has some risk factors for coronary artery disease, his presentation is atypical, he is now pain free, there is no sign of heart failure, and his ECG and cardiac enzymes are unremarkable.

The management strategies we are considering include admitting him to a hospital for overnight monitoring or sending him home with the appropriate follow-up, including an exercise test. Another way of thinking about the issue, however, is that we need to know the consequences of sending him home. Would discharge be a safe course of action, with an acceptably low likelihood of adverse events? Thinking of our question that way, the exposure of interest is time. Time is usually the exposure of interest in studies about patients' prognosis.

What would be our objective in admitting the patient to a coronary care unit? By doing this, we will not be able to prevent more distant events (such as a myocardial infarction a month later). We are interested primarily in events that might occur during the next 72 hours, the maximum time the patient is likely to be monitored in the absence of complications. What adverse events might we prevent if the patient is in a hospital bed with cardiac monitoring? Should he develop severe chest pain, cardiac failure, or myocardial infarction, we would be able to treat him immediately. Most important, should he develop ventricular fibrillation or another life-threatening arrhythmia we would be able to administer cardioversion and save his life.

Improved (Searchable) Question: A searchable question would specify the relevant patient population, the management strategy and exposure, and the patient-relevant consequences of that exposure as follows:

- *Patients:* Young men with atypical symptoms and normal ECG and cardiac enzymes presenting with possible unstable angina

- *Intervention/Exposure:* Either admission to a monitored bed vs discharge home, or time

- *Outcomes:* Severe angina, myocardial infarction, heart failure, or arrhythmia, all within the next 72 hours

Example 3: Squamous Cell Carcinoma

A 60-year-old, 40-pack-year smoker presents with hemoptysis. A chest radiograph shows a parenchymal mass with a normal mediastinum, and a fine needle aspiration of the mass shows squamous cell carcinoma. Aside from the hemoptysis, the patient is asymptomatic and physical examination is entirely normal.

Initial Question: What investigations should we undertake before deciding whether to offer this patient surgery?

Digging Deeper: The key defining features of this patient are his non-small-cell carcinoma and the fact that his history, physical examination, and chest radiograph show no evidence of intrathoracic or extrathoracic metastatic disease. Alternative investigational strategies address two separate issues: Does the patient have occult mediastinal disease, and does he have occult extrathoracic metastatic disease? For this discussion, we will focus on the former issue. Investigational strategies for addressing the possibility of occult mediastinal disease include undertaking a mediastinoscopy or performing a computed tomographic (CT) scan of the chest and proceeding according to the results of this investigation.

What outcomes are we trying to influence in our choice of investigational approach? We would like to prolong the patient's life, but the extent of his underlying tumor is likely to be the major determinant of survival and our investigations cannot change that. The reason we wish to detect occult mediastinal metastases if they are present is that if the cancer has spread to the mediastinum, resectional surgery is very unlikely to benefit the patient. Thus, in the presence of mediastinal disease, patients will usually receive palliative approaches and avoid an unnecessary thoracotomy. Thus, the primary outcome of interest is an unnecessary thoracotomy.

Improved (Searchable) Question: A searchable question would specify the relevant patient population, the management strategy and exposure, and the patient-relevant consequences of that exposure as follows:

- *Patients:* Newly diagnosed non-small-cell lung cancer with no evidence of extrapulmonary metastases

- *Intervention*: Mediastinoscopy for all or chest CT-directed management

- *Outcome:* Unnecessary thoracotomy

Another way of structuring this question is as an examination of the test properties of the chest CT scan. Looking at the problem this way, the patient population is the same, but the exposure is the CT scan and the outcome is the presence or absence of the target condition, mediastinal metastatic disease. As we will subsequently discuss (see Part 1C2, "Diagnostic Tests"), this latter way of structuring the question is less likely to provide strong guidance about optimal management.

These examples illustrate that constructing a searchable question that allows you to use the medical literature to generate an answer is often no simple matter. It requires an in-depth understanding of the clinical issues involved in patient management. The three examples above illustrate that each patient may trigger a large number of clinical questions, and that clinicians must give careful thought to what they really want to know. Bearing the structure of the question in mind—patient, intervention or exposure, and outcome—is extremely helpful in arriving at an answerable question.

Once the question is posed, the next step in the process is translating the question into an effective search strategy. By first looking at the components of the question, putting the search strategy together is easier.

SEARCHING FOR THE ANSWER

In this section, we will introduce you to the electronic resources available for quickly finding the answers to your clinical questions. We will demonstrate how the careful definition of the question, including specification of the population, the intervention, and the outcome, can help you develop a workable search strategy. However, you must also consider a fourth component. What sort of study do you hope to find? By sort of study, we mean the way the study is organized or constructed—the study design.

Determining Question Type

To fully understand issues of study design, we suggest that you read the entire Part 1 of this book. Following is a brief introduction.

There are four fundamental types of clinical questions. They involve:

- **Therapy:** determining the effect of different treatments on improving patient function or avoiding adverse events

- **Harm:** ascertaining the effects of potentially harmful agents (including the very therapies we would be interested in examining in the first type of question) on patient function, morbidity, and mortality

- **Diagnosis:** establishing the power of an intervention to differentiate between those with and without a target condition or disease

- **Prognosis:** estimating the future course of a patient's disease

To answer questions about a therapeutic issue, we identify studies in which a process analogous to flipping a coin determines participants' receipt of an experimental treatment or a control or standard treatment, the so-called *randomized controlled trial* or *RCT* (see Part 1B1, "Therapy"). Once the investigator allocates participants to treatment or control groups, he or she follows them forward in time looking for whether they have, for instance, a stroke or heart attack—what we call the *outcome* of interest (Figure 1A-2).

FIGURE 1A–2

Randomized Controlled Trial

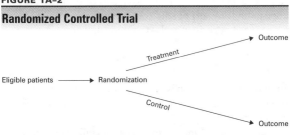

Eligible patients ⟶ Randomization

Treatment ⟶ Outcome

Control ⟶ Outcome

Ideally, we would also look to randomized trials to address issues of harm. However, for many potentially harmful exposures, randomly allocating patients is neither practical nor ethical. For instance, one could not suggest to potential study participants that an investigator will decide by the flip of a coin whether or not they smoke during the next 20 years or whether they will be exposed to potentially harmful ionizing radiation. For exposures like smoking and radiation, the best one can do is identify studies in which personal choice, or happenstance, determines whether people are exposed or not exposed. These observational studies provide weaker evidence than randomized trials.

Figure 1A-3 depicts a common observational study design in which patients with and without the exposure of interest are followed forward in time to determine whether they experience the outcome of interest. For smoking or radiation exposure, one important outcome would likely be the development of cancer.

FIGURE 1A-3

Observational Study: Assessing Exposure

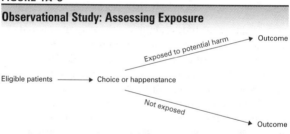

For establishing how well a diagnostic test works (what we call its properties or operating characteristics) we need yet another study design. In diagnostic test studies, investigators identify a group of patients who may or may not have the disease or condition of interest (such as tuberculosis, lung cancer, or iron-deficiency anemia), which we will call the *target condition*. Investigators begin by collecting a group of patients whom they suspect may have the target condition. These patients undergo both the new diagnostic test and a *gold standard* (that is, the test considered to be the diagnostic standard for a particular disease of condition; synonyms include *criterion standard, diagnostic standard*, or *reference standard*). Investigators evaluate the diagnostic test by comparing its classification of patients with that of the gold standard (Figure 1A-4).

FIGURE 1A-4

Study Design to Assess a Diagnostic Test

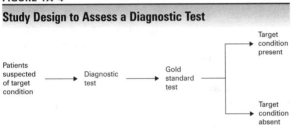

A final type of study examines patients' prognosis and may identify factors that modify that prognosis. Here, investigators identify patients who belong to a particular group (such as pregnant women, patients undergoing surgery, or patients with cancer) with or without factors that may modify their prognosis (such as age or comorbidity). The exposure here is time, and investigators follow patients to determine if they experience the target outcome, such as a problem birth at the end of a pregnancy, a myocardial infarction after surgery, or survival in cancer (Figure 1A-5).

FIGURE 1A-5

Observational Study Assessing Prognosis

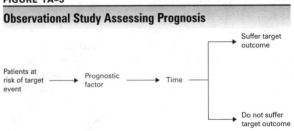

One of the clinician's tasks in searching the medical literature is to correctly identify the category of study that will address her question. For example, if you look for a randomized trial to inform you of the properties of a diagnostic test (as opposed to whether patients benefit from its application), you are unlikely to find the answer you seek.

Think back to the questions we identified in the previous section. Determining the best strategy for managing hypertension is clearly a treatment issue. However, we may also be interested in rare and delayed adverse effects of the medications we use to lower blood pressure, which is an issue of harm.

Considering the second scenario we presented, we can formulate the question in two ways. If we ask, How likely is myocardial infarction or death among young men with symptoms suggestive but atypical of unstable angina? the issue is one of prognosis. If we ask, What is the impact of alternative management strategies, such as admission to a coronary care unit or discharge? we are interested in treatment and would look for a randomized trial that allocated patients to the alternative approaches.

We can also formulate the question from the third scenario in two ways. If we ask, How well does CT scanning of the chest distinguish between non-small-cell lung cancer patients with and without mediastinal metastases? we would look for a study design that can gauge the power of a diagnostic test (see Figure 1A-4). We might also ask, "What is the rate of unnecessary thoracotomy in non-small-cell lung cancer patients who go straight to mediastinoscopy vs those who have CT scan-directed management?" For this treatment issue, we will seek a randomized trial (see Figure 1A-2).

Is Searching the Medical Literature Worthwhile?

Because our time for searching is limited, we would like to ensure that there is a good chance that our search will be productive. Consider the following clinical questions:

Example: In patients with pulmonary embolism, to what extent do those with pulmonary infarction have a poorer outcome than those without pulmonary infarction?

Before formulating our search strategy and beginning our literature search to answer this question, we should think about how investigators would differentiate between those with and without infarction. Since there is no reliable way, short of autopsy, of making this differentiation, our literature search is doomed before we even begin.

Example: Consider also a 50-year-old woman who has suffered an uncomplicated myocardial infarction 4 days previously and who asks, before discharge home, when she can resume sexual intercourse.

Were we to formulate a question that would allow us to address her inquiry, its components would look something like this:

- *Patients:* Women after uncomplicated myocardial infarction

- *Intervention:* Advice to resume intercourse as soon as so inclined vs waiting, say, 8 weeks

- *Outcomes:* Recurrent infarction, unstable angina, cardiovascular and total mortality, health-related quality of life

- *Type of question:* Therapy, therefore we would look for a randomized trial.

How likely is it that investigators have conducted a randomized trial of this question? Highly improbable. It is slightly less implausible that investigators have conducted an observational study of timing of return to sexual intercourse (here, patients would report when they had returned to sexual intercourse and investigators would compare outcomes in those who had started early vs those who had waited until later).

These two examples illustrate situations in which you will not want to use the medical literature to solve your patient management problems. The medical literature will not help you when there is no feasible study design that investigators could use to resolve the issue. Your search will also be fruitless if there is a feasible design, but it is very unlikely that anyone has taken the time and effort to carry out the necessary study. Before embarking on a search, carefully consider whether the yield is likely to be worth the time expenditure.

SOURCES OF EVIDENCE

You can look to local specialists, subspecialists, and more experienced clinical colleagues not only for opinion, but also for evidence to address your clinical problem (see Part 1A, "The Philosophy of Evidence-Based Medicine"). Their experience and advice are particularly crucial when the medical literature is unlikely to be helpful. Furthermore, experts who stay current on the latest evidence in their field may be able to quickly provide you with the most relevant citations.

Clinicians will not need this book to advise them to consult respected colleagues—they do not neglect this source of data. Where clinicians might need help is in the use of online resources. We focus on online rather than print products because they are generally easier to search and more current than print products (Table 1A-3).[4] With the relatively recent appearance of many of the resources we recommend, however, little research specifically addresses their relative merits. The approaches we describe reflect our own experiences and those of our colleagues working individually or with medical trainees.

TABLE 1A-3

Online Medical Information Resource Contact Information

Resource	Internet Address	Annual Cost*
ACP Journal Club	www.acponline.org/journals/acpjc/jcmenu.htm	$65
Best Evidence	www.acponline.org/catalog/electronic/best_evidence.htm	$85
Cochrane Library	www.update-software.com/cochrane/cochrane-frame.html	$225
UpToDate	www.uptodate.com	$495
MEDLINE PubMed Internet Grateful Med Other sources	www.ncbi.nlm.nih.gov/PubMed igm.nlm.nih.gov www.medmatrix.org/info/medlinetable.asp	Free Free Free
Scientific American Medicine	www.samed.com	$245 ($159 for online access alone)
Clinical Evidence	www.evidence.org	$115
Harrison's Online	www.harrisonsonline.com	$89
emedicine	www.emedicine.com	Free

Resource	Internet Address	Annual Cost*
Medscape	www.medscape.com/Home/Topics/homepages.html	Free
Medical Matrix	www.medmatrix.org/index.asp	Free
ScHARR Netting the Evidence	www.shef.ac.uk/~scharr/ir/netting/	Free
Medical World Search	www.mwsearch.com	Free
Journal listings	www.nthames-health.tpmde.ac.uk/connect/journals.htm www.pslgroup.com/dg/medjournals.htm	Free
Clinical practice guidelines	www.guidelines.gov www.cma.ca/cpgs	Free
MD Consult	www.mdconsult.com	$200
Evidence-based Medicine Reviews (OVID)	www.ovid.com/products/clinical/ebmr.cfm (available through many medical libraries)	$1995

* Costs as of 2000

Selecting the Best Medical Information Resource

What is the optimal medical information resource? To a large extent, it depends on the type of question that you have and the time you have available.[5] During the late 1980s, observational studies suggested that clinicians could identify one to two unanswered questions per patient in an outpatient setting[6] and up to five per patient in a hospital setting.[7] More recent studies in family practice in the United Kingdom[8] and the United States[9] have found the rate of questions arising in patient care to be 0.32 question per patient.

Be sure to match your question to the source of information that could likely provide the most appropriate answer. To take extreme examples, MEDLINE is not the best source of information on gross anatomy, and the hospital information system is the best place to provide laboratory data for a specific patient. Table 1A-4 summarizes the types of questions that clinicians ask, along with the optimal study designs, online sources of data, and MEDLINE searching terms to match the methodologic type.

To answer focused foreground clinical questions, the most efficient approach is to begin with a prefiltered evidence-based medicine resource such as Best Evidence, the Cochrane Library, or Clinical Evidence (see Table 1A-3). By prefiltered, we mean that someone has reviewed the literature and chosen only the methodologically strongest studies. The authors of these products have designed them in such a way as to make searching easy. The sources are updated regularly—from months to a couple of years—with methodologically sound and clinically important studies.

Textbooks. To find answers to general background medical questions, prefiltered evidence-based medicine resources are unlikely to be helpful. Referring to a textbook that is well referenced and updated frequently is likely to be faster and more rewarding. UpToDate and *Scientific American Medicine* are updated regularly—from months to years, depending on the rapidity with which important new evidence is accumulating; they are heavily referenced so that you can assess how current the material is and you can even read the original articles. Other textbooks available in electronic formats, such as *Harrison's Principles of Internal Medicine*, can also provide valuable general background information. Additionally, new textbooks that are entirely Internet based, such as *emedicine*,

TABLE 1A-4

Asking Focused and Answerable Clinical Questions

Question Type	Population	Intervention/ Exposure	Outcome	Best Feasible Study Designs	Suitable Databases	Best Single MEDLINE Search Term for Appropriate Study Type
Diagnosis	In patients with lung cancer	What is the test performance of CT scan	For detecting mediastinal metastatic disease	Cross-sectional analytic study	Best Evidence, UpToDate, MEDLINE	Sensitivity.tw
Harm	In men	Does vasectomy	Cause testicular cancer	Cohort study, population-based case-control study	Best Evidence, UpToDate, MEDLINE	Risk.tw
Prognosis	In young men with atypical chest pain	Sent home from the emergency department, in the next 72 hours	Suffer appreciable rates of unstable angina, heart failure, arrhythmia, myocardial infarction, or sudden death	Cohort study	Best Evidence, UpToDate, MEDLINE	Explode cohort studies
Treatment	In patients with hypertension and type 2 diabetes mellitus	Does a target DBP of 80 compared with DBP of 90 mm Hg	Lower risk of stroke, MI, cardiovascular death, and all-cause mortality	RCT or systematic review of RCTs	Cochrane Library, Best Evidence, UpToDate, MEDLINE	Meta-analysis.pt (for systematic reviews) or Clinical trial.pt (for RCTs)

CT indicates computed tomographic; DBP, diastiric blood pressure; MI, myocardial infarction; RCT, randomized controlled trial.

are now available. As texts become more evidence based and routinely are updated as new evidence is published, they will provide an increasingly important source of answers to foreground as well as background questions. Our own experience suggests that UpToDate and Clinical Evidence are already well along the path to becoming evidence-based sources to answer foreground questions.

MEDLINE. MEDLINE, the bibliographic database maintained by the US National Library of Medicine, is useful primarily to answer focused foreground questions. The size and complexity of this database, however, make searching somewhat more difficult and time consuming. As a result, we recommend using MEDLINE only when searching prefiltered sources has proved fruitless (or when prior knowledge suggests, before beginning the search, that prefiltered sources will prove barren).

We will now review the databases suitable for answering a specific clinical question, illustrating their use with the example of the optimal blood pressure target level in patients with diabetes.

Using Prefiltered Medical Information Resources

A good starting point in the evidence-seeking process is to look for a systematic review article on your topic. A systematic review addresses a targeted clinical question using strategies that decrease the likelihood of bias. The authors of a rigorous systematic review will have already done the work of accumulating and summarizing the best of the published (and ideally unpublished) evidence. You will find both Best Evidence and the Cochrane Library useful for finding high-quality systematic reviews quickly and effectively. Both are also good sources to consult for original studies.

Best Evidence

Best Evidence is one of the quickest available routes to systematic reviews and original studies that address focused clinical questions. Available in CD-ROM format or on the Internet through OVID Technology's Evidence-Based Medicine Reviews, Best Evidence is the cumulative electronic version of two paper-based secondary journals: *ACP Journal Club* and *Evidence-Based Medicine*. (These journals were combined into one journal, *ACP Journal Club*, in North, South, and Central America in January 2000. *Evidence-Based Medicine* is available only outside the United States.) The editorial team for these journals systematically searches 170 medical journals on a regular basis to identify original studies and systematic reviews that are both methodologically sound and clinically relevant, especially for the more common diseases and conditions. By methodologically sound, we mean that they meet validity criteria (see Part 1B1, "Therapy"; Part 1B2, "Harm"; Part 1C, "The Process of Diagnosis"; Part 1C1, "Differential Diagnosis"; Part 1C2, "Diagnostic Tests"; and Part 1D, "Prognosis"). For example, the treatment section includes only randomized trials with 80% follow-up, and the diagnosis section includes only studies that make an independent, blind comparison of a test with a gold standard.

ACP Journal Club and *Evidence-Based Medicine* present structured abstracts of studies that meet these criteria, along with an accompanying commentary by an expert who offers a clinical perspective on the study results. In a section of Best Evidence entitled "Other Articles Noted," clinicians can find other studies that meet methodologic criteria but have been judged less relevant. Best Evidence is updated annually and now includes over 2000 abstracted articles that relate to general internal medicine, dating back to 1991. The editors review each article every 5 years to make sure that it has not become dated in view of more recent evidence. In addition to general internal medicine, Best Evidence includes a broader range of articles since 1995 that encompass obstetrics and gynecology, family medicine, pediatrics, psychiatry, and surgery.

Because Best Evidence includes only articles that reviewers have decided meet basic standards of methodologic quality, it is substantially smaller than many other medical literature databases, and thus is easier to search. The downside of this small size is that it is not comprehensive; a search restricted to Best Evidence will not be complete and will put you at risk for receiving a biased selection of articles. However, we believe that the uniformly relatively high methodologic quality of the articles, and the very quick searches that Best Evidence allows, compensate for this limitation.

Example of Best Evidence Search. To locate information on blood pressure control in people with type 2 diabetes mellitus, we used the "Search" option in Best Evidence 4 (Figure 1A-6). We entered the phrase representing the question aspects,

"hypertension AND diabetes AND mortality"

resulting in a list of 109 articles. Many of these citations, however, dealt with the prognosis of patients with diabetes and were not directly relevant to our question. Therefore, we returned to the search option, entered the same terms but changed the search strategy from "All topics" to "Selected topics," and clicked on the "Therapeutics" option before completing the search. This yielded a shorter list of 27 articles, all pertaining to therapy (Figure 1A-7). Five were review articles but none of these addressed our topic. Of the 22 original studies, the first was entitled "Tight Blood Pressure Control Reduced Diabetes Mellitus-Related Death and Complications and Was Cost-effective in Diabetes" (Figure 1A-8). Double-clicking on this title

produced a structured abstract[10] describing a randomized
trial that enrolled persons with type 2 diabetes mellitus and
hypertension and evaluated the effect of aiming for either a
blood pressure of less than 150/85 mm Hg or a blood pressure of less than 180/105 mm Hg (Figure 1A-9). After an
average of 9 years of follow-up, the tight blood pressure
control arm had a 32% reduction in the risk of death
related to diabetes (95% confidence interval, 8%-50%;
P=.019) (Figure 1A-10).

FIGURE 1A–6

Best Evidence—Title Page (CD-ROM version)

Reproduced with permission from the American College of Physicians-Society of
Internal Medicine.

FIGURE 1A–7

Best Evidence—Selected Topic Search

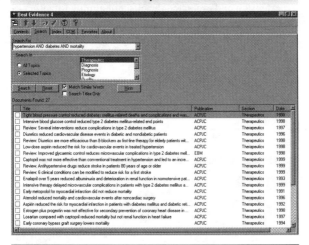

Searching Best Evidence will not always provide an article that answers your question. High-quality evidence is not available or may not have been published in one of the 170 Best Evidence target journals. A relevant trial may have been published after the most recent edition of Best Evidence was released, or before 1991. Rigorous studies published since 1991 will not appear in Best Evidence if the editors believe that they pertain more to subspecialty care than to general internal medicine. Despite these limitations, searching Best Evidence will often be rewarding, especially if you are searching for one of the more common diseases and conditions. And if your search is not rewarding, Best Evidence searches occur so quickly that you will have plenty of time to look elsewhere.

FIGURE 1A–8

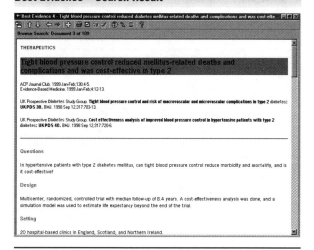

Best Evidence—Search Result

> + Best Evidence 4 · Tight blood pressure control reduced diabetes mellitus-related deaths and complications and was cost-effe...
>
> Browse Search: Document 3 of 189
>
> THERAPEUTICS
>
> **Tight blood pressure control reduced mellitus-related deaths and complications and was cost-effective in type 2**
>
> ACP Journal Club. 1999 Jan-Feb;130:4-5.
> Evidence-Based Medicine. 1999 Jan-Feb;4:12-13.
>
> UK Prospective Diabetes Study Group. **Tight blood pressure control and risk of macrovascular and microvascular complications in type 2** diabetes: **UKPDS 38.** BMJ. 1998 Sep 12;317:703-13.
>
> UK Prospective Diabetes Study Group. **Cost effectiveness analysis of improved blood pressure control in hypertensive patients with type 2** diabetes: **UKPDS 40.** BMJ. 1998 Sep 12;317:720-6.
>
> ___
>
> Questions
>
> In hypertensive patients with type 2 diabetes mellitus, can tight blood pressure control reduce morbidity and mortality, and is it cost-effective?
>
> Design
>
> Multicenter, randomized, controlled trial with median follow-up of 8.4 years. A cost-effectiveness analysis was done, and a simulation model was used to estimate life expectancy beyond the end of the trial.
>
> Setting
>
> 20 hospital-based clinics in England, Scotland, and Northern Ireland.

Reproduced with permission from the American College of Physicians-Society of Internal Medicine.

Cochrane Library

The Cochrane Collaboration, an international organization that prepares, maintains, and disseminates systematic reviews of health care interventions, offers another electronic resource for locating high-quality information quickly. They publish the Cochrane Library, which focuses primarily on systematic reviews of controlled trials of therapeutic interventions. It provides little help in addressing other aspects of medical care, such as the value of a new diagnostic test or a patient's prognosis.

Updated quarterly, the Cochrane Library is available in CD-ROM format or over the Internet. It contains three main sections. The first of these, the Cochrane Database of

FIGURE 1A–9

Best Evidence—Abstract

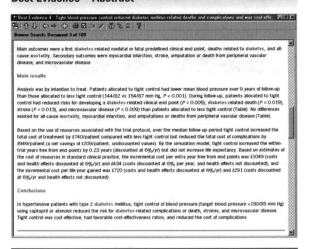

Reproduced with permission from the American College of Physicians-Society of Internal Medicine.

Systematic Reviews (CDSR), includes the complete reports for all of the systematic reviews that have been prepared by members of the Cochrane Collaboration (716 were in the first issue for 2000) and the protocols for Cochrane systematic reviews that are under way. A second part of the Cochrane Library, the Database of Reviews of Effectiveness (DARE), includes systematic reviews that have been published outside of the collaboration; the first issue for 2000 included 2565 such reviews. Database of Reviews of Effectiveness is searchable outside the Cochrane Library (at http://nhscrd.york.ac.uk); this site also includes access to a database of economic evaluations and health technology assessments.

FIGURE 1A–10

Best Evidence—Results Table

Best Evidence 4 - Tight blood pressure control reduced diabetes mellitus-related deaths and complications and was cost-effe...

Browse Search: Document 3 of 189

Tight vs less tight blood pressure control in hypertensive patients with type 2 diabetes mellitus*

Outcomes over 8.4 y of follow-up	Tight control	Less tight control	RRR (95% CI)	NNT (CI)
Any diabetes-related clinical end point	34%	44%	22% (9 to 32)	11 (6 to 29)
Diabetes-related death	11%	16%	32% (8 to 50)	20 (10 to 100)
All-cause mortality	18%	21%	17% (-6 to 35)	Not significant
Myocardial infarction	14%	18%	20% (-5 to 39)	Not significant
Stroke	5%	9%	42% (10 to 63)	27 (14 to 141)
Peripheral vascular stroke	1%	2%	49% (-32 to 60)	Not significant
Microvascular disease	9%	14%	35% (9 to 54)	21 (11 to 94)

*Abbreviations defined in Glossary ; RRR, NNT, and CI calculated from data in article.

Commentary

The UKPDS shows that meticulous blood pressure reduction is important in patients with type 2 diabetes. This finding has major implications for health care because of the projected dramatic increase in diabetes in the future and the clear relation between diabetes and hypertension. The Systolic Hypertension in the Elderly Program (SHEP) has shown that antihypertensive treatment reduces cardiovascular events in elderly patients with and without diabetes (1). The present trial consolidates this information and extends the findings to younger patients and to patients with newly detected diabetes. The results are consistent with the recently published Hypertension Optimal Treatment (HOT) study, in which intensive blood

Reproduced with permission from the American College of Physicians-Society of Internal Medicine.

The third section of the Library, the Cochrane Controlled Trials Registry (CCTR), contains a growing list of over 268,000 references to clinical trials that Cochrane investigators have found by searching a wide range of sources. The sources include the MEDLINE and EMBASE (Excerpta Medica) bibliographic databases, hand searches, and the reference lists of potentially relevant original studies and reviews. Although most citations refer to randomized trials, the database also includes a small number of observational studies. Studies of diagnostic tests will likely be included soon. In addition to the three main sections, the Cochrane Library also includes information about the Cochrane

Collaboration and information on how to conduct a systematic review and related methodologic issues.

To search the Cochrane Library, you can enter terms in the first screen that appears after selecting "Search" (Figure 1A-11). If you have access to the CD-ROM version, using the Advanced Search option you can create more complex search strategies that include Medical Subject Headings and logical operators (see the section on MEDLINE for an introduction to Medical Subject Headings and logical operators).

Example of Cochrane Library Search. To find information about blood pressure control in people with diabetes, we entered the search terms

"diabetes AND hypertension AND mortality"

using the 2000 version of the Cochrane Library (Issue 1) (Figure 1A-12). This yielded 36 reports in the CDSR, six citations in the DARE, and 130 citations in the CCTR (Figure 1A-13). A Cochrane review entitled "Antihypertensive therapy in diabetes mellitus"[11] appeared promising (Figure 1A-14). Double-clicking on this item, we found an entire Cochrane Collaboration systematic review, including information on the methodology for the review, the inclusion and exclusion criteria, the results, and a discussion (Figure 1A-15). The results presented the findings in both textual and graphical forms. As was the case with the review article found in Best Evidence, however, this review did not help to resolve the issue of the optimal blood pressure goal for people with diabetes mellitus.

FIGURE 1A–11

The Cochrane Database of Systematic Reviews

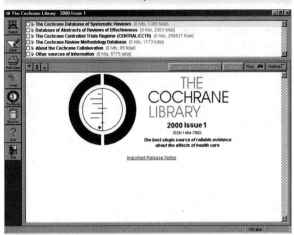

Reproduced with permission from Update Software.

Turning to the CCTR (we double-clicked on the CCTR option to make the citation titles appear), we found both the United Kingdom Prospective Diabetes Study Group (UKPDS)[10] and the Hypertension Optimal Treatment (HOT) trial[12] within the first 26 citations. The HOT trial was a randomized trial that compared three different blood pressure management strategies in persons with hypertension. Subgroup analyses showed that patients with diabetes who reduced their blood pressure to 81.1 mm Hg vs 85.2 mm Hg because of being in the groups randomized to lower target blood pressures had lower rates of cardiovascular events and cardiovascular death.

FIGURE 1A–12

The Cochrane Database of Systematic Reviews— Search Strategy

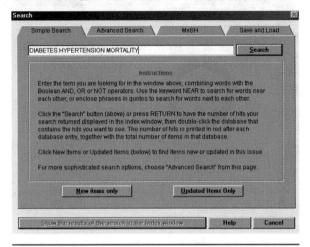

Reproduced with permission from Update Software.

A second search further illustrates the usefulness of the CCTR database. Recall the patient with non-small-cell lung cancer for whom we were considering alternative investigational strategies of mediastinoscopy for all, or a selective approach based on the results of CT scanning. Using the search term "mediastinoscopy," we found that the clinical trials database yielded 20 citations, of which the fourth and fifth were MEDLINE and EMBASE records of a study a randomized trial in 685 patients with apparently operable non-small-cell carcinoma of the lung. The investigators randomized patients to an arm in which all patients underwent mediastinoscopy or an

FIGURE 1A–13

The Cochrane Database of Systematic Reviews— Search Results

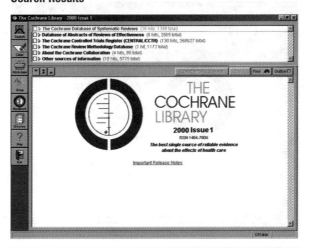

Reproduced with permission from Update Software.

arm in which all patients underwent CT scanning, with patients with small nodes going straight to thoracotomy and those with larger nodes undergoing mediastinoscopy. The relative risk of an unnecessary thoracotomy in patients in the CT scanning arm was 0.88 (95% confidence interval, 0.71-1.10). The mediastinoscopy strategy cost $708 more per patient (95% confidence interval, $723-$2140). The authors concluded that "the computed tomography strategy is likely to produce the same number of or fewer unnecessary thoracotomies in comparison with doing mediastinoscopy on all patients and is also likely to be as or less expensive."[13]

FIGURE 1A–14

The Cochrane Database of Systematic Reviews—Article

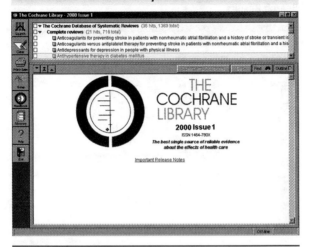

Reproduced with permission from Update Software.

UpToDate

UpToDate is a well-referenced online textbook that is carefully updated every 4 months. It exists in digital format because it is too large to print. Although UpToDate, unlike Best Evidence and the Cochrane Database of Systematic Reviews, does not have a set of explicit methodologic quality criteria that included articles must meet, it does reference many high-quality studies chosen by its section authors.

Example of UpToDate Search. To locate information on blood pressure control in people with type 2 diabetes mellitus, we entered the term "diabetes" in the search window for

FIGURE 1A–15

The Cochrane Database of Systematic Reviews— Review Article

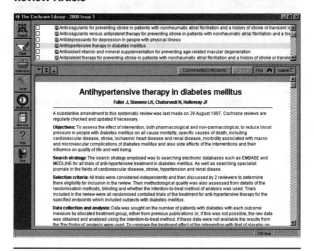

Reproduced with permission from Update Software.

version 8.3 (Figure 1A-16). This resulted in a list of 21 key word options and we selected "diabetes mellitus, type 2." This yielded 64 articles, including one entitled "Treatment of Hypertension in Diabetes" that reviewed pathogenesis and included a section on the goal of blood pressure reduction (Figures 1A-17 and 1A-18). This section provided a detailed description of the two large randomized trials, the HOT[12] and UKPDS,[10] trials, that specifically addressed the clinical outcomes associated with more aggressive compared with less aggressive blood pressure management strategies. The text summarized the design and findings, and we were able to retrieve the study abstracts by clicking on the references.

FIGURE 1A–16

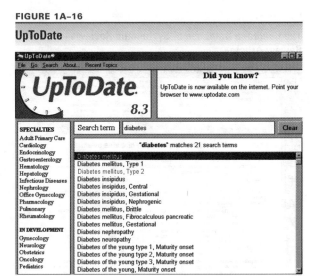

Reproduced with permission from UpToDate.

Clinical Evidence

Clinical Evidence, published by the *BMJ* Publishing Group
and American College of Physicians/American Society of
Internal Medicine, is similar to UpToDate, although less
oriented to provide bottom-line clinical advice from experts.
Clinical Evidence is text based and available online. By
design the producers have not written a textbook; instead,
they aim to provide a concise account of the current state of
knowledge, ignorance, and uncertainty about the prevention
and treatment of common and important clinical conditions. It is published biannually and online products are now
available (www.evidence.org).

FIGURE 1A-17

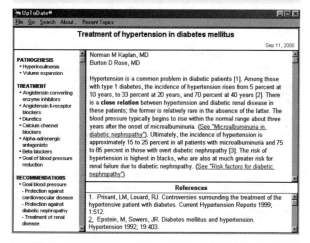

UpToDate—Search Results

Treatment of hypertension in diabetes mellitus

Sep 11, 2000

PATHOGENESIS
• Hyperinsulinemia
• Volume expansion

TREATMENT
• Angiotensin converting enzyme inhibitors
• Angiotensin II-receptor blockers
• Diuretics
• Calcium channel blockers
• Alpha-adrenergic antagonists
• Beta blockers
• Goal of blood pressure reduction

RECOMMENDATIONS
• Goal blood pressure
  - Protection against cardiovascular disease
  - Protection against diabetic nephropathy
  - Treatment of renal disease

Norman M Kaplan, MD
Burton D Rose, MD

Hypertension is a common problem in diabetic patients [1]. Among those with type 1 diabetes, the incidence of hypertension rises from 5 percent at 10 years, to 33 percent at 20 years, and 70 percent at 40 years [2]. There is a **close relation** between hypertension and diabetic renal disease in these patients; the former is relatively rare in the absence of the latter. The blood pressure typically begins to rise within the normal range about three years after the onset of microalbuminuria. (See "Microalbuminuria in diabetic nephropathy"). Ultimately, the incidence of hypertension is approximately 15 to 25 percent in all patients with microalbuminuria and 75 to 85 percent in those with overt diabetic nephropathy [3]. The risk of hypertension is highest in blacks, who are also at much greater risk for renal failure due to diabetic nephropathy. (See "Risk factors for diabetic nephropathy").

References

1. Prisant, LM, Louard, RJ. Controversies surrounding the treatment of the hypertensive patient with diabetes. Current Hypertension Reports 1999; 1:512.
2. Epstein, M, Sowers, JR. Diabetes mellitus and hypertension. Hypertension 1992; 19:403.

Reproduced with permission from UpToDate.

Example of Clinical Evidence Search. For the question of target blood pressure in people with diabetes, a search using the terms

"target blood pressure AND diabetes"

took us directly to the section entitled "Which interventions improve cardiovascular outcomes in patients with diabetes?" (Figure 1A-19). A subsection on treatment of hypertension includes a discussion of target levels backed up by evidence from the trials we have found in the other resources (HOT and UKPDS trials).

FIGURE 1A–18

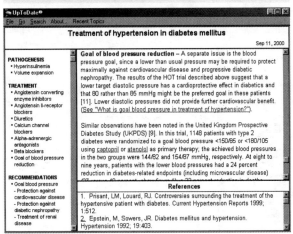

UpToDate—Search Results (continued)

Reproduced with permission from UpToDate.

Using Unfiltered Medical Information Sources

MEDLINE

If a search of Best Evidence, the Cochrane Library, UpToDate, and Clinical Evidence does not provide a satisfactory answer to a focused clinical question, it is time to turn to MEDLINE. The US National Library of Medicine maintains this impressive bibliographic database, which includes over 11,000,000 citations of both clinical and preclinical studies. A complementary database known as PreMEDLINE includes citations and abstracts for studies that have been published recently but not yet indexed. MEDLINE is an attractive database for finding medical information because of its relatively comprehensive coverage of medical journals

FIGURE 1A–19

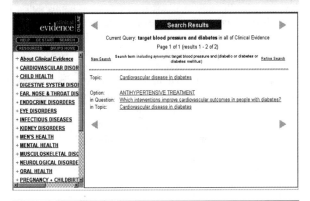

Reproduced with permission from the BMJ Publishing Group.

and because it is readily accessible. Anyone with Internet access can search MEDLINE free of charge using PubMed or Internet Grateful Med. In addition, most health sciences or hospital libraries provide access to MEDLINE through a commercial vendor such as OVID, Knowledge Finder, or Silver Platter.

These positive features are balanced with a disadvantage that relates to MEDLINE's size and to the range of publications that it encompasses. Searching MEDLINE effectively often requires careful thought, along with a thorough knowledge of how the database is structured and how publications are indexed. Understanding how to use Medical Subject Headings is essential, as is text word searching and exploding and use of the logical operators AND and OR to combine different search results.

If you are unfamiliar with MEDLINE searching techniques, an article by Greenhalgh[14] presents a good introduction. If you suspect that you may have gaps in your searching skills, strongly consider spending some time with an experienced medical librarian or taking a course on MEDLINE searching. Another potential source for information on searching techniques is to visit an Internet Web site designed to introduce the topic. A listing of tutorials designed to assist users of different MEDLINE systems and at different experience levels is available (www.docnet.org.uk/drfelix/medtut.html). More detailed information on searching MEDLINE and a number of other large bibliographic databases, including EMBASE (Excerpta Medica), is also available in a reference book.[15] In this section, we present only the most crucial and basic MEDLINE searching advice.

The MEDLINE indexers choose Medical Subject Headings (MeSH) for each article. These headings provide one strategy for searching. Note, however, that indexers reference articles under the most specific subject heading available (for example, "ventricular dysfunction, left" rather than the more general term "ventricular dysfunction"). As a result, if you choose the more general heading ("ventricular dysfunction") you risk missing out on many articles of interest. To deal with this problem, use a command known as *explode*. This command identifies all articles that have been indexed using a given MeSH term, as well as articles indexed using more specific terms. For example, in the PubMed MEDLINE system for the 1966 to 2000 file, the MeSH heading "sports" contains 10,806 indexed articles, whereas "explode sports," which picks up more than 20 specific sports from baseball and basketball through weight lifting and wrestling, contains 37,043 indexed articles.

Another fundamental search strategy substitutes reliance on the decisions made by MEDLINE indexers with the choices of study authors regarding terminology. Using "text word" searching makes it possible to identify all articles in which either the study title or abstract includes a certain term. Experience with MEDLINE allows a clinician to develop preferred search strategies. Comprehensive searches will usually utilize both MeSH headings and text words.

Example of MEDLINE Search. To search for information pertaining to blood pressure control targets in people with type 2 diabetes mellitus, we used the National Library of Medicine's PubMed MEDLINE searching system. We began by entering the term "diabetes mellitus" and clicking the "Go" button. This yielded a total of 143,691 citations dating back to 1966 (Figure 1A-20). Notice that before searching MEDLINE and PreMEDLINE, the PubMed system processed our request. Rather than simply completing a text word search, PubMed developed a more comprehensive strategy that also included the most appropriate MeSH term. To further increase the yield of citations, PubMed also automatically exploded the MeSH term. PubMed searched MEDLINE and PreMEDLINE using the strategy:

> diabetes mellitus (text word) OR explode
> diabetes mellitus (MeSH term).

The "OR" in the strategy is called a logical operator. It asks MEDLINE to combine the publications found using either the first search term or the second search term to make a more comprehensive list of publications in which diabetes is a topic of discussion.

FIGURE 1A-20

PubMed—Diabetes Mellitus Search

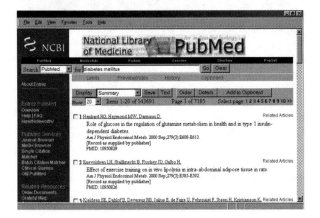

We then searched using the term "hypertension" (180,333
references) and the term "mortality" (320,133 references).
To combine these three searches, we initially clicked on the
"History" button, which showed us a summary. By entering
the phrase

"#1 AND #2 AND #3"

into the search window, we were able to ask PubMed to
locate only those citations that addressed all of diabetes
mellitus, hypertension, and mortality (Figure 1A-21).

FIGURE 1A–21

PubMed—Combining Search Terms

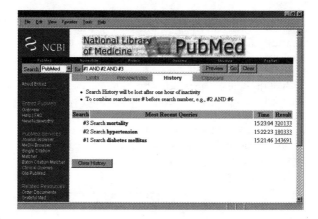

Reproduced with permission from the National Library of Medicine.

Unfortunately, the list of publications that concern all of diabetes, hypertension, and mortality still included 1965 references (Figure 1A-22), prompting us to take advantage of another searching technique designed to help identify particular types of clinical studies. Search hedges or search filters are systematically tested search strategies that help identify methodologically sound studies pertaining to questions of therapy, diagnosis, prognosis, or harm (Figure 1A-23). For example, to retrieve studies related to prognosis, the sensitive search strategy is

incidence (MeSH) OR explode mortality (MeSH)
OR follow-up studies (MeSH) OR mortality (subheading)
OR prognos: (text word) OR predict: (text word)
OR course (text word)

and the specific search strategy is

prognosis (MeSH) OR survival analysis (MeSH).

Sensitive search strategies have comprehensive retrieval with some irrelevant citations, whereas a specific search strategy is not as comprehensive but is less likely to retrieve irrelevant citations. A complete listing of the strategies is available, along with the sensitivities and specificities for each of the different approaches.[16–18] Although the strategies tend to be complex, many MEDLINE searching systems now have them automatically available for use. The PubMed system has a special section with these strategies entitled "Clinical Queries." Access to this option is on the left side of the main searching screen.

FIGURE 1A–22

PubMed—Combining Search Terms (Results)

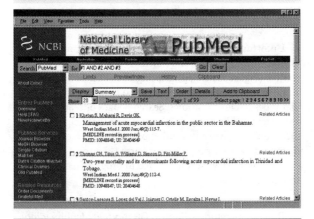

FIGURE 1A–23

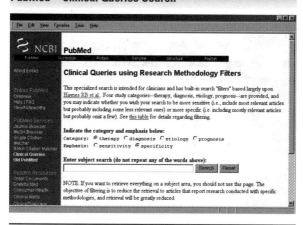

PubMed—Clinical Queries Search

Reproduced with permission from the National Library of Medicine.

As an alternative to the hedges, clinicians can use "single best terms" for finding higher-quality studies. These terms include "clinical trial" (publication type) for treatment; "sensitivity" (text word) for diagnosis; "explode cohort studies" (MeSH) for prognosis; and "risk" (text word) for harm (see Table 1A-4).

Combining our previous strategy with the term "clinical trial" (publication type) yielded a list of 117 publications (Figure 1A-24). Once again, we found references to the UKPDS trial and the HOT trial in the citation list.

FIGURE 1A–24

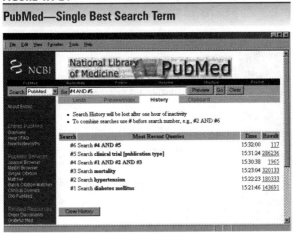

Reproduced with permission from the National Library of Medicine.

One other useful feature of PubMed is its easy-to-use search-ing system, which makes knowledge of how to use the various subject heading features and logical operators described above less crucial. The searcher can enter a set of words or phrases into the first window. For example, thinking back to our young man with atypical—possible unstable—angina, we could type

"unstable angina monitor* discharg*"

in the first searching window, and would find 26 citations. The "*" indicates truncation to pick up similar words with varying endings: monitor* picks up "monitor," monitoring, and monitored. The 11th article is a narrative review.[19] By clicking on the "See related" button, the searcher finds another 238 related citations presented in order from the most to least relevant (according to the computer algorithm).

The World Wide Web

The World Wide Web is rapidly becoming an important source of medical information. A vast number of resources can now be accessed using the Internet—some for a fee, others free of charge. To make these resources more accessible, certain Web sites have been designed specifically to provide links to medical information locations or to facilitate searching for medical information on the Internet. Examples of such Web sites include Medical Matrix, Medscape, ScHARR, and Medical World Search. Clinicians can also use the Internet to access medical journals and clinical practice guidelines.

We must, however, issue a user beware caveat: some of these guidelines may fail to meet *Users' Guides* criteria for evidence-based guidelines (see Part 1F, "Moving From Evidence to Action"). An example of a site that provides access to many resources, including journals, textbooks, and guidelines, albeit for a fee, is MD Consult.

Finally, Web sites produced and maintained by reputable organizations such as the American Cancer Society (www.cancer.org) or the American Diabetes Association (www.diabetes.org) provide another approach for finding information.

CLINICAL APPLICATION

The health sciences literature is enormous and continues to expand rapidly. To the extent that this reflects ongoing research and the identification of potential improvements for patient care, this is very promising. At the same time, however, it makes the task of locating the best and most current therapy or diagnostic test more challenging. The emergence of new information products specifically designed to provide ready access to high-quality, clinically relevant, and current information is timely and encouraging.

Finding the articles that address your clinical question requires 5 to 30 minutes, depending on the resource you use or your experience with systematic searching.[3] A full assessment of the validity and applicability requires an additional half-hour. The UKPDS study[10] and the HOT study[12] are the closest matches to your patient and the clinical situation. The studies show a clear reduction of diabetes-related mortality with tight blood pressure control in persons with type 2 diabetes mellitus and hypertension. You decide to set target systolic blood pressure at < 150 mm Hg and target diastolic blood pressure at < 80 mm Hg.

References

1. Haynes RB. Loose connections between peer reviewed clinical journals and clinical practice. *Ann Intern Med.* 1990;113:724-728.

2. Oxman AD, Sackett DL, Guyatt GH, for the Evidence-based Medicine Working Group. Users' guides to the medical literature, I: How to get started. *JAMA.* 1993;270:2093-2095.

3. Richardson WS, Wilson MC, Nishikawa J, Hayward RSA. The well-built clinical question: a key to evidence-based decisions. *ACP Journal Club.* Nov-Dec 1995;123:A-12.

4. McKibbon KA, Richardson WS, Walker Dilks C. Finding answers to well built clinical questions. *Evidence-Based Medicine.* 1999;6:164-167.

5. Sackett DL, Straus SE. Finding and applying evidence during clinical rounds: the "evidence cart." *JAMA.* 1998;280:1336-1338.

6. Covell DG, Uman GC, Manning PR. Information needs in office practice: are they being met? *Ann Intern Med.* 1985;103:596-599.

7. Osheroff JA, Forsythe DE, Buchanan BG, Bankowitz RA, Blumenfeld BH, Miller RA. Physicians' information needs: analysis of questions posed during clinical teaching. *Ann Intern Med.* 1991;114:576-581.

8. Barrie AR, Ward AM. Questioning behaviour in general practice: a pragmatic study. *BMJ.* 1997;315:1515.

9. Ely JW, Osheroff JA, Ebell MH, et al. Analysis of questions asked by family doctors regarding patient care. *BMJ.* 1999;319:358-361.

10. Tight blood pressure control and risk of macrovascular and microvascular complications in Type 2 diabetes mellitus: UKPDS 38. *BMJ.* 1998;317:703-713.

11. Fuller J, Stevens LK, Chaturvedi N, Holloway JF. Antihypertensive therapy in diabetes mellitus (Cochrane Review). In: The Cochrane Library, Issue 4, 1999. Oxford: Update Software.

12. Hansson L, Zanchetti A, Carruthers SG, et al, for the HOT Study Group. Effects of intensive blood-pressure lowering and low-dose aspirin in patients with hypertension: principal results of the Hypertension Optimal Treatment (HOT) randomized trial. *Lancet.* 1998;351:1755-1762.

13. The Canadian Lung Oncology Group. Investigation for mediastinal disease in patients with apparently operable lung cancer. *Ann Thorac Surg.* 1995;60:1382-1389.

14. Greenhalgh T. How to read a paper: the Medline database. *BMJ.* 1997;315:180-183.

15. McKibbon A. *Evidence-based Principles and Practice.* Hamilton: Decker; 1999.

16. Haynes RB, Wilczynski N, McKibbon KA, et al. Developing optimal search strategies for detecting clinically sound studies in MEDLINE. *J Am Med Informatics Assoc.* 1994;1:447-458.

17. Wilczynski NL, Walker CJ, McKibbon KA, Haynes RB. Assessment of methodologic search filters in MEDLINE. *Proc Annu Symp Comp Appl Med Care.* 1994;17:601-605.

18. Devillé WL, Bezemer PD, Bouter LM. Publications on diagnostic test evaluation in family medicine journals: an optimal search strategy. *J Clin Epidemiol.* 2000;53:65-69.

19. Bankwala Z, Swenson LJ. Unstable angina pectoris: what is the likelihood of further cardiac events? *Postgrad Med.* 1995;98:155-158,161-162,164-165.

THERAPY AND HARM: AN INTRODUCTION

Gordon Guyatt

Peter Wyer also made substantive contributions to this section

IN THIS SECTION

Clinicians' most compelling questions involve choosing the optimal management strategy for their patients. For example, what are the benefits of prescribing pharmacologic treatment or mandating dietary change to lower blood pressure, cholesterol level, or a patient's weight. What are the benefits of screening women for breast cancer or screening men for prostate cancer, or of instituting a smoking cessation program? What symptomatic benefit or increased longevity might patients anticipate from treatment of their chronic heart failure, asthma, or diabetes? Equally important, what short-term or long-term adverse effects might they expect as a result of their intervention?

These questions address two related issues. First, what risks, if any, will result for patients if they smoke or are overweight, if their blood pressure, cholesterol level, or glucose level is elevated, or if their heart function is abnormal? These are issues of harm. Second, if we intervene to modify their behavior or their bodies' physiology, what benefits will ensue, and will these benefits outweigh any deleterious consequences? These are issues of therapy.

When we address questions of both therapy and harm, we are confronting issues of causation. There are myriad examples. In a particular group of people (healthy men or women, patients with diabetes, or patients with heart failure, for example) is there a causal relationship between an exposure (smoking, obesity, or high blood pressure) or intervention (an antismoking or weight loss program, or a drug that lowers blood pressure) and a particular anticipated outcome (lung cancer, myocardial infarction, or stroke) or unanticipated outcome (eg, the profound visual loss resulting from one antihypertensive medication[1]).

For each of these questions, there is an underlying true answer. If our inferences about the underlying truth are wrong, the consequences may be disastrous. Consider how many lives must have been lost over the course of several hundred years when physicians were convinced that blood-letting was an effective treatment for an extraordinarily wide variety of illnesses. It is impossible to estimate the numbers. By contrast, records of the number of prescriptions and an evaluation of the magnitude of harm from a randomized trial make it possible to estimate the thousands of lives lost resulting from the much more recent administration of class I antiarrhythmia drugs—agents that physicians believed would prevent lethal arrhythmias when, in fact, they were causing them.[2]

Why has the medical community made such disastrous blunders, and what can we do to prevent their repetition? The answer lies in clinicians learning rules of evidence that allow them to differentiate false claims from valid ones. If you are content with a practical approach to determining when you can believe study results and when you cannot, read on. If, however, you would like a deeper conceptual understanding of the foundation of our *Users' Guides to the Medical Literature,* turn now to Part 2A, "Therapy and Harm, Why Study Results Mislead—Bias and Random Error."

THREE STEPS IN USING AN ARTICLE FROM THE MEDICAL LITERATURE

When using the medical literature to answer a clinical question, approach the study using three discrete steps.

In the first step, ask, "***Are the results of the study valid?***" This question has to do with the believability or credibility of the results. In answering this question, you consider whether the estimate of the treatment effect reported in the article faithfully represents the direction and magnitude of the underlying true effect. Another way to state this question is: "Do these results represent an unbiased estimate of the treatment effect, or have they been influenced in some systematic fashion to lead to a false conclusion?" If the results are valid and the study likely yields an unbiased assessment of the treatment effect, then the results are worth examining further.

In the second step, ask, "*What are the results?*" to consider the size and precision of the treatment's effect. The best estimate of that effect will be the study findings themselves; the precision of the estimate may be superior in larger studies.

Once you understand the results, ask yourself the third question, "*How can I apply these results to patient care?*" This question has two parts. First, can you generalize (or, to put it another way, particularize) the results to your patient? For instance, you should hesitate to institute a treatment if your patient is too dissimilar from those who participated in the trial. Second, if the results are generalizable to your patient, what is the net impact of the treatment? Have the investigators measured all outcomes of importance to patients? The impact depends on both benefits and risks (side effects and toxicity) of treatment and the consequences of withholding treatment. Thus, even therapy that is effective might be withheld when a patient's prognosis is already good without treatment, especially when the treatment is accompanied by important side effects and toxicity.

THERAPY AND HARM: STUDY DESIGNS

Randomized Controlled Trials to Assess Treatment

When investigating an issue of treatment, researchers have much more control than when exploring a question of harm. For instance, they can determine who receives the experimental intervention and who receives the control (eg, no treatment or placebo). Ideally, they will allocate patients to groups according to a process analogous to a coin flip, called *randomization,* and they will conduct a randomized controlled trial. In addition, they can design their study so that neither patients nor caregivers are aware of which patients receive the experimental treatment.

Observational Studies to Assess Harm

By contrast, researchers looking at issues of harm generally do not have this sort of control. They cannot dictate to people whether they should live in high- or low-pollution environments; neither can they allocate them to groups living in spacious or overcrowded settings. Investigators cannot conceal from study participants their living environment—or whether or not they smoke. As a result, investigators use observational study designs. They may follow patients who, as a result of preference or circumstances, have been exposed to a harmful stimulus. They follow them forward in time to determine if they suffer the outcome about which they are concerned, the target outcome (a *cohort* study). Alternatively, researchers may select individuals who have already suffered the target outcome. In addition, they select another group that has not yet suffered the target outcome, and compare the extent to which the two groups had been exposed to the putative harmful agent (a *case-control study*) (see Part 1B2, "Harm").

Applying Appropriate Criteria

Inferences from studies investigating harm are generally much weaker than those from studies of therapy. As a user of the medical literature, you must apply different criteria to a study of a therapeutic question than to one investigating a harmful exposure. We therefore provide separate *Users' Guides* for coverage of issues of therapy and harm (see Part 1B1, "Therapy," and Part 1B2, "Harm").

There are exceptions to this general rule. Sometimes, the harmful exposure may be a medical intervention, such as a drug, and researchers will perceive the putative harmful effect as occurring quickly and frequently. Under these circumstances, investigators may be able to use the study design usually associated with therapy to determine if there is a causal relation between the drug and the toxic effect.

Similarly, there may be no randomized trials available—or even feasible—addressing a particular therapeutic issue. Investigations of rare conditions, community interventions, the care delivered in different hospitals, or the quality of care within a hospital do not easily lend themselves to randomized trials. Randomizing health care systems to rely more on primary care physicians or specialists, or to base reimbursement on fee-for-service or capitation, or to public funding vs user-pay, seems, for the foreseeable future at least, improbable.

In all situations when clinicians addressing issues of therapy find that randomized trials are unavailable, they need to rely on cohort and case-control studies—the strongest evidence available. In doing so, they must apply the appropriate criteria for the evaluation of these studies, criteria that ordinarily would be associated with investigations of potentially harmful exposures. When relying on cohort or case-control studies to address issues of therapeutic benefit, however, clinicians must bear in mind that the strength of any inferences about the causal relation between the intervention and the outcome become much weaker than they would if evidence came from a randomized trial.

References

1. Wright P. Untoward effects associated with practolol administration: oculomucocutaneous syndrome. *BMJ.* 1975;1:595-598.

2. Moore TJ. *Deadly Medicine*. New York, NY: Simon & Schuster; 1995.

THERAPY

Gordon Guyatt, Deborah Cook, PJ Devereaux,
Maureen Meade, and Sharon Straus

The following EBM Working Group members also made
substantive contributions to this section: Peter Wyer,
Roman Jaeschke, Daren Heyland, Anne Holbrook,
and Luz Maria Letelier

IN THIS SECTION

Finding the Evidence

Are the Results Valid?

Were Patients Randomized?

Was Randomization Concealed?

Were Patients Analyzed in the Groups to Which They
Were Randomized?

Were Patients in the Treatment and Control Groups
Similar With Respect to Known Prognostic Variables?

Were Patients Aware of Group Allocation?

Were Clinicians Aware of Group Allocation?

Were Outcome Assessors Aware of Group Allocation?

Was Follow-up Complete?

What Are the Results?

How Large Was the Treatment Effect?

How Precise Was the Estimate of the Treatment Effect?

When Authors Do Not Report the Confidence Interval

How Can I Apply the Results to Patient Care?

Were the Study Patients Similar to the Patient in
My Practice?

Were All Clinically Important Outcomes Considered?

Are the Likely Treatment Benefits Worth the Potential
Harm and Costs?

Clinical Resolution

CLINICAL SCENARIO

The Internet Tells Me Spironolactone Will Prolong My Life: Doctor, Should I Take It?

You are a general internist reviewing a 66-year-old man with idiopathic dilated cardiomyopathy whom you have been following for 3 years. The patient, who has been very involved in decision making with regard to his care, presents you with an Internet summary of a new study stating, "Spironolactone saves lives in heart failure." He is very encouraged by the summary and believes that spironolactone will prolong his life.

For the preceding 18 months, the patient has been stable with mild symptoms that you classify as New York Heart Association (NYHA) class II. His echocardiogram 3 months ago demonstrated unchanged global left-sided ventricular dysfunction with an ejection fraction of 30%. His current medications include enalapril 10 mg twice a day, metoprolol 50 mg twice a day, and furosemide 20 mg once a day. His blood pressure is 110/70 mm Hg and his heart rate is 60 bpm. His blood work from the previous week reveals a creatinine level of 100 mmol/L and potassium level of 4.1 mmol/L. Since enalapril suppresses aldosterone, you wonder how spironolactone, an aldosterone antagonist, could provide additional benefit. You check the *Physician's Desk Reference* (PDR) and read that simultaneous use of enalapril and spironolactone is relatively contraindicated because of the risk of hyperkalemia.[1] You share with the patient your concerns about spironolactone as well as your determination not to overlook its potential benefits, you inform him that you will review the evidence and offer a recommendation when he returns to see you in 1 week.

FINDING THE EVIDENCE

You begin by formulating your question:

> In patients with NYHA class II heart failure
> and a decreased ejection fraction, what is the
> impact of spironolactone therapy on
> mortality and quality of life?

Since the study you are seeking was published during the past couple of months, you know that it will not yet be included in Best Evidence, the database you would normally use to begin such a search. You therefore begin with a MED-LINE search using OVID and the following search strategy: "heart failure, congestive" (MH)—which stands for "MeSH heading"—and "spironolactone" (MH) limited to "clinical trials" and the year "1999." This search yields only four articles, one of which is evidently your target.[2]

The article you retrieve reports a trial in which investigators randomized 1663 patients with NYHA class III and class IV heart failure to receive spironolactone 25 mg once daily. In this trial, patients were followed for an average of 2 years. You immediately discern that the patient you are seeing with class II heart failure would not have been eligible for the study. However, you still suspect the trial might be relevant to this patient's care and you decide to review the report carefully before the patient returns to see you.

Although this book discusses evaluation of articles about therapy, we caution that our definition of therapy is a broad one. The principles apply to therapies designed to ameliorate symptoms or reduce morbidity and mortality in those who are acutely or chronically ill (eg, the therapeutic use of spironolactone for patients with heart failure); to interventions designed to prevent chronologically distant morbid or mortal events in patients with known underlying pathology (eg, beta blockade after myocardial infarction); to interventions designed to prevent morbidity and mortality in those at risk but without current evident illness (eg, treatment of high blood pressure); to interventions designed to improve patient outcome by improving the process of care; to diagnostic tests designed to reduce morbidity or mortality (eg, gastroscopy in those with acute gastrointestinal bleeding); and to the combination of diagnostic testing and subsequent therapy that make up screening programs (eg, screening for fecal occult blood). In each of these situations, you risk doing more harm than good when you intervene. Before acting, therefore, ascertain the benefits and risks of the therapy and seek assurance that the societal resources (usually valued in dollars) consumed in the intervention will not be exorbitant.

ARE THE RESULTS VALID?

As described in "How to Use This Book," we suggest a three-step approach to using an article from the medical literature to guide patient care. We recommend that you first determine whether the study provides valid results, that you next review the results, and, finally, that you consider how the results can be applied to the patients in your practice (Table 1B-1).

Whether the study will provide valid results depends on whether it was designed and conducted in a way that justifies claims about the benefits or risks of a therapeutic regimen. Tests of study methods break down into two sets of four questions. The first set helps you decide whether persons exposed to the experimental therapy had a similar prognosis to patients exposed to a control intervention at the beginning of the study. The second set helps you confirm that the two groups were still similar with respect to prognostic factors throughout the study.

TABLE 1B–1

Users' Guides for an Article About Therapy

Are the results valid?

Did experimental and control groups begin the study with a similar prognosis?

- Were patients randomized?
- Was randomization concealed (blinded or masked)?
- Were patients analyzed in the groups to which they were randomized?
- Were patients in the treatment and control groups similar with respect to known prognostic factors?

Did experimental and control groups retain a similar prognosis after the study started?

- Were patients aware of group allocation?
- Were clinicians aware of group allocation?
- Were outcome assessors aware of group allocation?
- Was follow-up complete?

What are the results?

- How large was the treatment effect?
- How precise was the estimate of the treatment effect?

How can I apply the results to patient care?

- Were the study patients similar to my patient?
- Were all clinically important outcomes considered?
- Are the likely treatment benefits worth the potential harm and costs?

Were Patients Randomized?

Consider the question of whether, in very sick people, hospital care prolongs life. A study finds that more sick people die in the hospital than in the community. We would easily reject the naive conclusion that hospital care kills because, intuitively, we understand that hospitalized patients are generally much sicker than patients in the community. This difference would lead to a biased assessment, a massive underestimation of the beneficial effect of hospital care. An unbiased comparison would require a comparison of those in the hospital with equally sick patients in the community, a study that an institutional review board is unlikely to approve.

During the 1970s and early 1980s, surgeons frequently performed extracranial-intracranial bypass (ie, anastomosis of a branch of the external carotid artery—the superficial temporal—to a branch of the internal carotid artery—the middle cerebral). They believed it prevented strokes in patients whose symptomatic cerebrovascular disease was otherwise surgically inaccessible. Comparisons of outcomes among nonrandomized cohorts of patients who, for various reasons, did or did not undergo this operation fueled their conviction. These studies suggested that patients who underwent surgery appeared to fare much better than those who did not undergo surgery. However, to the surgeons' surprise, a large multicenter randomized controlled trial (RCT) in which patients were allocated to surgical or medical treatment using a process analogous to flipping a coin demonstrated that the only effect of surgery was to increase adverse outcomes in the immediate postsurgical period.[3]

Other surprises generated by randomized trials that contradicted the results of less rigorous trials include the demonstration that steroid injections do not ameliorate facet-joint back pain,[4] that plasmapheresis does not benefit patients with polymyositis,[5] and that a variety of initially promising drugs increase mortality in patients with heart failure.[6-10] Such surprises occur frequently when treatments are assigned by random allocation, rather than by the conscious decisions of clinicians and patients.

The reason that studies in which patient or physician preference determines whether a patient receives treatment or control (*observational studies*) often yield biased outcomes is that morbidity and mortality result from many causes, of which treatment is only one. Treatment studies attempt to determine the impact of an intervention on such events as stroke, myocardial infarction, or death—occurrences that we call the trial's *target outcomes* or *target events*. A patient's age, the underlying severity of illness, the presence of comorbid conditions, and a host of other factors typically determine the frequency with which a trial's target outcome occurs (*prognostic factors* or determinants of outcome). If prognostic factors—either those we know about or those we don't know about—prove unbalanced between a trial's treatment and control groups, the study's outcome will be biased, either under- or overestimating the treatment's effect. Because known prognostic factors often influence clinicians' recommendations and patients' decisions about taking treatment, observational studies often yield misleading results. Typically, observational studies tend to show larger treatment effects than do randomized trials,[11-14] although systematic underestimation of treatment effects also may occur.[15] Observational studies can theoretically match patients, either in selecting patients for study or in the subsequent statistical analysis, for known prognostic factors (see Part 1B2, "Harm"; and see Part 2A, "Therapy and Harm, Why Study Results Mislead—Bias and Random Error"). The power of randomization is that treatment and control groups are far more likely to be balanced with respect to both the known and the unknown determinants of outcome.

Randomization does not always succeed in its goal of achieving groups with similar prognosis. Investigators may make mistakes that compromise randomization—if those who determine eligibility are aware of the arm of the study to which the patient will be allocated, or if patients are not analyzed in the group to which they were allocated—or they may encounter bad luck.

Was Randomization Concealed?

Some years ago, a group of Australian investigators undertook a randomized trial of open vs laparoscopic appendectomy.[16] The trial ran smoothly during the day. At night, however, the attending surgeon's presence was required for the laparoscopic procedure but not the open one; and the limited operating room availability made the longer laparoscopic procedure an annoyance. Reluctant to call in a consultant, and particularly reluctant with specific senior colleagues, the residents sometimes adopted a practical solution. When an eligible patient appeared, the residents checked the attending staff and the lineup for the operating room and, depending on the personality of the attending surgeon and the length of the lineup, held the translucent envelopes containing orders up to the light. As soon as they found one that dictated an open procedure, they opened that envelope. The first eligible patient in the morning would then be allocated to a laparoscopic appendectomy group according to the passed-over envelope (D. Wall, written communication, June 9, 2000). If patients who presented at night were sicker than those who presented during the day, the residents' behavior would bias the results against the open procedure.

This story demonstrates that if those making the decision about patient eligibility are aware of the arm of the study to which the patient will be allocated—if randomization is unconcealed (unblinded or unmasked)—they may systematically enroll sicker—or less sick—patients to either treatment or control groups. This behavior will defeat the purpose of randomization and the study will yield a biased result.[17,18] Careful investigators will ensure that randomization is concealed, for example, through (a) preparation of blinded medication in a pharmacy, (b) remote randomization, in which the individual recruiting the patient makes a call to a methods center to discover the arm of the study to which the patient is allocated, or (c) (in our view a much less secure approach) ensuring that the envelope containing the code is sealed.

Were Patients Analyzed in the Groups to Which They Were Randomized?

Investigators can also corrupt randomization by systematically omitting from the results patients who do not take their assigned treatment. Readers might initially agree that such patients who never actually received their assigned treatment should be excluded from the results. Their exclusion, however, will bias the results.

The reasons people do not take their medication are often related to prognosis. In a number of randomized trials, patients who did not adhere to their treatment regimens have fared worse than those who took their medication as instructed, even after taking into account all known prognostic factors and even when their medications were placebos.[19-24] Excluding noncompliant patients from the analysis leaves behind those who may be destined to have a better outcome and destroys the unbiased comparison provided by randomization.

The situation is similar with surgical therapies. Some patients randomized to surgery never have the operation because they are too sick or because they suffer the outcome of interest (eg, stroke or myocardial infarction) before they get to the operating room. If investigators include such poorly destined patients in the control arm but not in the surgical arm of a trial, even a useless surgical therapy will appear to be effective. However, the apparent effectiveness of surgery will come not from a benefit to those who have surgery, but from the systematic exclusion from the surgical group of those with the poorest prognosis.

This principle of attributing all patients to the group to which they were randomized results in an *intention-to-treat analysis,* which is analysis of outcomes based on the treatment arm to which patients were randomized, rather than which treatment they actually received. This strategy preserves the value of randomization: prognostic factors that we know about—and those we do not know about—will be, on average, equally distributed in the two groups; and the effect we see will result simply from the treatment assigned.

In conclusion, when reviewing a report of a randomized trial, look for evidence that the investigators analyzed all patients in the groups to which they were randomized.

Were Patients in the Treatment and Control Groups Similar With Respect to Known Prognostic Factors?

The purpose of randomization is to create groups whose prognosis, with respect to the target outcome, is similar. Sometimes, through bad luck, randomization will fail to achieve this goal. The smaller the sample size, the more likely the trial will suffer from prognostic imbalance.

Picture a trial testing a new treatment for heart failure enrolling patients in New York Heart Association functional class III and class IV. Patients in class IV have a much worse prognosis than those in class III. The trial is small, with only eight patients. One would not be terribly surprised if all four class III patients were allocated to the treatment group and all four class IV patients were allocated to the control group. Such a result of the allocation process would seriously bias the study in favor of the treatment. Were the trial to enroll 800 patients, one would be startled if randomization placed all 400 class III patients in the treatment arm. The larger the sample size, the more likely randomization will achieve its goal of prognostic balance.

Investigators can check how well randomization has done its job by examining the distribution of all prognostic factors in treatment and control groups. Clinicians should look for a display of prognostic features of the treatment and control patients at the study's commencement—the baseline or entry prognostic features. Although we never will know whether similarity exists for the unknown prognostic factors, we are reassured when the known prognostic factors are well balanced.

The issue here is not whether there are statistically significant differences in known prognostic factors between treatment groups (eg, in a randomized trial, one knows in advance that any differences that did occur happened by chance, making the frequently cited P values unhelpful), but, rather, the magnitude of these differences. If the differences are large, the validity of the study may be compromised. The stronger the relationship between the prognostic factors and outcome, and the greater the differences in distribution between groups, the more the differences will weaken the strength of any inference about treatment impact (ie, you will have less confidence in the study results).

All is not lost if the treatment groups are not similar at baseline. Statistical techniques permit adjustment of the study result for baseline differences. Accordingly, clinicians should look for documentation of similarity for relevant baseline characteristics; if substantial differences exist, they should note whether the investigators conducted an analysis that adjusted for those differences. When both unadjusted and adjusted analyses generate the same conclusion, readers justifiably gain confidence in the validity of the study result.

Were Patients Aware of Group Allocation?

Patients who take a treatment that they believe is efficacious may feel and perform better than those who do not, even if the treatment has no biologic action. Although we know relatively little about the magnitude and consistency of this *placebo effect*,[25] its possible presence can mislead clinicians interested in determining the biologic impact of a pharmacologic treatment. Even in the absence of placebo effects, patients might answer questions or perform functional tests differently, depending on whether they believe they are taking active medication.

The best way to avoid these problems is to ensure that patients are unaware of whether they are receiving the experimental treatment. For instance, in a trial of a new drug, control group patients can receive an inert tablet or capsule that is identical in color, taste, and consistency to the active medication administered to the treatment group patients. These placebos can ensure that control group patients benefit from placebo effects to the same extent as actively treated patients.

Were Clinicians Aware of Group Allocation?

If randomization succeeds, treatment and control groups in a study begin with a very similar prognosis. However, randomization provides no guarantees that the two groups will remain prognostically balanced. Differences in patient care other than the intervention under study can bias the results. For example, returning to the spironolactone trial described earlier in this section, if treatment group patients received more intensive treatment with angiotensin-converting enzyme inhibitors or beta blockers than control group patients did, the results would yield an overestimate of the treatment effect. The reason is that both of these classes of cointervention drugs prolong life in heart failure patients.

Clinicians gain greatest confidence in study results when investigators document that all cointerventions that may plausibly impact on the outcome are administered more or less equally in treatment and control groups. The absence of such documentation is a much less serious problem if clinicians are blind to whether patients are receiving active treatment or are part of a control group. Effective blinding eliminates the possibility of either conscious or unconscious differential administration of effective interventions to treatment and control groups.

Were Outcome Assessors Aware of Group Allocation?

If either the treatment or the control group receives closer follow-up, target outcome events may be reported more frequently. In addition, unblinded study personnel who are measuring or recording outcomes such as physiologic tests, clinical status, or quality of life may provide different interpretations of marginal findings or may offer differential encouragement during performance tests, either one of which can distort results.[26] The study personnel assessing outcome can almost always be kept blind to group allocation, even if (as is the case for surgical therapies or health services interventions) patients and treating clinicians cannot. Investigators can take additional precautions by constructing a blinded adjudication committee to review clinical data and decide issues such as whether a patient has had a stroke or myocardial infarction, or whether a death can be attributed to cancer or cardiovascular disease. The more judgment is involved in determining whether a patient has suffered a target outcome (blinding is less crucial in studies in which the outcome is all-cause mortality, for instance) the more important blinding becomes.

Was Follow-up Complete?

Ideally, at the conclusion of a trial investigators will know the status of each patient with respect to the target outcome. We often refer to patients whose status is unknown as lost to follow-up. The greater the number of patients who are *lost to follow-up*, the more a study's validity is potentially compromised. The reason is that patients who are lost often have different prognoses from those who are retained; these patients may disappear because they suffer adverse outcomes (even death) or because they are doing well (and so did not return to be assessed). The situation is completely analogous to the reason for the necessity for an intention-to-treat analysis: patients who discontinue their medication may be less or (usually) more likely to suffer the target adverse event of interest.

When does loss to follow-up seriously threaten validity? Rules of thumb (you may run across thresholds such as 20%) are misleading. Consider two hypothetical randomized trials, each of which enters 1000 patients into both treatment and control groups, of whom 30 (3%) are lost to follow-up (Table 1B-2). In trial A, treated patients die at half the rate of the control group (200 vs 400), a reduction in relative risk of 50%. To what extent does the loss to follow-up potentially threaten our inference that treatment reduces the death rate by half? If we assume the worst, ie, that all treated patients lost to follow-up died, the number of deaths in the experimental group would be 230 (23%). If there were no deaths among the control patients who were lost to follow-up, our best estimate of the effect of treatment in reducing the risk of death drops from 200/400, or 50%, to (400 − 230) or 170/400, or 43%. Thus, even assuming the worst makes little difference in the best estimate of the magnitude of the treatment effect. Our inference is therefore secure.

TABLE 1B–2

When Does Loss to Follow-up Seriously Threaten Validity?

| | Trial A | | Trial B | |
	Treatment	Control	Treatment	Control
Number of patients randomized	1000	1000	1000	1000
Number (%) lost to follow-up	30 (3%)	30 (3%)	30 (3%)	30 (3%)
Number (%) of deaths	200 (20%)	400 (40%)	30 (3%)	60 (6%)
RRR not counting patients lost to follow-up	0.2/0.4 = 0.50		0.03/0.06 = 0.50	
RRR for worst-case scenario*	0.17/0.4 = 0.43		0.00/0.06 = 0	

* The worst-case scenario assumes that all patients allocated to the treatment group and lost to follow-up died and all patients allocated to the control group and lost to follow-up survived.

RRR indicates relative risk reduction.

Contrast this with trial B. Here, the reduction in the relative risk of death is also 50%. In this case, however, the total number of deaths is much lower; of the treated patients, 30 die—and the number of deaths in control patients is 60. In trial B, if we make the same worst-case assumption about the fate of the patients lost to follow-up, the results would change markedly. If we assume that all patients initially allocated to treatment—but subsequently lost to follow-up—die, the number of deaths among treated patients rises from 30 to 60, which is exactly equal to the number of control group deaths. Let us assume that this assumption is accurate. Since we would have 60 deaths in both treatment and control groups, the effect of treatment drops to 0. Because of this dramatic change in the treatment effect (50% relative risk reduction if we ignore those lost to follow-up; 0% relative risk reduction if we assume all patients in the treatment group who were lost to follow-up died), the 3% loss to follow-up in trial B threatens our inference about the magnitude of the relative risk reduction.

Of course, this worst-case scenario is unlikely. When a worst-case scenario, were it true, substantially alters the results, you must judge the plausibility of a markedly different outcome event rate in the treatment and control group patientswho have not been followed. Investigators' demonstration that patients lost to follow-up are similar with respect to important prognostic variables such as age and disease severity decreases—but does not eliminate—the possibility of a different rate of target events.

USING THE GUIDE

Returning to our opening clinical scenario, how well did the study of spironolactone achieve the goal of creating groups with similar prognostic factors? The investigators tell us the study was randomized, but they do not explicitly address the issue of concealment. Of the 822 treated patients, 214 discontinued treatment because of a lack of response, adverse events, or administrative reasons, as did 200 of 841 patients in the control group. The investigators appear to have included all these patients in the analysis, which they state followed intention-to-treat principles. They document the two groups' similarity with respect to age, sex, race, blood pressure, heart rate, ejection fraction, cause of heart failure, and medication use. The one variable for which there was some imbalance is the severity of underlying heart failure: 31% of control patients, vs 27% of treated patients, had NYHA class IV symptoms. This could potentially bias the results in favor of the treatment group. However, the effect is likely to be small, and we are reassured by the investigators' report of an analysis that adjusted for baseline differences in known prognostic factors.

As in many reports of randomized trials, the authors describe their study as "double-blind." Unfortunately, neither clinical epidemiologists nor readers are certain what this term signifies in terms of who is blind to allocation.[27] We will therefore avoid its use and instead, we will specify which groups were unaware of treatment allocation. The spironolactone report implies that patients, care-givers, and those adjudicating outcome were all blinded to allocation, and the editors of Best Evidence have conferred with the authors and reassure us that this is the case.[28]

The authors make no explicit statement about loss to follow-up and their presentation of the data suggests they did not lose any patients. While this is possible for other outcomes, for the outcome of mortality, it seems unlikely.

The final assessment of validity is never a "yes" or "no" decision. Rather, think of validity as a contin-uum ranging from strong studies that are very likely to yield an accurate estimate of the treatment effect to weak studies that are very likely to yield a biased estimate of effect. Inevitably, the judgment as to where a study lies in this continuum involves some subjectivity. In this case, despite uncertainty about loss to follow-up, we judge that overall, the methods

> were strong. The study is thus high on the contin-
> uum between very low and very high validity, likely
> provides a minimally biased assessment of spirono-
> lactone's impact on heart failure patients, and can
> help us decide whether to recommend spironolac-
> tone to the patient under consideration.

In conclusion, loss to follow-up potentially threatens a study's validity. If assuming a worst-case scenario does not change the inferences arising from study results, then loss to follow-up is not a problem. If such an assumption would significantly alter the results, validity is compromised. The extent of that compromise remains a matter of judgment and will depend on how likely it is that treatment patients lost to follow-up did poorly, while control patients lost to follow-up did well.

WHAT ARE THE RESULTS?

How Large Was the Treatment Effect?

Most frequently, randomized clinical trials carefully monitor how often patients experience some adverse event or outcome. Examples of these *dichotomous outcomes* ("yes" or "no" outcomes—ones that either happen or do not happen) include cancer recurrence, myocardial infarction, and death. Patients either do or do not suffer an event, and the article reports the proportion of patients who develop such events. Consider, for example, a study in which 20% of a control group died, but only 15% of those receiving a new treatment died. How might these results be expressed?

One way would be as the absolute difference (known as the *absolute risk reduction,* or risk difference), between the proportion who died in the control group (x) and the proportion who died in the treatment group (y), or $x - y = 0.20 - 0.15 = 0.05$. Another way to express the impact of treatment would be as a *relative risk*: the risk of events among patients on the new treatment, relative to that risk among patients in the control group, or $y/x = 0.15 / 0.20 = 0.75$.

The most commonly reported measure of dichotomous treatment effects is the complement of this relative risk, and is called the *relative risk reduction* (RRR). It is expressed as a percent: $(1 - y/x) \times 100 = (1 - 0.75) \times 100 = 25\%$. An RRR of 25% means that the new treatment reduced the risk of death by 25% relative to that occurring among control patients; and the greater the relative risk reduction, the more effective the therapy. Investigators may compute the relative risk over a period of time, as in a *survival analysis*, and call it a *hazard ratio* (see Part 2D, "Therapy and Understanding the Results, Measures of Association"). When people do not specify whether they are talking about relative or absolute risk reduction—for instance, "Drug X was 30% effective in reducing the risk of death," or "The efficacy of the vaccine was 92%," they are almost invariably talking about relative risk reduction. Pharmaceutical advertisements, whether they make it explicit or not, almost invariably cite relative risk. See Part 2D, "Therapy and Understanding the Results, Measures of Association," for more detail about how the relative risk reduction results in a subjective impression of a larger treatment effect than do other ways of expressing treatment effects.

How Precise Was the Estimate of the Treatment Effect?

Realistically, the true risk reduction can never be known. The best we have is the estimate provided by rigorous controlled trials, and the best estimate of the true treatment effect is that observed in the trial. This estimate is called a point estimate, a single value calcuated from observations of the sample that is used to estimate a population value or parameter. The *point estimate* reminds us that, although the true value lies somewhere in its neighborhood, it is unlikely to be precisely correct. Investigators often tell us the neighborhood within which the true effect likely lies by the statistical strategy of calculating *confidence intervals,* a range of values within which one can be confident that that a population parameter is estimated to lie.[29]

We usually (though arbitrarily) use the 95% confidence interval (see Part 2C, "Therapy and Understanding the Results, Confidence Intervals"). You can consider the 95% confidence interval as defining the range that includes the true relative risk reduction 95% of the time. You will seldom find the true RRR toward the extremes of this interval, and you will find the true RRR beyond these extremes only 5% of the time, a property of the confidence interval that relates closely to the conventional level of "statistical significance" of $P < .05$ (see Part 2B, "Therapy and Understanding the Results, Hypothesis Testing"). We illustrate the use of confidence intervals in the following examples.

Example 1. If a trial randomized 100 patients each to treatment and control groups, and there were 20 deaths in the control group and 15 deaths in the treatment group, the authors would calculate a point estimate for the RRR of 25% ($x = 20/100$ or 0.20, $y = 15/100$ or 0.15, and $1 - y/x = [1 - 0.75] \times 100 = 25\%$). You might guess, however, that the true RRR might be much smaller or much greater than this 25%, based on a difference of only five deaths. In fact, you might surmise that the treatment might provide no benefit (an RRR of 0%) or might even do harm (a negative RRR). And you would be right—in fact, these results are consistent with both an RRR of –38% (that is, patients given the new treatment might be 38% more likely to die than control patients) and an RRR of nearly 59% (that is, patients subsequently receiving the new treatment might have a risk of dying almost 60% less than that of those who are not treated). In other words, the 95% confidence interval on this RRR is –38% to 59%, and the trial really has not helped us decide whether or not to offer the new treatment.

Example 2. What if the trial enrolled 1000 patients per group rather than 100 patients per group, and the same event rates were observed as before, so that there were 200 deaths in the control group ($x = 200/1000 = 0.20$) and 150 deaths in the treatment group ($y = 150/1000 = 0.15$)? Again, the point estimate of the RRR is 25% ($1 – y/x = 1 – [0.15/0.20] \times 100 = 25\%$). In this larger trial, you might think that the true reduction in risk is much closer to 25% and, again, you would be right. The 95% confidence interval on the RRR for this set of results is all on the positive side of zero and runs from 9% to 41%.

What these examples show is that the larger the sample size of a trial, the larger the number of outcome events, and the greater our confidence that the true relative risk reduction (or any other measure of efficacy) is close to what we have observed. In the second example above, the lowest plausible value for the RRR was 9% and the highest value was 41%. The point estimate—in this case, 25%—is the one value most likely to represent the true RRR. As one considers values farther and farther from the point estimate, they become less and less consistent with the observed RRR. By the time one crosses the upper or lower boundaries of the 95% confidence interval, the values are extremely unlikely to represent the true RRR, given the point estimate (that is, the observed RRR).

Figure 1B-1 represents the confidence intervals around the point estimate of a RRR of 25% in these two examples, with a risk reduction of 0 representing no treatment effect. In both scenarios, the point estimate of the RRR is 25%, but the confidence interval is far narrower in the second scenario.

FIGURE 1B–1

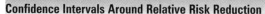

Confidence Intervals Around Relative Risk Reduction

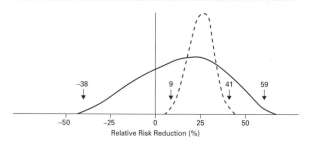

Two studies with the same point estimate, a 25% relative risk reduction, but different sample sizes and correspondingly different confidence intervals. The solid line represents the confidence interval around the first example, in which there were 100 patients per group and the numbers of events in active and control were 15 and 20, respectively. The broken line represents the confidence interval around the first example in which there were 1000 patients per group, and the numbers of events in active and control were 150 and 200, respectively.

It is evident that the larger the sample size, the narrower the confidence interval. When is the sample size big enough[30] (see Part 2C, "Therapy and Understanding the Results, Confidence Intervals")? In a *positive study*—a study in which the authors conclude that the treatment is effective—one can look at the lower boundary of the confidence interval. In the second example, this lower boundary was +9%. If this RRR (the lowest RRR that is consistent with the study results) is still important (that is, it is large enough for you to recommend the treatment to the patient), then the investigators have enrolled sufficient patients. If, on the other hand, you do not consider an RRR of 9% important, then the study cannot be considered definitive, even if its results are statistically significant (that is, they exclude a risk reduction of 0). Keep in mind that the probability of the true value being less than the lower boundary of the confidence interval is only 2.5%, and that a different criterion for the confidence interval (a 90% confidence interval, for instance) might be as or more appropriate.

The confidence interval also helps us interpret *negative studies* in which the authors have concluded that the experimental treatment is no better than control therapy. All we need do is look at the upper boundary of the confidence interval. If the RRR at this upper boundary would, if true, be clinically important, the study has failed to exclude an important treatment effect. For example, consider the first example we presented in this section—the study with 100 patients in each group. This study does not exclude the possibility of harm (indeed, it is consistent with a 38% increase in relative risk), the associated *P* value would be greater than .05, and the study would be considered negative in that it failed to show a convincing treatment effect (see Figure 1B-1). Recall, however, that the upper boundary of the confidence interval was an RRR of 59%. Clearly, if this large relative risk reduction represented the truth, the benefit of the treatment would be substantial. We can conclude that, although the investigators have failed to prove that experimental treatment was better than placebo, they have also failed to prove that it is not; they have not excluded a large, positive treatment effect. Once again, you must bear in mind the proviso that the choice of a 95% confidence interval is arbitrary. A reasonable alternative, a 90% confidence interval, would be somewhat narrower.

When Authors Do Not Report the Confidence Interval

What can you do if the confidence interval around the RRR is not reported in the article? The easiest approach is to examine the *P* value. If it is exactly .05, then the lower bound of the 95% confidence limit for the RRR has to lie exactly at zero (a relative risk of 1), and you cannot exclude the possibility that the treatment has no effect. As the *P* value decreases below .05, the lower bound of the 95% confidence limit for the RRR rises above zero.

A second approach involves calculating the confidence intervals yourself[31] or asking the help of someone else (a statistician, for instance) to do so. Once you obtain the confidence intervals, you know how high and low the RRR might be (that is, you know the precision of the estimate of the treatment effect) and can interpret the results as described above.

Not all randomized trials have dichotomous outcomes, nor should they. For example, the authors of the spironolactone study might have reported changes in exercise capacity or quality of life with the drug. In a study of respiratory muscle training for patients with chronic airflow limitation, one primary outcome measured how far patients could walk in 6 minutes in an enclosed corridor.[32] This 6-minute walk improved from an average of 406 to 416 m (up 10 m) in the experimental group receiving respiratory muscle training, and from 409 to 429 m (up 20 m) in the control group. The point estimate for improvement in the 6-minute walk due to respiratory muscle training therefore was negative, at −10 m (or a 10-m difference in favor of the control group).

Here, too, you should look for the 95% confidence intervals around this difference in changes in exercise capacity and consider their implications. The investigators tell us that the lower boundary of the 95% confidence interval was −26 (that is, the results are consistent with a difference of 26 m in favor of the control treatment) and the upper boundary was

+5 m. Even in the best of circumstances, adding 5 m to the 400 m recorded at the start of the trial would not be important to the patient, and this result effectively excludes an important benefit of respiratory muscle training as applied in this study.

Having determined the magnitude and precision of the treatment effect, clinicians can turn to the final question of how to apply the article's results to patients in their clinical practice.

HOW CAN I APPLY THE RESULTS TO PATIENT CARE?

Were the Study Patients Similar to the Patient in My Practice?

Often, the patient before you has different attributes or characteristics from those enrolled in the trial. She may be older, sicker or less sick, or may suffer from comorbid disease that would have excluded her from participation in the research study. If the patient had qualified for enrollment in the study—that is, if she had met all inclusion criteria and had violated none of the exclusion criteria—you can apply the results with considerable confidence.

Even here, however, there is a limitation. Treatments are not uniformly effective in every individual. Typically, some patients respond extremely well, whereas others achieve no benefit whatsoever. Conventional randomized trials estimate average treatment effects. Applying these average effects means that the clinician will likely be exposing some patients to the cost and toxicity of the treatment without benefit.

Randomized trials in individual patients offer a solution to this dilemma. In these trials, clinicians use the same strategies that minimize bias in conventional trials of therapy

USING THE GUIDE

Of the 822 treated patients, 284 died during the mean 2-year follow-up (35%), as did 386 of 841 control patients (46%). The investigators conducted a survival analysis that takes into account not only the number of people who died by the end of the trial, but the timing of their deaths along the way. Using only the raw death rate, we would compute a relative risk of 76% and a relative risk reduction of 24%. Because patients in the control group not only died more often but at an earlier point than those in the treatment group, the survival analysis yields a relative risk reduction (or hazard ratio) of 35% (95% confidence interval, 18%-48%). The survival curves started to diverge after 6 months of follow-up and showed increasing separation thereafter.

The numbers of patients hospitalized for cardiac causes in the treatment and control groups were, respectively, 336 and 260 (relative risk [RR] 0.70, 95% confidence interval [CI] 0.59-0.82). In the placebo group, about 33% of the patients improved by one or more NYHA functional classes, about 18% were unchanged, and about 48% deteriorated. In the spironolactone group, the comparable percentages were 41%, 21%, and 38%. Chance is a very unlikely explanation for the difference in changes in NYHA functional class ($P < .001$).

In terms of adverse events, nine (1%) of the patients in the control group and 61 (10%) of the treated men developed gynecomastia or breast pain ($P < .001$), and serious hyperkalemia occurred in 10 (1%) and 14 (2%) of the control and treated patients, respectively. The difference in the frequency of serious hyperkalemia was not significant.

involving multiple patients to guard against misleading results in studies involving single patients.[33] In the N of 1 randomized controlled trial, a single patient undertakes a pair of treatment periods in which the patient receives a target treatment in one period of each pair and a placebo or alternative in the other. The patient and clinician are blinded to allocation, the order of the target treatment and control are randomized, and the patient makes quantitative ratings of his or her symptoms during each period. The N of 1 RCT continues until both the patient and clinician conclude that the patient is, or is not, obtaining benefit from the target intervention. When the conditions are right, N of 1 RCTs (a) are feasible,[34, 35] (b) can provide definitive evidence of treatment effectiveness in individual patients, and (c) may lead to long-term differences in treatment administration.[36]

On the other hand, N of 1 RCTs are unsuitable for short-term problems, for therapies that cure, or for ascertaining effects on long-term outcomes or those that occur infrequently. Furthermore, they are possible only when patients and clinicians have the interest and time required. In most instances, clinicians must content themselves with applying results of conventional trials of other patients to the individual before them.

What if that individual does not meet a study's eligibility criteria? The study result probably applies even if, for example, she was 2 years too old for the study, had more severe disease, had previously been treated with a competing therapy, or had a comorbid condition. A better approach than rigidly applying the study's inclusion and exclusion criteria is to ask whether there is some compelling reason why the results should not be applied to the patient. A compelling reason usually will not be found, and most often you can generalize the results to the patient with confidence.

A related issue has to do with the extent to which we can generalize findings from a study using a particular drug to another closely (or not so closely) related agent. This is the issue of drug class effects. The issue of how conservative one should be in assuming class effects is controversial.

A final issue arises when a patient fits the features of a subgroup of patients in the trial report. In articles reporting the results of a trial (especially when the treatment does not appear to be efficacious for the average patient), the authors may have examined a large number of subgroups of patients at different stages of their illness, with different comorbid conditions, with different ages at entry, and the like. Quite often these subgroup analyses were not planned ahead of time, and the data are simply dredged to see what might turn up. Investigators may sometimes overinterpret these data-dependent analyses as demonstrating that the treatment really has a different effect in a subgroup of patients. For example, those who are older or sicker may be held up as benefiting substantially more or less than other subgroups of patients in the trial.

We encourage you to be skeptical of subgroup analyses.[37] The treatment is really likely to benefit the subgroup more or less than the other patients only if the difference in the effects of treatment in the subgroups is large and very unlikely to occur by chance. Even when these conditions apply, the results may be misleading if investigators did not specify their hypotheses before the study began, if they had a very large number of hypotheses, or if other studies fail to replicate the finding.

Were All Clinically Important Outcomes Considered?

Treatments are indicated when they provide important benefits. Demonstrating that a bronchodilator produces small increments in forced expired volume in patients with chronic airflow limitation, that a vasodilator improves cardiac output in heart failure patients, or that a lipid-lowering agent improves lipid profiles does not necessarily provide a sufficient reason for administering these drugs. What is required is evidence that the treatments improve outcomes that are important to patients, such as reducing shortness of breath during the activities required for daily living, avoiding hospitalization for heart failure, or decreasing the risk of myocardial infarction. We can consider forced expired volume in 1 second, cardiac output, and the lipid profile as substitute or *surrogate endpoints* or outcomes. That is, investigators have chosen to substitute these variables for those that patients would consider important, usually because to confirm benefit on the latter, they would have had to enroll many more patients and follow them for far longer periods of time.

Trials of the impact of antiarrhythmic drugs following myocardial infarction provide a dramatic example of the danger of using substitute endpoints. Because such drugs have been shown to reduce abnormal ventricular depolarizations (the substitute endpoints) in the short run, it made sense that they should reduce the occurrence of life-threatening arrhythmias in the long run. A group of investigators performed randomized trials on three agents (encainide, flecainide, and moricizine) previously shown to be effective in suppressing the substitute endpoint of abnormal ventricular depolarizations to determine whether they reduced mortality in patients with asymptomatic or mildly symptomatic arrhythmias following myocardial infarction. The investigators had to stop the trials when they discovered that mortality was substantially higher in patients receiving antiarrhythmic treatment than in those receiving placebo.[38, 39] Clinicians relying on the substitute endpoint of arrhythmia suppression would have continued to administer the three drugs to the considerable detriment of their patients.

Even when investigators report favorable effects of treatment on one clinically important outcome, you must consider whether there may be deleterious effects on other outcomes. For instance, it is likely that a class of lipid-lowering agents, while reducing cardiovascular mortality, increases mortality from other causes.[40] Cancer chemotherapy may lengthen life but decreases its quality. Surgical trials often document prolonged life for those who survive the operation (yielding a higher 3-year survival rate in those receiving surgery), but an immediate risk of dying during or shortly after surgery. Accordingly, users of the reports of surgical trials should look for information on immediate and early mortality (typically higher in the surgical group) in addition to longer-term results. The most common limitation of randomized trials with regard to reporting important outcomes is the omission of documentation of drug toxicity or adverse effects.

Another long-neglected outcome is the resource implications of alternative management strategies. Few randomized trials measure either direct costs, such as drug or program expenses and health care worker salaries, or indirect costs, such as patients' loss of income due to illness. Nevertheless, the increasing resource constraints that health care systems face mandate careful attention to economic analysis, particularly of resource-intense interventions.

Are the Likely Treatment Benefits Worth the Potential Harm and Costs?

If you can apply the study's results to a patient, and its outcomes are important, the next question concerns whether the probable treatment benefits are worth the effort that you and the patient must put into the enterprise. A 25% reduction in the relative risk of death may sound quite impressive, but its impact on the patient and your practice may nevertheless be minimal. This notion is illustrated using a concept called *number needed to treat* (NNT), the number of patients who must receive an intervention of therapy during a specific period of time to prevent one adverse outcome or produce one positive outcome.[41]

The impact of a treatment is related not only to its relative risk reduction, but also to the risk of the adverse outcome it is designed to prevent. One large trial suggests that tissue plasminogen activator (tPA) administration reduces the relative risk of death following myocardial infarction by approximately 12% in comparison to streptokinase in the setting of acute myocardial infarction.[42] Table 1B-3 considers two patients presenting with acute myocardial infarction associated with elevation of ST segments on their electrocardiograms.

TABLE 1B-3

Considerations in the Decision to Treat Two Patients With Myocardial Infarction With Tissue Plasminogen Activator or Streptokinase

	Risk of Death Year After Myocardial Infarction (MI) With Streptokinase	Risk With tPA (Absolute Risk Reduction)	Number Needed to Treat
40-year-old man with small MI	2%	1.76% (0.24% or 0.0024)	417
70-year-old man, large MI and heart failure	40%	35.2% (4.8% or 0.048)	21

MI indicates myocardial infarction; tPA, tissue plasminogen activator.

In the first case, a 40-year-old man presents with electrocardiographic findings suggesting an inferior myocardial infarction. You find no signs of heart failure, and the patient is in normal sinus rhythm with a rate of 90 beats per minute. This individual's risk of death in the first year after infarction may be as low as 2%. In comparison to streptokinase, tPA would reduce this risk by 12% to 1.76%, an absolute risk reduction of 0.24% (0.0024). The inverse of this absolute risk reduction (ARR) (that is, 1 divided by the ARR) is equal to the number of such patients we would have to treat to prevent one event (in this case, to prevent one death following a mild heart attack in a low-risk patient)—the number needed to treat (NNT). In this case, we would have to treat approximately 417 such patients to save a single life (1 / 0.0024 = 417). Given the small increased risk of intracerebral hemorrhage associated with tPA, and its additional cost, many clinicians might prefer streptokinase in this patient.

In the second case, a 70-year-old man presents with electrocardiographic signs of anterior myocardial infarction with pulmonary edema. His risk of dying in the next year is approximately 40%. A 12% RRR of death in such a high-risk patient generates an ARR of 4.8% (0.048), and we would have to treat only 21 such individuals to avert a premature death (1 / 0.048 = 20.8). Many clinicians would consider tPA the preferable agent in this man.

A key element of the decision to start therapy, therefore, is to consider the patient's risk of the adverse event if left untreated. For any given RRR, the higher the probability that a patient will experience an adverse outcome if we do not treat, the more likely the patient will benefit from treatment and the fewer such patients we need to treat to prevent one adverse outcome (see Part 2D, "Therapy and Understanding the Results, Measures of Association"). Knowing the NNT helps clinicians in the process of weighing the benefits and downsides associated with the management options.

Trading off benefit and risk requires an accurate assessment of medication adverse effects. Randomized trials, with relatively small sample sizes, are unsuitable for detecting rare but catastrophic adverse effects of therapy. Although RCTs are the correct vehicle for reporting commonly occurring side effects, reports regularly neglect to include these outcomes. Clinicians must often look to other sources of information—often characterized by weaker methodology—to obtain an estimate of the adverse effects of therapy.

The preferences or values that determine the correct choice when weighing benefit and risk are those of the individual patient. Clinicians should attend to the growing literature concerning patients' response to illness. Great uncertainty about how best to communicate information to patients, and how to incorporate their values into clinical decision making, remains. Vigorous investigation of this frontier of evidence-based decision making is, however, under way.

CLINICAL RESOLUTION

The spironolactone study addressed a wide variety of relevant endpoints, including mortality, hospitalization rate, and day-to-day function. In addition, the study documents substantial increases in gynecomastia and breast pain in treated men, and a small and nonsignificant increase in episodes of serious hyperkalemia is reported.

For the group as a whole, the ARR of dying from 46% to 35% corresponds to an NNT of 1 / 0.11, or approximately 9. However, not all patients with heart failure have the same prognosis. Class IV patients may have a mortality rate over 2 years of as high as 60%, whereas approximately 40% of class III patients may die during this time period. We would anticipate the mortality rate in class II patients to be approximately 20% during the same period.

Table 1B-4 presents some of the benefits and risks that patients with heart failure might anticipate with spironolactone. Using the point estimate of the RRR, the NNT for those with class IV failure and a higher mortality would be 6; class III and class II, with a lower baseline risk, have higher NNTs of 9 and 17, respectively. This table also highlights the smallest RRR consistent with the data (RRR, 18%), the extreme boundary of the 95% confidence interval and, hence, the largest plausible NNT. For the NYHA class IV, III, and II patients, these NNTs prove to be 9, 14, and 27, respectively. Since breast pain and gynecomastia are likely independent of NYHA functional class, given an incidence of 9%, the number needed to harm (NNH) would be 11 in all three groups (we calculate the NNH in the same way as the NNT: 1 divided by the risk difference; in this case, 1 divided by 0.09). Finally, the drug is inexpensive; the cost of a year's treatment is approximately $25.

TABLE 1B-4

Trading Off Benefits and Risks of Spironolactone Treatment in Three Different Patients With Heart Failure

NYHA Classification for Heart Failure	Risk of Dying During 2 Years if Untreated	Likely Absolute Risk Reduction and NNT During 2 Years if Treated (30% RRR)	Smallest Plausible Absolute Risk Reduction (18% RRR)*	Risk of Breast Pain or Gynecomastia in Men and NNH
Class IV	60%	18% NNT 6	11% NNT 9	9% NNH 11
Class III	40%	12% NNT 9	7% NNT 14	9% NNH 11
Class II	20%	6% NNT 17	3.6% NNT 27	9% NNH 11

* Calculated using lower boundary of 95% confidence interval around the RRR of 18%.

NNT indicates number needed to treat; RRR, relative risk reduction; NNH, number needed to harm.

We anticipate that, given these risks and benefits, most patients would choose spironolactone treatment. This is particularly so since, if breast pain or gynecomastia develops, men can always stop the medication. However, there were virtually no class II patients who participated in this trial. Can we assume that we would see the same reduction in relative risk in these class II patients as in those with worse heart failure?

There are a number of reasons to think we might. The biology of heart failure remains similar throughout its course. The authors of the study postulate that spironolactone prevented progressive heart failure by reducing sodium retention and myocardial fibrosis, and that it prevented sudden death by averting potassium loss and increasing the myocardial uptake of norepinephrine. Spironolactone may prevent myocardial fibrosis by blocking the effects of aldosterone on the formation of collagen. There is little reason to think these mechanisms, if they indeed explain the results, would not be important in patients with NYHA class II heart failure.

Further reassurance comes from the fact that the RRR appeared similar in participating subgroups of patients with ischemic and nonischemic etiology of their heart failure and those receiving and not receiving beta blockers. Finally, other drugs that lower mortality in heart failure—angiotensin-converting enzyme inhibitors and beta blockers—appear to have similar reductions in relative risk across subgroups of patients with NYHA class II, III, and IV heart failure.[43]

The patient before you is very interested in actively participating in decisions regarding his care. Salient points you must communicate to him include his risk of breast pain or gynecomastia of 9% during a 2-year period and his likely reduction in mortality from 20% to 14%. You must also convey the uncertainty associated with this estimate that arises both from the confidence interval around the estimate of RRR in mortality with spironolactone (which suggests his mortality may drop from 20% to 16%, rather than 14%) and from the exclusion of NYHA class II patients from the trial. When you are satisfied that the patient understands these key concepts, you will be in a position to help him arrive at a final decision about whether he wishes to take the medication.

References

1. Vasotec tablets: enalapril maleate. In: *Physician's Desk Reference.* 52nd ed. Montvale, NJ: Medical Economics; 1998:1771-1774.

2. Pitt B, Zannad F, Remme WJ, et al. The effect of spironolactone on morbidity and mortality in patients with severe heart failure. *N Engl J Med.* 1999;341:709-717.

3. Haynes RB, Mukherjee J, Sackett DL, et al. Functional status changes following medical or surgical treatment for cerebral ischemia: results in the EC/IC Bypass Study. *JAMA.* 1987;257:2043-2046.

4. Carette S, Marcoux S, Truchon R, et al. A controlled trial of corticosteroid injections into facet joints for chronic low back pain. *N Engl J Med.* 1991;325:1002-1007.

5. Miller FW, Leitman SF, Cronin ME, et al. Controlled trial of plasma exchange and leukapheresis in polymyositis and dermatomyositis. *N Engl J Med.* 1992;326:1380-1384.

6. The Xamoterol in Severe Heart Failure Group. Xamoterol in severe heart failure. *Lancet.* 1990;336:1-6.

7. Packer M, Carver JR, Rodeheffer RJ, et al, for the PROMISE Study Research Group. Effects of oral milrinone on mortality in severe chronic heart failure. *N Engl J Med.* 1991;325:1468-1475.

8. Packer M, Rouleau JL, Svedberg K, Pitt B, Fisher L, and the Profile investigators. Effect of flosequinan on survival in chronic heart failure: preliminary results of the PROFILE study [abstract]. *Circulation.* 1993;88(suppl I):I-301.

9. Hampton JR, van Veldhuisen DJ, Kleber FX, et al, for the Second Prospective Randomized Study of Ibopamine on Mortality and Efficacy (PRIME II) Investigators. Randomised study of effect of Ibopamine on survival in patients with advanced severe heart failure. *Lancet.* 1997;349:971-977.

10. Califf RM, Adams KF, McKenna WJ, et al. A randomized controlled trial of epoprostenol therapy for severe congestive heart fialure: the Flolan International Randomized Survival Trial (FIRST). *Am Heart J.* 1997;134:44-54.

11. Sacks HS, Chalmers TC, Smith H Jr. Sensitivity and specificity of clinical trials: randomized v historical controls. *Arch Intern Med.* 1983;143:753-755.

12. Chalmers TC, Celano P, Sacks HS, Smith H Jr. Bias in treatment assignment in controlled clinical trials. *N Engl J Med.* 1983;309:1358-1361.

13. Colditz GA, Miller JN, Mosteller F. How study design affects outcomes in comparisons of therapy, I: medical. *Stat Med*. 1989;8:441-454.

14. Emerson JD, Burdick E, Hoaglin DC, et al. An empirical study of the possible relation of treatment differences to quality scores in controlled randomized clinical trials. *Controlled Clin Trials*. 1990;11:339-352.

15. Kunz R, Oxman AD. The unpredictability paradox: review of empirical comparisons of randomised and non-randomised clinical trials. *BMJ*. 1998;317:1185-1190.

16. Hansen JB, Smithers BM, Schache D, Wall DR, Miller BJ, Menzies BL. Laparoscopic versus open appendectomy: prospective randomized trial. *World J Surg*. 1996;20:17-20.

17. Schulz KF, Chalmers I, Hayes RJ, Altman DG. Empirical evidence of bias: dimensions of methodological quality associated with estimates of treatment effects in controlled trials. *JAMA*. 1995;273:408-412.

18. Moher D, Jones A, Cook DJ, et al. Does quality of reports of randomised trials affect estimates of intervention efficacy reported in meta-analyses? *Lancet*. 1998;352:609-613.

19. Coronary Drug Project Research Group. Influence of adherence treatment and response of cholesterol on mortality in the Coronary Drug Project. *N Engl J Med*. 1980;303:1038-1041.

20. Asher WL, Harper HW. Effect of human chorionic gonadotropin on weight loss, hunger, and feeling of well-being. *Am J Clin Nutr*. 1973;26:211-218.

21. Hogarty GE, Goldberg SC. Drug and sociotherapy in the aftercare of schizophrenic patients. *Arch Gen Psychiatry*. 1973;28:54-64.

22. Fuller R, Roth H, Long S. Compliance with disulfiram treatment of alcoholism. *J Chronic Dis*. 1983;36:161-170.

23. Pizzo PA, Robichaud KJ, Edwards BK, Schumaker C, Kramer BS, Johnson A. Oral antibiotic prophylaxis in patients with cancer: a double-blind randomized placebo-controlled trial. *J Pediatr*. 1983;102:125-133.

24. Horwitz RI, Viscoli CM, Berkman L, et al. Treatment adherence and risk of death after myocardial infarction. *Lancet*. 1990;336:542-545.

25. Kaptchuk TJ. Powerful placebo: the dark side of the randomised controlled trial. *Lancet*. 1998;351:1722-1725.

26. Guyatt GH, Pugsley SO, Sullivan MJ, et al. Effect of encouragement on walking test performance. *Thorax*. 1984;39:818-822.

27. Devereaux PJ, Manns BJ, Ghali WA, et al. In the dark: physician interpretation of blinding terminology in randomized controlled trials. *JAMA*. In press.

28. Henderson M, Mulrow CD. Commentary on "The effect of spironolactone on morbidity and mortality in patients with severe heart failure." ACP J Club. 2000 Jan-Feb; 132(1):2.

29. Altman DG, Gore SM, Gardner MJ, Pocock SJ. Statistical guidelines for contributors to medical journals. In: Gardner MJ, Altman DG, eds. *Statistics With Confidence: Confidence Intervals and Statistical Guidelines.* London: British Medical Journal; 1989:83-100.

30. Detsky AS, Sackett DL. When was a "negative" trial big enough? How many patients you needed depends on what you found. *Arch Intern Med*. 1985;145:709-715.

31. Sackett DL, Haynes RB, Guyatt GH, Tugwell P. *Clinical Epidemiolog: A Basic Science for Clinical Medicine*. 2nd ed. Boston: Little Brown & Co Inc; 1991:218.

32. Guyatt GH, Keller J, Singer J, Halcrow S, Newhouse M. Controlled trial of respiratory muscle training in chronic airflow limitation. *Thorax*. 1992;47:598-602.

33. Guyatt GH, Sackett DL, Taylor DW, et al. Determining optimal therapy: randomized trials in individual patients. *N Engl J Med*. 1986;314:889-892.

34. Guyatt GH, Keller JL, Jaeschke R, et al. The n-of-1 randomized control trial: clinical usefulness. Our three year experience. *Ann Intern Med*. 1990;112:293-299.

35. Larson EB, Ellsworth AJ, Oas J. Randomized clinical trials in single patients during a 2-year period. *JAMA*. 1993;270:2708-2712.

36. Mahon J, Laupacis A, Donner A, Wood T. Randomised study of n of 1 trials versus standard practice. *BMJ*. 1996;312:1069-1074.

37. Oxman AD, Guyatt GH. A consumer's guide to subgroup analysis. *Ann Intern Med*. 1992;116:78-84.

38. Echt DS, Liebson PR, Mitchell LB, et al. Mortality and morbidity in patients receiving encainide, flecainide, or placebo: the Cardiac Arrhythmia Suppression Trial. *N Engl J Med*. 1991;324:781-788.

39. The Cardiac Arrhythmia Suppression Trial II Investigators. Effect of the antiarrhythmic agent moricizine on survival after myocardial infarction. *N Engl J Med*. 1992;327:227-233.

40. Muldoon MF, Manuck SB, Matthews KA. Lowering cholesterol concentrations and mortality: a quantitative review of primary prevention trials. *BMJ*. 1990;301:309-314.

41. Laupacis A, Sackett DL, Roberts RS. An assessment of clinically useful measures of the consequences of treatment. *N Engl J Med*. 1988;318:1728-1733.

42. The GUSTO Investigators. An international randomized trial comparing four thrombolytic strategies for acute myocardial infarction. *N Engl J Med*. 1993;329:673-682.

43. Garg R, Yusuf S. Overview of randomized trials of angiotensin-converting enzyme inhibitors on mortality and morbidity in patients with heart failure. *JAMA*. 1995;273:1450-1456.

HARM

Mitchell Levine, David Haslam, Stephen Walter,
Robert Cumming, Hui Lee, Ted Haines, Anne Holbrook,
Virginia Moyer, and Gordon Guyatt

The following EBM Working Group members also made
substantive contributions to this section: Peter Pronovost
and Sharon Straus

IN THIS SECTION

CLINICAL SCENARIO

Do SSRIs Cause Gastrointenstinal Bleeding?

You are a general practitioner considering the optimal choice of antidepressant medication. Your patient is a 55-year-old previously cheerful and well-adjusted individual who, during the past 2 months, has become sad and distressed for the first time in his life. He has developed difficulty concentrating and experiences early morning wakening, but lacks thoughts of self-harm. The patient has attended your practice for the past 20 years and you know him well. You believe he is suffering from a major depressive episode and that he might benefit from antidepressant medication.

During recent years, you have been administering a selective serotonin reuptake inhibitor (SSRI), paroxetine, as your first-line antidepressant agent. However, recent reviews suggesting that the SSRIs are no more effective[1-3] and do not have lower discontinuation rates[1-4] than tricyclic antidepressants (TCAs) have led you to revert to your previous first choice, nortriptyline, in some patients. Patients in your practice usually consider the adverse effects in some depth before agreeing to any treatment decisions and many choose SSRIs on the basis of a preferable side-effect profile.

However, for the past 5 years the patient you are seeing today has been taking ketoprofen (a nonsteroidal anti-inflammatory drug, or NSAID), 50 mg three times per day, which has controlled the pain from his hip osteoarthritis. Your mind jumps to a review article suggesting that SSRIs may be associated with an increased risk of bleeding, and you become concerned about the risk of gastrointestinal bleeding when you consider that the patient is also receiving an NSAID. Unfortunately, an abstract from *Evidence Based Mental Health*,[5] which you have used to obtain a summary of side effects of antidepressant medications, provides no information regarding this issue.

You remember the review article[6] and locate a copy in your files, but at a glance you realize that it will not help answer your question for three reasons: It did not use explicit inclusion and exclusion criteria, it failed to conduct a systematic and comprehensive search, and it did not evaluate the methodologic quality of the original research it summarized. In addition, it did not cite any original studies specific to an association between SSRI treatment and gastrointestinal bleeding.

You consider that it is worth following up this issue before you make a final recommendation to the patient. You inform him that he will need antidepressant medication, but you explain your concern about the possible bleeding risk and your need to acquire more definitive information before making a final recommendation. You schedule a follow-up visit 2 days later and you commit to presenting a strategy at that time.

FINDING THE EVIDENCE

You formulate the following focused question:

> Do adults suffering from depression and taking SSRI medications, compared to patients not taking antidepressants, suffer an increased risk of serious upper gastrointestinal bleeding?

Later that day, you begin your search using prefiltered evidence-based medicine resources—the journal *Evidence Based Mental Health*, Best Evidence4, Clinical Evidence, and the Cochrane Library. For each database, you enter the term "serotonin reuptake inhibitor." Search of *Evidence Based Mental Health* yields eight reviews in volumes 1 (1998) and 2 (1999). Four of these deal with adverse effects associated with SSRI use, but none addresses gastrointestinal bleeding. Searching Best Evidence4 yields 17 equally unhelpful articles. A Clinical Evidence search identifies only a review on treatment of depressive disorders in adults. The Cochrane Library search locates four complete reviews and two abstracts of systematic reviews, but none addresses the issue of gastrointestinal bleeding in SSRI users.

You now turn to the PubMed version of MEDLINE and PreMEDLINE searching system (www.ncbi.nlm.nih.gov/entrez/query.fcgi). For optimum search efficiency, you click on "Clinical queries" under "PubMed Services" to access systematically tested search strategies, or you go to "Search hedges," which will help you identify methodologically sound studies pertaining to your question on harm (see Part 1A1, "Finding the Evidence"). You enter the following: "selective serotonin reuptake inhibitor" AND "bleeding" for the subject search term; and you click on "Etiology" for study category and "Specificity" for emphasis. Your MEDLINE search (from 1966 through 2000) identifies one citation, an epidemiologic study assessing the association between SSRIs and upper gastrointestinal bleeding.[7] This study describes a threefold increased risk of upper gastrointestinal bleeding associated with the use of SSRIs. Thinking that this article may answer your question, you download the full text free of charge from the *British Medical Journal* (*BMJ*) Web site (www.bmj.com) as a portable document format (PDF) file, an electronic version of a printed page or pages.

ARE THE RESULTS VALID?

Clinicians often encounter patients who are facing potentially harmful exposures, either to medical interventions or environmental agents, and important questions arise. Are pregnant women at increased risk of miscarriage if they work in front of video display terminals? Do vasectomies increase the risk of prostate cancer? Do hypertension management programs at work lead to increased absenteeism? When examining these questions, physicians must evaluate the validity of the data, the strength of the association between the assumed cause and the adverse outcome, and the relevance to patients in their practice.

As when answering any clinical question, our first goal should be to identify a systematic review of the topic that can provide an objective summary of all the available evidence (see Part 1E, "Summarizing the Evidence"). However, interpreting a systematic review requires an understanding of the rules of evidence for observational (nonrandomized) studies. The tests for judging the validity of observational study results, like the validity tests for randomized controlled trials, help you decide whether experimental and control groups began the study with a similar prognosis and whether similarity with respect to prognostic factors persisted after the study was started (see Table 1B-5).

TABLE 1B–5

Users' Guides for an Article About Harm

Are the results valid?

Did experimental and control groups begin the study with a similar prognosis?

- Did the investigators demonstrate similarity in all known determinants of outcome; did they adjust for differences in the analysis?

- Were exposed patients equally likely to be identified in the two groups?

Did experimental and control groups retain a similar prognosis after the study started?

- Were the outcomes measured in the same way in the groups being compared?

- Was follow-up sufficiently complete?

What are the results?

- How strong is the association between exposure and outcome?

- How precise is the estimate of the risk?

How can I apply the results to patient care?

- Were the study patients similar to the patient under consideration in my practice?

- Was the duration of follow-up adequate?

- What was the magnitude of the risk?

- Should I attempt to stop the exposure?

Did the Investigators Demonstrate Similarity in All Known Determinants of Outcome? Did They Adjust for Differences in the Analysis?

Studies of potentially harmful exposures will yield biased results if the group exposed to the putative harmful agent and the unexposed group begin with a different prognosis. Let us say we are interested in the impact of hospitalization on mortality rate. To investigate this question, we compare mortality in hospitalized individuals to that in people of similar age and sex in the community. Although an examination of the results would lead us to stay clear of hospitals, few would take these results seriously. The reason for skepticism is that people are admitted to hospitals because they are sick and, therefore, are at greater risk of dying. This higher risk results in a spurious (that is, noncausal) association between exposure (hospitalization) and outcome (death). In general, people who seek health care or who take medicine are sicker than people who do not. If clinicians fail to take this into account, they are at high risk of making inaccurate inferences about causal relations between medications and adverse effects.

How can investigators ensure that their comparison groups start a study with a similar likelihood of suffering the target outcome? Randomized controlled trials provide less biased estimates of potentially harmful effects than other study designs because randomization is the best way to ensure that groups are balanced with respect to both known and unknown determinants of outcome (see Part 1B1, "Therapy"). Although investigators conduct RCTs to determine whether therapeutic agents are beneficial, RCTs can also demonstrate harm. The unexpected results of some randomized trials (for example, drugs that investigators expected to show benefit sometimes are associated with increased mortality) have demonstrated the potential of this study design for demonstrating harm.

There are two reasons that we cannot usually find RCTs to help us determine if a putative harmful agent truly has deleterious effects. First, we consider it unethical to randomize patients to exposures that may be harmful (not beneficial). Even if we did not hold these scruples, informed patients would not consent to such an experiment.

Second, we are often concerned about rare and serious adverse effects that occur over prolonged periods of time—ones that become evident only after tens of thousands of patients have consumed the medication. For instance, even a very large randomized trial[8] failed to detect an association between clopidogrel and thrombotic thrombocytopenic purpura, which was detected by a subsequent observational study.[9] Randomized trials specifically addressing side effects may be feasible for adverse event rates as low as 1%[10,11] and meta-analyses may be very helpful when event rates are low.[12] The randomized trials we would need to explore harmful events that occur in less than one in 100 exposed patients—trials characterized by huge sample size and lengthy follow-up—are logistically difficult and prohibitively expensive.

Given that clinicians will not find RCTs to answer most questions about harm, they must understand alternative strategies for ensuring a balanced prognosis in the groups being compared. This understanding requires a familiarity with observational study designs, which we will now describe (Table 1B-6).

TABLE 1B-6

Directions of Inquiry and Key Methodologic Strengths and Weaknesses for Different Study Designs

Design	Starting Point	Assessment	Strengths	Weaknesses
Cohort	Exposure status	Outcome event status	Feasible when randomization of exposure not possible	Susceptible to bias, limited validity
Case-Control	Outcome event status	Exposure status	Overcomes temporal delays, may only require small sample size	Susceptible to bias, limited validity
RCT	Exposure status	Adverse event status	Low susceptibility to bias	Feasibility, generalizability

RCT indicates randomized controlled trial.

Cohort Studies

In a *cohort study*, the investigator identifies exposed and nonexposed groups of patients, each a cohort, and then follows them forward in time, monitoring the occurrence of the predicted outcome. In one such study, for example, investigators assessed perinatal outcomes among infants of men exposed to lead and organic solvents in the printing industry by means of a cohort of all males who had been members of printers' unions in Oslo.[13] The investigators used job classification to categorize fathers as being either exposed to lead and solvents or not exposed to those substances. In this study, exposure was associated with an eightfold increase in preterm births, but it was not linked with birth defects.

Investigators may rely on cohort designs when harmful outcomes occur infrequently. For example, clinically apparent upper gastrointestinal hemorrhage in patients using NSAIDs occurs approximately 1.5 times per 1000 person-years of exposure, in comparison with 1.0 per 1000 person-years in those not taking NSAIDs.[14] Because the event rate in unexposed patients is so low (0.1%), a randomized trial to study an increase in risk of 50% would require huge numbers of patients (sample size calculations suggest about 75,000 patients per group) for adequate power to test the hypothesis that NSAIDs cause the additional bleeding.[15] Such a randomized trial would not be feasible, but a cohort study, in which the information comes from a large administrative database, would be possible.

The danger in using observational studies to assess a possible harmful exposure is that exposed and unexposed patients may begin with a different risk of the target outcome. For instance, in the association between NSAIDs and the increased risk of upper gastrointestinal bleeding, age may be associated both with exposure to NSAIDs and with gastrointestinal bleeding. In other words, since patients taking NSAIDs will be older and older patients are more likely to bleed, this *confounding variable* makes attribution of an increased risk of bleeding to NSAID exposure problematic.

There is no reason patients who self-select (or who are selected by their physician) for exposure to a potentially harmful agent should be similar, with respect to other important determinants of outcome, to the nonexposed patients. Indeed, there are many reasons to expect they will not be similar. Physicians are reluctant to prescribe medications they perceive will put their patients at risk and will selectively prescribe low-risk medications. In one study, for instance, 24.1% of patients who were given a then-new NSAID, ketoprofen, had received peptic ulcer therapy during the previous 2 years in comparison to 15.7% of the control population.[16] The likely reason is that the ketoprofen manufacturer succeeded in persuading clinicians that ketoprofen was less likely to cause gastrointestinal bleeding than other agents. A subsequent comparison of ketoprofen to other agents would be subject to the risk of finding a spurious increase in bleeding with the new agent because higher-risk patients would have been receiving the drug.

The prescription of benzodiazepines to elderly patients provides another example of the way that selective physician prescribing practices can lead to a different distribution of risk in patients receiving particular medications. This is referred to as the *channeling effect*.[17,18] Ray and colleagues[19] found an association between long-acting benzodiazepines and risk of falls (relative risk [RR], 2.0; 95% CI, 1.6-2.5) in data from 1977 to 1979, but not in data from 1984 to 1985 (RR, 1.3; 95% CI, 0.9-1.8). The most plausible explanation for the change is that patients at high risk for falls (those with dementia and anxiety or agitation) selectively received benzodiazepines during the earlier time period. Reports of associations between benzodiazepine use and falls led to greater caution, and the apparent association disappeared when physicians began to avoid benzodiazepine use in those at high risk of falling.

Therefore, investigators must document the characteristics of the exposed and nonexposed participants and either demonstrate their comparability or use statistical techniques to adjust for differences. Since investigators cannot recruit groups that are age-balanced, they must use statistical techniques that correct or adjust for the imbalances.

Effective adjustment for prognostic factors requires the accurate measurement of those prognostic factors. Large administrative databases, while providing a sample size that allows ascertainment of rare events, sometimes have limited quality of data concerning relevant patient characteristics. For example, Jollis and colleagues[20] wondered about the accuracy of information about patient characteristics in an insurance claims database. To investigate this issue, they compared the insurance claims data with prospective data collection by a cardiology fellow. They found that a high degree of chance corrected agreement between the fellow and the administrative database for the presence of diabetes: kappa, a measure of chance-corrected agreement, was 0.83. They also found a high degree of agreement for myocardial infarction (kappa, 0.76), and moderate agreement for hypertension (kappa, 0.56). However, agreement was poor for heart failure (kappa, 0.39) and very poor for tobacco use (kappa, 0.19).

Even if investigators document the comparability of potentially confounding variables in exposed and nonexposed cohorts and even if they use statistical techniques to adjust for differences, important prognostic factors that the investigators do not know about or have not measured may be unbalanced between the groups and, thus, may be responsible for differences in outcome. Returning to our earlier example, for instance, it may be that the illnesses that require NSAIDs, rather than the NSAIDs themselves, are responsible for the increased risk of bleeding. Thus, the strength of inference from a cohort study will always be less than that of a rigorously conducted RCT.

Case-Control Studies

Rare outcomes, or those that take a long time to develop, threaten cohort studies' feasibility. An alternative design relies on the initial identification of *cases*—that is, patients who have already developed the target outcome. The investigators then choose *controls*—persons who, as a group, are reasonably similar to the cases with respect to important determinants of outcome such as age, sex, and concurrent medical conditions, but who have not suffered the target outcome. Using this *case-control* design, investigators then assess the relative frequency of exposure to the putative harmful agent in the cases and controls, adjusting for differences in the known and measured prognostic variables.

This design permits the simultaneous exploration of multiple exposures that have a possible association with the target outcome.

For example, investigators used a case-control design to demonstrate the association between diethylstilbestrol (DES) ingestion by pregnant women and the development of vaginal adenocarcinomas in their daughters many years later.[21] An RCT or prospective cohort study designed to test this cause-and-effect relationship would have required at least 20 years from the time when the association was first suspected until the completion of the study. Further, given the infrequency of the disease, either an RCT or a cohort study would have required hundreds of thousands of participants. By contrast, using the case-control strategy, the investigators delineated two groups of young women. Those who had suffered the outcome of interest (vaginal adenocarcinoma) were designated as the cases (n = 8) and those who did not experience the outcome were designated as the controls (n = 32). Then, working backward in time, they determined exposure rates to DES for the two groups. The investigators found a strong association between in utero DES exposure and vaginal adenocarcinoma, which was extremely unlikely to be attributable to the play of chance ($P < .00001$). They found their answer without a delay of 20 years and by studying outcomes in only 40 women.

In another example, investigators used a case-control design relying on computer record linkages between health insurance data and a drug plan to investigate the possible relationship between use of beta-adrenergic agonists and mortality rates in patients with asthma.[22] The database for the study included 95% of the population of the province of Saskatchewan in western Canada. The investigators matched 129 cases of fatal or near-fatal asthma with 655 controls who also suffered from asthma but who had not had a fatal or near-fatal asthma attack.

The tendency of patients with more severe asthma to use more beta-adrenergic medications could create a spurious association between drug use and mortality rate. The investigators attempted to control for the confounding effect of disease severity by measuring the number of hospitalizations in the 24 months prior to death (cases) or the index date of entry in to the study (control group) and by using an index of the aggregate use of medications. They found an association between the routine use of large doses of beta-adrenergic agonist metered-dose inhalers and death from asthma (odds ratio [OR], 2.6 per canister per month; 95% CI, 1.7-3.9), even after correcting for their measures of disease severity.

As with cohort studies, case-control studies are susceptible to unmeasured confounding variables, particularly when exposure varies over time. For instance, previous hospitalization and medication use may not adequately capture all the variability in underlying disease severity in asthma. In addition, adverse lifestyle behaviors of asthmatic patients who use large amounts of beta agonists could contribute to the association. Furthermore, choice of controls may inadvertently create spurious associations. For instance, in a study that examined the association between coffee and pancreatic cancer, the investigators chose control patients from the practices of the physicians looking after the patients with pancreatic cancer.[23] These control patients had a variety of gastrointestinal problems, some of which were exacerbated by coffee ingestion. The control patients had learned to avoid coffee; as a result, the investigators found an association between coffee (which the pancreatic cancer patients consumed at general population levels) and cancer. Subsequent investigations, using more appropriate controls, refuted the association.[24, 25] These problems illustrate why clinicians can draw inferences of only limited strength from the results of observational studies, even after adjustment for known determinants of outcome.

Case Series and Case Reports

Case series (descriptions of a series of patients) and *case reports* (descriptions of individual patients) do not provide any comparison group, and are therefore unable to satisfy the requirement that treatment and control groups share a similar prognosis. Although descriptive studies occasionally demonstrate dramatic findings mandating an immediate change in physician behavior (eg, recall the consequences when a link was associated between thalidomide and birth defects[26]), there are potentially undesirable consequences when actions are taken in response to weak evidence. Consider the case of the drug Bendectin (a combination of doxylamine, pyridoxine, and dicyclomine used as an antiemetic in pregnancy), whose manufacturer withdrew it from the market as a result of case reports suggesting it was teratogenic.[27] Later, even though a number of comparative studies demonstrated the drug's relative safety,[28] they could not eradicate the prevailing litigious atmosphere—which prevented the manufacturer from reintroducing Bendectin. Thus, many pregnant women who potentially could have benefited from the drug's availability were denied the symptomatic relief it could have offered.

In general, clinicians should not draw conclusions about cause-and-effect relationships from case series but, rather, should recognize that the results may generate questions for regulatory agencies and clinical investigators to address.

Design Issues—Summary

Just as is true for the resolution of questions of therapeutic effectiveness, clinicians should look first for randomized trials to resolve issues of harm. They will often be disappointed in this search and must make use of studies of weaker design. Regardless of the design, however, they should look for an appropriate control population before making a strong inference about a putative harmful agent. For RCTs and cohort studies, the control group should have a similar baseline risk of outcome, or investigators should use statistical techniques to adjust or correct for differences. Similarly, in case-control studies the derived exposed and nonexposed groups should be similar with respect to determinants of outcome other than the exposure under study. Alternatively, investigators should use statistical techniques to adjust for differences. Even when investigators have taken all the appropriate steps to minimize bias, clinicians should bear in mind that residual differences between groups may always bias the results of observational studies.[29] Since prescribing in the real world is carried out on the basis of evidence, clinician values, and patient values, exposure opportunities in nonrandomized medication studies are likely to differ among patients (channeling bias or effect).

Were Exposed Patients Equally Likely to Be Identified in the Two Groups?

In case-control studies, ascertainment of the exposure is a key issue. For example, when patients with leukemia are asked about prior exposure to solvents, they may be more likely to recall exposure than would control group members, either because of increased patient motivation (*recall bias*) or because of greater probing by an interviewer (*interviewer bias*). Clinicians should note whether investigators used bias-minimizing strategies such as blinding participants and interviewers to the hypothesis of the study. For example, a case-control study found a twofold increase in risk of hip fracture associated with psychotropic drug use. In this study, investigators established drug exposure by examining computerized claims files of the Michigan Medicaid program, a strategy that avoided both recall and interviewer bias.[30] The study of beta-adrenergic agonist use in patients with asthma suggesting an association with mortality also relied on an administrative database to ascertain exposure.[9] In both cases, the assurance of unbiased exposure status increases our confidence in the studies' findings.

Were the Outcomes Measured in the Same Way in the Groups Being Compared?

In RCTs and cohort studies, ascertainment of outcome is a key issue. For example, investigators have reported a threefold increase in the risk of malignant melanoma in individuals working with radioactive materials. One possible explanation for some of the increased risk might be that physicians, aware of a possible risk, search more diligently and, therefore, detect disease that might otherwise go unnoticed (or they may detect disease at an earlier point in time). This could result in the exposed cohort having an apparent, but spurious, increase in risk—a situation we refer to as *surveillance bias*.[31]

Was Follow-up Sufficiently Complete?

As we pointed out in Part 1B1, "Therapy," loss to follow-up can introduce bias because the patients who are lost may have very different outcomes from those still available for assessment. The longer the required follow-up period, the greater the possibility that the follow-up will be incomplete.

For example, in a well-executed study, investigators determined the vital status of 1235 of 1261 white males (98%) employed in a chrysotile asbestos textile operation between 1940 and 1975.[32] The relative risk for lung cancer death over time increased from 1.4 to 18.2 in direct proportion to the cumulative exposure among asbestos workers with at least 15 years since first exposure. Because the 2% missing data were unlikely to affect the results, the loss to follow-up does not threaten the validity of the inference that asbestos exposure causes lung cancer deaths.

USING THE GUIDE

Returning to our earlier discussion, the study that we retrieved investigating the association between SSRIs and risk of upper gastrointestinal bleeding used a case-control design.[6] Data came from a general practitioner electronic medical record database in the United Kingdom, which included data from more than 3 million people, most of whom had been entered prospectively during a 5-year period.[33-35] The investigators identified cases of upper gastrointestinal bleeding ($n=1651$) and ulcer perforation ($n=248$) among patients aged 40 to 79 years between 1993 and 1997. They then randomly selected 10,000 controls from the at-risk source population that gave rise to cases, choosing their sample so that age, sex, and the year patients were identified were similar among the cases and control groups.

The analysis controlled for a number of possible prognostic factors: previous dyspepsia, gastritis, peptic ulcer and upper gastrointestinal bleeding or perforation, smoking status, and current use of NSAIDs, anticoagulants, corticosteroids, and aspirin. The database included prescription drugs only. The investigators examined the relative frequency of SSRI prescription use in the 30 days before the *index date* (that is, the date of the reported bleeding or perforation) in patients with and without bleeding and perforation after controlling for the prognostic variables. Control patients received a random date as their index date.

Although the investigators controlled for a number of prognostic factors, there are other potential important determinants of bleeding for which they did not control. For example, more patients being treated for depression or anxiety suffer from painful medical conditions than those without depression and anxiety. Patients may have been using over-the-counter NSAIDs for these problems. The database the investigators used does not capture the use of self-medication with over-the-counter analgesics.

Alcohol use is another potential confounder. Although the investigators excluded patients with known alcoholism, many persons afflicted with alcoholism remain unrevealed to their primary care physician, and alcoholism is associated with an increased prevalence of depression and anxiety that could lead to the prescription of SSRIs. Since alcoholism is associated with increased bleeding risk, this prognostic variable fulfills all the criteria for a confounding variable that could bias the results of the study. Finally, it is possible that patients returning for prescription of SSRIs would be more likely to have their bleeding diagnosed in comparison to patients under less intense surveillance (a state of affairs known as *detection bias*).

These biases should apply to all three classes of antidepressants (ie, SSRIs, nonselective serotonin reuptake inhibitors, and a miscellaneous group of other drugs) that the investigators considered. The results of the study, which we will discuss later in this section, showed an association only between gastrointestinal bleeding and SSRIs, rather than between gastrointestinal bleeding and other antidepressant medications. One would expect all these biases to influence the association between any antidepressant agent and bleeding. Thus, the fact that the investigators found the association only with

SSRIs decreases our concern about the threats to validity from possible differences in prognostic factors in those receiving—and not receiving—SSRIs.

At the same time, most physicians make decisions regarding the prescription of SSRIs or tricyclic antidepressant agents based on particular patient characteristics. Thus, it remains possible that these characteristics include some that are associated with the incidence of gastrointestinal bleeding. This would be true, for instance, if clinicians differentially used SSRI rather than other antidepressant medications in patients in whom they suspected alcohol abuse.

The major strength of the use of a large database for this study is that it eliminates the possibility of biased assessment of exposure (or recall bias) to SSRIs in the patients who suffered the outcomes as well as in those who did not. The outcomes and exposures were probably measured in the same way in both groups, as most clinicians are unaware that UGI bleeding may be associated with SSRI use. We have no idea, however, about the number of patients lost to follow-up. Although the investigators included only those patients who stayed in the practices of the participating primary care physicians from the beginning to the end of the study, we do not know, for instance, how many people in the database began to receive SSRIs but subsequently left those practices.

In summary, the study suffers from the limitation inherent in any observational study: that exposed and unexposed patients may differ in prognosis at baseline. In this case, at least two unmeasured variables, over-the-counter NSAID use and alcohol consumption, might create a spurious association between SSRIs and gastrointestinal bleeding.

> The other major limitation of the study is the lack of
> information regarding completeness of follow-up.
> That said, although these limitations weaken any
> inferences we might make, we are likely to conclude
> that the study is strong enough to warrant a review
> of the results.

WHAT ARE THE RESULTS?

How Strong Is the Association Between Exposure and Outcome?

We have described the alternatives for expressing the association between the exposure and the outcome, the relative risk and the odds ratio, in other sections of this book (see Part 1B1, "Therapy"; see also Part 2D, "Therapy and Understanding the Results, Measures of Association"). In a cohort study assessing in-hospital mortality after noncardiac surgery in male veterans, 23 of 289 patients with a history of hypertension died, compared with three of 185 patients without the condition. The relative risk for hypertension and mortality, (23/289)/(3/185), was 4.9.[36] The relative risk tells us that death after noncardiac surgery occurs almost five times more often in patients with hypertension than in normotensive patients.

The estimate of relative risk depends on the availability of samples of exposed and unexposed patients, where the proportion of the patients with the outcome of interest can be determined. The relative risk is therefore not applicable to case-control studies in which the number of cases and controls—and, therefore, the proportion of individuals with the outcome—is chosen by the investigator. For case-control studies, instead of using a ratio of risks (*relative risk*), we use a ratio of odds (*odds ratio*): the odds of a case-patient being exposed, divided by the odds of a control patient being exposed (see Part 2D, "Therapy and Understanding the Results, Measures of Association").

When considering both study design and strength of association, we may be ready to interpret a small increase in risk as representing a true harmful effect when the study design is strong (such as in a RCT). A much higher increase in risk might be required of weaker designs (such as cohort or case-control studies), as subtle findings are more likely to be caused by the inevitably higher risk of bias. Very large values of relative risk or odds ratio represent strong associations that are less likely to be caused by confounding variables or bias.

In addition to showing a large magnitude of relative risk or odds ratio, a second finding will strengthen an inference that we are dealing with a true harmful effect. If, as the quantity or the duration of exposure to the putative harmful agent increases, the risk of the adverse outcome also increases (that is, the data suggest a dose-response gradient), we are more likely to be dealing with a causal relationship between exposure and outcome. The fact that the risk of dying from lung cancer in male physician smokers increases by 50%, 132%, and 220% for 1 to 14, 15 to 24, and 25 or more cigarettes smoked per day, respectively, strengthens our inference that cigarette smoking causes lung cancer.[37]

How Precise Is the Estimate of the Risk?

Clinicians can evaluate the precision of the estimate of risk by examining the confidence interval around that estimate (see Part 1B1, "Therapy"; see also Part 2C, "Therapy and Understanding the Results, Confidence Intervals"). In a study in which investigators have shown an association between an exposure and an adverse outcome, the lower limit of the estimate of relative risk associated with the adverse exposure provides a minimal estimate of the strength of the association. By contrast, in a study in which investigators fail to demonstrate an association (a negative study), the upper boundary of the confidence interval around the relative risk tells the clinician just how big an adverse effect may still be present, despite the failure to show a statistically significant association (see Part 2C, "Therapy and Understanding the Results, Confidence Intervals").

USING THE GUIDE

Returning to our earlier discussion, the investigators calculated odds ratios (ORs) of the risk of bleeding in those exposed to SSRIs vs those not exposed, but they reported the results as relative risks (RR). Unfortunately, this practice is not unusual. Fortunately, when event rates are low, relative risks and odds ratios closely approximate one another (see Part 2D, "Therapy and Understanding the Results, Measures of Association"). The investigators found an association between current use of SSRIs and upper gastrointestinal bleeding (adjusted OR, 3.0; 95% CI, 2.1-4.4). They noted a weak association with nonselective serotonin reuptake inhibitors (adjusted OR, 1.4; 95% CI, 1.1-1.9), but found no association with antidepressant medications that had no action on the serotonin reuptake mechanism. The investigators found that the association between NSAID use and bleeding (adjusted OR, 3.7; 95% CI, 3.2-4.4) was of similar magnitude to the association between bleeding and SSRIs. The current use of SSRIs with prescription NSAID drugs further increased the risk of upper gastrointestinal bleeding (adjusted OR, 15.6; 95% CI, 6.6-36.6). The dose and duration of SSRI use had little influence on the risk of this adverse outcome.

HOW CAN I APPLY THE RESULTS TO PATIENT CARE?

Were the Study Patients Similar to the Patient in My Practice?

If possible biases in a study are not sufficient to dismiss the study out of hand, you must consider the extent to which they might apply to the patient in your office. Is the patient before you similar to those described in the study with respect to morbidity, age, sex, race, or other potentially important factors? If not, is the biology of the harmful exposure likely to differ in the patient you are attending? Are there important differences in the treatments or exposures between the patients you see and the patients studied? For example, the risk of thrombophlebitis associated with oral contraceptive use described in the 1970s may not be applicable to the patient of the 1990s because of the lower estrogen dose in oral contraceptives used in the 1990s. Similarly, increases in uterine cancer secondary to postmenopausal estrogen replacement do not apply to women who are also taking concomitant progestins tailored to produce monthly withdrawal bleeding with chronic, noncyclic use.

Was the Duration of Follow-up Adequate?

Let us return for a moment to the study that showed that workers employed in chrysotile asbestos textile operation between 1940 and 1975 showed an increased risk for lung cancer death, a risk that increased from 1.4 to 18.2 in direct relation to cumulative exposure among asbestos workers with at least 15 years since first exposure.[32] The fact that the follow-up was sufficiently long to capture a large proportion of the lung cancers destined to occur enhances our confidence in application of the results to patients in our practice.

By contrast, excessively short follow-up may fail to detect harmful effects that emerge with longer observation.

What Was the Magnitude of the Risk?

The relative risk and the odds ratio do not tell us how frequently the problem occurs; they tell us only that the observed effect occurs more or less often in the exposed group compared to the unexposed group. Thus, we need a method for assessing clinical importance. In our discussion of therapy (see Part 1B1, "Therapy"; see also Part 2D, "Therapy and Understanding the Results, Measures of Association"), we described the way to calculate the number of patients who must be treated to prevent an adverse event. When the issue is harm, we can use data from a randomized trial or cohort study, but not a case-control study, to make an analogous calculation to determine how many people must be exposed to the harmful agent to cause an adverse outcome.

For example, over an average of 10 months of follow-up, investigators conducting the Cardiac Arrhythmia Suppression Trial (CAST), a RCT of antiarrhythmic agents,[38,39] found that the mortality rate was 3.0% for placebo-treated patients and 7.7% for those treated with either encainide or flecainide. The *absolute risk* increase was 4.7%, the reciprocal of which tells us that, on average, for every 21 patients we treat with encainide or flecainide for about a year, we will cause one excess death. This contrasts with our example of the association between NSAIDs and upper gastrointestinal bleeding. Of 2000 unexposed patients, two will suffer a bleeding episode each year. Of 2000 patients taking NSAIDs, three will suffer such an episode each year. Thus, if we treat 2000 patients with NSAIDs, we can expect a single additional bleeding event.[7]

Should I Attempt to Stop the Exposure?

After evaluating the evidence that an exposure is harmful and after establishing that the results are potentially applicable to the patient in your practice, determining subsequent actions may not be simple. There are at least three aspects to consider in making a clinical decision.

First is the strength of inference: how strong was the study or studies that demonstrated harm in the first place? Second, what is the magnitude of the risk to patients if exposure to the harmful agent continues? Third, what are the adverse consequences of reducing or eliminating exposure to the harmful agent—that is, the magnitude of the benefit that patients will no longer receive?

Clinical decision making is simple when both the likelihood of harm and its magnitude are great. Because the evidence of increased mortality from encainide and flecainide came from a randomized trial,[38] we can be confident of the causal connection. Since treating only 21 people will result in an excess death, it is no wonder that clinicians quickly curtailed their use of these antiarrhythmic agents when the study results became available.

The clinical decision is also made easier when an acceptable alternative for avoiding the risk is available. For example, beta blockers prescribed for the treatment of hypertension can result in symptomatic increase in airway resistance in patients with asthma or chronic airflow limitation. This risk mandates the use of an alternative drug, such as a thiazide diuretic, in susceptible patients.[40]

Even if the evidence is relatively weak, the availability of an alternative can result in a clear decision. The early case-control studies demonstrating the association between aspirin use and Reye syndrome, for example, were relatively weak and left considerable doubt about the causal relationship. Although the strength of inference was not great, the availability of a safe, inexpensive, and well-tolerated alternative, acetaminophen, justified use of this alternative agent in children at risk of Reye syndrome.[41]

In contrast to the early studies regarding aspirin and Reye syndrome, multiple well-designed cohort and case-control studies have consistently demonstrated an association between NSAIDs and upper gastrointestinal bleeding; therefore, our inference about harm has been relatively strong. However, the risk of an upper gastrointestinal bleeding episode is quite low, and until recently we have not had safer and equally efficacious anti-inflammatory alternatives available. We were therefore probably right in continuing to prescribe NSAIDs for the appropriate clinical conditions. Depending on both their safety profile after longer experience and cost-effectiveness considerations, COX 2-inhibiting NSAIDs may prove to be an appropriate alternative class of agents.

CLINICAL RESOLUTION

To decide on your course of action, you proceed through the three steps of using the medical literature to guide your clinical practice. First, you consider the validity of the study before you. The antidepressant and upper gastrointestinal bleeding study addressed multiple classes of antidepressant agents and the risk of upper gastrointestinal bleeding or ulcer perforation. You decide that the limitations of the case-control design, along with the lack of information about loss to follow-up, leave you uncertain about a causal relationship between SSRIs and gastrointestinal bleeding. Furthermore, this is a single study and, as we have previously mentioned, in other areas of medicine subsequent investigations[11, 12, 42-45] have failed to confirm many apparent harmful associations.[10, 46, 47]

Turning to the results, you note the very strong association between the combined use of SSRIs and NSAIDs. Despite the methodologic limitations of this single study, you believe the association is too strong to ignore. You therefore proceed to the third step and consider the implications of the results for the patient before you.

The primary care database from which the investigators drew their sample suggests that the results are readily applicable to the patient before you. You consider the magnitude of the risk to which you would be exposing this patient if you prescribed an SSRI and it actually did cause bleeding. Using the baseline risk reported by Carson et al in a similar population,[14] you calculate that you would need to treat about 625 patients with SSRIs for a year to cause a single bleeding episode in patients not using NSAIDs, and about 55 patients a year taking NSAIDs along with an SSRI for a year to cause a single bleeding episode.

From previous experience with the patient before you, you know that he is risk averse. When he returns to your office, you note the equal effectiveness of the SSRIs and tricyclic antidepressants that you can offer him, and you describe the side-effect profile of the alternative agents. You note, among the other considerations, the possible increased risk of gastrointestinal bleeding with the SSRIs. The patient decides that, on balance, he would prefer a tricyclic antidepressant and leaves your office with a prescription for nortriptyline.

References

1. Geddes JR, Freemantle N, Mason J, Eccles MP, Boynton J. SSRIs versus other antidepressants for depressive disorder. *Cochrane Database of Systematic Reviews*. 2000:1-26.

2. Trindale E, Menon D. *Selective Serotonin Reuptake Inhibitors (SSRIs) for Major Depression.* Ottawa: Canadian Coordinating Office for Health Technology Assessment; 1997.

3. Mulrow CD, Williams JW Jr, Trivedi M. *Treatment of Depression: Newer Pharmacotherapies*. San Antonio, Texas: San Antonio Evidence-based Practice Centre; 1999.

4. Hotopf M, Hardy R, Lewis G. Discontinuation rates of SSRIs and tricyclic antidepressants: a meta-analysis and investigation of heterogeneity. *Br J Psychiatry*. 1997;170:120-127.

5. Trindale E, Menon D. Review: selective serotonin reuptake inhibitors differ from tricyclic antidepressants in adverse events. *Evidence Based Mental Health*. 1998;1:50.

6. Goldberg RJ. Selective serotonin reuptake inhibitors: infrequent medical adverse effects. *Arch Fam Med*. 1998;7:78-84.

7. de Abajo FJ, Rodriguez LA, Montero D. Association between selective serotonin reuptake inhibitors and upper gastrointestinal bleeding: population based case-control study. *BMJ.* 1999;319:1106-1109.

8. CAPRIE Steering Committee. A randomised, blinded, trial of clopidogrel versus aspirin in patients at risk of ischaemic events (CAPRIE). *Lancet*. 1996;348:1329-1339.

9. Bennett CL, Connors JM, Carwile JM, et al. Thrombotic thrombo-cytopenic purpura associated with clopidogrel. *N Engl J Med*. 2000;342:1773-1777.

10. Silverstein FE, Graham DY, Senior JR, et al. Misoprostol reduces serious gastrointestinal complications in patients with rheuma-toid arthritis receiving nonsteroidal anti-inflammatory drugs: a randomized, double-blind, placebo-controlled trial. *Ann Intern Med*. 1995;123:241-249.

11. Merck and Co. VIGOR Study Summary. Paper presented at: Digestive Disease Week Congress; May 24, 2000; San Diego.

12. Langman MJ, Jensen DM, Watson DJ, et al. Adverse upper gas-trointestinal effects of rofecoxib compared with NSAIDs. *JAMA*. 1999;282:1929-1933.

13. Kristensen P, Irgens LM, Daltveit AK, Andersen A. Perinatal outcome among children of men exposed to lead and organic solvents in the printing industry. *Am J Epidemiol*. 1993;137:134-143.

14. Carson JL, Strom BL, Soper KA, et al. The association of nonsteroidal anti-inflammatory drugs with upper gastrointestinal tract bleeding. *Arch Intern Med*. 1987;147:85-88.

15. Walter SD. Determination of significant relative risks and optimal sampling procedures in prospective and retrospective comparative studies of various sizes. *Am J Epidemiol*. 1977;105:387-397.

16. Leufkens HG, Urquhart J, Stricker BH, Bakker A, Petri H. Channelling of controlled release formulation of ketoprofen (Oscorel) in patients with history of gastrointestinal problems. *J Epidemiol Community Health*. 1992;46:428-432.

17. Joseph KS. The evolution of clinical practice and time trends in drug effects. *J Clin Epidemiol*. 1994;47:593-598.

18. Leufkens HG, Urquhart J. Variability in patterns of drug usage. *J Pharm Pharmacol*. 1994;46(suppl 1):433-437.

19. Ray WA, Griffin MR, Downey W. Benzodiazepines of long and short elimination half-life and risk of hip fracture. *JAMA*. 1989;262:3303-3307.

20. Jollis JG, Ancukiewicz M, DeLong ER, Pryor DB, Muhlbaier LH, Mark DB. Discordance of databases designed for claims payment versus clinical information systems: implications for outcomes research. *Ann Intern Med*. 1993;119:844-850.

21. Herbst AL, Ulfelder H, Poskanzer DC. Adenocarcinoma of the vagina: association of maternal stilbestrol therapy with tumor appearance in young women. *N Engl J Med*. 1971;284:878-881.

22. Spitzer WO, Suissa S, Ernst P, et al. The use of beta-agonists and the risk of death and near death from asthma. *N Engl J Med*. 1992;326:501-506.

23. MacMahon B, Yen S, Trichopoulos D, Warren K, Nardi G. Coffee and cancer of the pancreas. *N Engl J Med*. 1981;304:630-633.

24. Baghurst PA, McMichael AJ, Slavotineck AH, Baghurst KI, Boyle P, Walker AM. A case-control study of diet and cancer of the pancreas. *Am J Epidemiol*. 1991;134:167-179.

25. Zheng W, McLaughlin JK, Gridley G, et al. A cohort study of smoking, alcohol consumption and dietary factors for pancreatic cancer. *Cancer Causes Control*. 1993;4:477-482.

26. Lenz W. Epidemiology of congenital malformations. *Ann NY Acad Sci*. 1965; 123:228-236.

27. Soverchia G, Perri PF. Two cases of malformation of a limb in infants of mothers treated with an antiemetic in a very early phase of pregnancy. *Pediatr Med Chir*. 1981;3:97-99.

28. Holmes LB. Teratogen update: Bendectin. *Teratology*. 1983;27:277-281.

29. Kellermann AL, Rivara FP, Rushforth NB, Banton JG, et al. Gun ownership as a risk factor for homicide in the home. *N Engl J Med*. 1993;329:1084-1091.

30. Ray WA, Griffin MR, Schaffner W, et al. Psychotropic drug use and the risk of hip fracture. *N Engl J Med*. 1987;316:363-369.

31. Hiatt RA, Fireman B. The possible effect of increased surveillance on the incidence of malignant melanoma. *Prev Med*. 1986;15:652-660.

32. Dement JM, Harris RL Jr, Symons MJ, Shy CM. Exposures and mortality among chrysotile asbestos workers. Part II: mortality. *Am J Ind Med*. 1983;4:421-433.

33. Jick H, Jick SS, Derby LE. Validation of information recorded on general practitioner based computerised resource in the United Kingdom. *BMJ*. 1991;302:766-768.

34. Garcia Rodriguez LA, Perez Gutthann S. Use of the UK general practice research database for pharmacoepidemiology. *Br J Clin Pharmacol*. 1998;45:419-425.

35. Jick H, Terris B, Derby LE, Jick SS. Further validation of information recorded on a general practitioner database resource in the United Kingdom. *Pharmacoepidemiol Drug Saf*. 1992;1:347-349.

36. Browner WS, Li J, Mangano DT. In-hospital and long-term mortality in male veteran following noncardiac surgery. *JAMA*. 1992;268:228-232.

37. Doll R, Hill AB. Mortality in relation to smoking: ten years' observation of British doctors. *BMJ*. 1964;1:1399-1410, 1460-1467.

38. Echt DS, Liebson PR, Mitchell LB, et al. Mortality and morbidity in patients receiving encainide, flecainide, or placebo: the Cardiac Arrhythmia Suppression Trial. *N Engl J Med*. 1991;324:781-788.

39. The Cardiac Arrhythmia Suppression Trial II Investigators. Effect of the antiarrhythmic agent moricizine on survival after myocardial infarction. *N Engl J Med*. 1992;327:227-233.

40. Ogilvie RI, Burgess ED, Cusson JR, Feldman RD, Leiter LA, Myers MG. Report of the Canadian Hypertension Society Consensus Conference, 3: pharmacologic treatment of essential hypertension. *Can Med Assoc J.* 1993;149:575-584.

41. Soumerai SB, Ross-Degnan D, Kahn JS. Effects of professional and media warnings about the association between aspirin use in children and Reye's syndrome. *Milbank Q.* 1992;70:155-182.

42. Danesh J, Appleby P. Coronary heart disease and iron status: meta-analyses of prospective studies. *Circulation.* 1999;99:852-854.

43. Klebanoff MA, Read JS, Mills JL, Shiono PH. The risk of childhood cancer after neonatal exposure to vitamin K. *N Engl J Med.* 1993;329:905-908.

44. Passmore SJ, Draper G, Brownbill P, Kroll M. Case-control studies of relation between childhood cancer and neonatal vitamin K administration: retrospective case-control study. *BMJ.* 1998;316:178-184.

45. Parker L, Cole M, Craft AW, Hey EN. Neonatal vitamin K administration and childhood cancer in the north of England. *BMJ.* 1998;316:189-193.

46. Salonen JT, Nyyssonen K, Korpela H, Tuomilehto J, Seppanen R, Salonen R. High stored iron levels are associated with excess risk of myocardial infarction in eastern Finnish men. *Circulation.* 1992;86:803-811.

47. Golding J, Greenwood R, Birmingham K, Mott M. Childhood cancer, intramuscular vitamin K, and pethidine given during labour. *BMJ.* 1992;305:341-346.

THE PROCESS OF DIAGNOSIS

W. Scott Richardson, Mark Wilson, and Gordon Guyatt

The following EBM Working Group members also made
substantive contributions to this section: Peter Wyer,
Jonathan Craig, Roman Jaeschke, Jeroen Lijmer,
Luz Maria Letelier, Virginia Moyer, C. David Naylor,
and Deborah Cook

IN THIS SECTION

CLINICAL SCENARIO

Generating a Differential Diagnosis

It is another busy day in the emergency department and one of your nurse colleagues tells you that a 60-year-old man has presented with a severe cough of 1 day's duration. Immediately, you think, "upper respiratory tract infection; perhaps pneumonia." When you enter the room, you find the patient appears short of breath and is in more distress than you were expecting. Other possible diagnoses spring to mind: could the patient be suffering from acute airflow obstruction, myocardial infarction with pulmonary edema, a pneumothorax, or a pulmonary embolus? You sit down beside the patient and begin taking a history. You ask the nurse to place him on cardiac and pulse oximetry monitors, to start an intravenous line, and to obtain a 12-lead electrocardiogram and a portable chest radiograph.

The patient appears moderately tachypneic but is able to speak in complete sentences. Vital signs show a regular heart rate of 96 bpm, a blood pressure of 140/90 mm Hg, and a respiratory rate of 24/min. In view of his tachypnea, you request a rectal temperature. Oximetry shows a saturation of 93% and you ask that he receive 4 L/minute of oxygen by nasal cannula.

The patient reports that he was previously in excellent health, but began to suffer from a cough about 24 hours previously. There was no preceding or accompanying fever, runny nose, sore throat, headache, or muscular discomfort. However, he did experience several hours of central chest discomfort at the time of the onset of the cough, a discomfort that subsequently resolved. The cough has been productive of only small amounts of clear sputum which, during the past 2 hours, has been flecked with small amounts of bright red blood. During the past 12 hours, the patient has felt increasingly short of breath on minimal activity and now feels short of breath at rest.

Cardiac auscultation reveals no extra heart sounds or murmurs. Abnormal findings on physical examination are limited to decreased breath sounds and crackles at the left base on chest auscultation. The electrocardiogram confirms mild sinus tachycardia, but is otherwise normal, and the chest radiograph shows only a small left pleural effusion with minimal associated opacification. The nurse reports the patient's temperature to be 38.1°C. You draw arterial blood gases and arrange for an urgent ventilation-perfusion scan. The room air blood gas results show a normal PCO_2 and a PO_2 of 70 mm Hg with a saturation of 93%.

While waiting for the results of the ventilation-perfusion scan, you consider how likely the diagnosis of pulmonary embolism is, given the available information. On the one hand, the patient lacks risk factors, cough is a very prominent symptom, and highly suggestive findings for clinical examination (such as pleuritic chest pain) or further investigation (such as a typical electrocardiographic pattern) are absent. On the other hand, you believe you have ruled out a number of competing diagnoses, including asthma, pulmonary edema, and pneumothorax, and the clinical picture is not typical of pneumonia. You ultimately decide the probability is intermediate, and you mentally commit yourself to a 30% likeli-hood of pulmonary embolus. When the ventilation-perfusion scan reveals an unmatched segmental defect that you know is associated with a likelihood ratio of 18,[1] you use your likelihood ratio card (see Part 1C2, "Diagnostic Tests") to generate a posttest probability of approximately 90%, and you begin anticoagulation.

THE DIAGNOSTIC PROCESS

Making a diagnosis is a complex cognitive task that involves both logical reasoning and pattern recognition.[2,3] Although the process happens largely at an unconscious level, we can identify two essential steps.

Step 1. In the first step, you enumerate the diagnostic possi-bilities and estimate their relative likelihood.[4] Experienced clinicians often group the findings into meaningful clusters, summarized in brief phrases about the symptom, body loca-tion, or organ system involved, such as "generalized pruri-tus," "painless jaundice," and "constitutional symptoms." These clusters, or clinical problems, may be of biologic, psy-chologic, or sociologic origin, and they are the object of the differential diagnosis. In the opening scenario, we considered a previously healthy 60-year-old man with a clinical problem encompassing a day-long history of cough and dyspnea. The differential diagnosis included a respiratory infection, acute airflow obstruction, myocardial infarction with pulmonary edema, a pneumothorax, and pulmonary embolus.

Step 2. In the second step in the diagnostic process, you incorporate new information to change the relative probabilities, rule out some of the possibilities, and, ultimately, choose the most likely diagnosis. For each diagnostic possibility, the additional information increases or decreases the likelihood. In our scenario, the absence of manifestations that usually accompany an infectious process reduces the likelihood of an upper respiratory tract infection or pneumonia. The central chest discomfort increased the possibility that we could be observing an atypical presentation of a myocardial infarction and prompted the timely electrocardiogram. Physical examination made heart failure a much less likely possibility; pneumonia and pulmonary embolus remained as the competing diagnoses. The chest radiograph failed to provide definitive evidence of pneumonia, necessitating an additional test, the ventilation-perfusion scan.

Thus, with each new finding, we moved, albeit intuitively and implicitly, from one probability, the *pretest probability,* to another probability—the *posttest probability*. Some findings, such as the absence of any sign of pneumothorax on the chest radiograph, eliminated one of the possibilities (a posttest probability of 0). Prior to the last test, our approach became explicitly quantitative: we committed to a pretest likelihood of 30% and subsequently used information from the literature to arrive at a final, 90% posttest likelihood of pulmonary embolus.

If we know the properties of each of piece of information (and, in the case of pulmonary embolism, if we have strong data for many elements of the diagnostic workup), we can be highly quantitative in our sequential move from pre- to posttest probability. Later in this section, we will show you how.

Because the properties of the individual items of history and physical examination often are not available, you must rely on clinical experience and intuition to predict the extent to which many pieces of information modify your differential diagnosis. For some clinical problems, including the diagnosis of pulmonary embolism, clinicians' intuition has proved remarkably accurate.[1]

CHOICES IN THE DIAGNOSTIC PROCESS

When considering a patient's differential diagnosis, how can you decide which disorders to pursue? If you were to consider all known causes to be equally likely and test for them all simultaneously (the possibilistic approach), then the patient would undergo unnecessary testing. Instead, the experienced clinician is selective, considering first those disorders that are more likely (a probabilistic approach), more serious if left undiagnosed and untreated (a prognostic approach), or more responsive to treatment if offered (a pragmatic approach).

Wisely selecting a patient's differential diagnosis involves all three considerations (probabilistic, prognostic, and pragmatic). Your single best explanation for the patient's clinical problem(s) can be termed the leading hypothesis or working diagnosis. In the opening scenario, a respiratory infection was the leading diagnosis until the final test result became available. A few (usually one to five) other diagnoses, termed active alternatives, may be worth considering at the time of initial workup because of their likelihood, seriousness if undiagnosed and untreated, or responsiveness to treatment. In the scenario, pulmonary embolus entered the differential diagnosis early because of its seriousness and responsiveness to treatment.

Additional causes of the clinical problem(s), termed other hypotheses, may be too unlikely to consider at the time of initial diagnostic workup, but remain possible and could be considered further if the working diagnosis and active alternatives are later disproved. In our scenario, remote possibilities such a pulmonary hemorrhage or collagen vascular disease never entered the active differential diagnosis, but might eventually have done so if we had not confirmed one of the active alternatives.

DIAGNOSTIC AND THERAPEUTIC THRESHOLDS

Consider a patient who presents with a painful eruption of grouped vesicles in the distribution of a single dermatome. In an instant, an experienced clinician would make a diagnosis of herpes zoster and would consider whether to offer the patient therapy. In other words, the probability of herpes zoster is so high (near 1.0, or 100%) that it is above a threshold where no further testing is required.

Next, consider a previously healthy athlete who presents with lateral rib cage pain after being accidentally struck by an errant baseball pitch. Again, an experienced clinician would recognize the clinical problem (posttraumatic lateral chest pain), identify a leading hypothesis (rib contusion) and an active alternative (rib fracture), and plan a test (radiograph) to exclude the latter. If asked, the clinician could also list disorders that are too unlikely to consider further (such as myocardial infarction). In other words, while not as likely as rib contusion, the probability of a rib fracture is above a threshold for testing, while the probability of myocardial infarction is below the threshold for testing.

These cases illustrate how you can estimate the probability of disease and then compare disease probabilities to two thresholds (Figure 1C-1). The probability above which the diagnosis is sufficiently likely to warrant therapy defines the upper threshold. That is, if a clinician believes that the diagnosis is sufficiently likely that she is ready to recommend treatment, she has crossed the upper threshold. This threshold is termed the *treatment threshold*.[5] In the case of shingles described above, the clinician judged the diagnosis of herpes zoster to be above this treatment threshold of probability. In our scenario, with the results of the ventilation-perfusion scan we crossed the treatment threshold only after we arrived at a probability of 90% for one of the competing causes, pulmonary embolus.

FIGURE 1C–1

Test and Treatment Thresholds in the Diagnostic Process

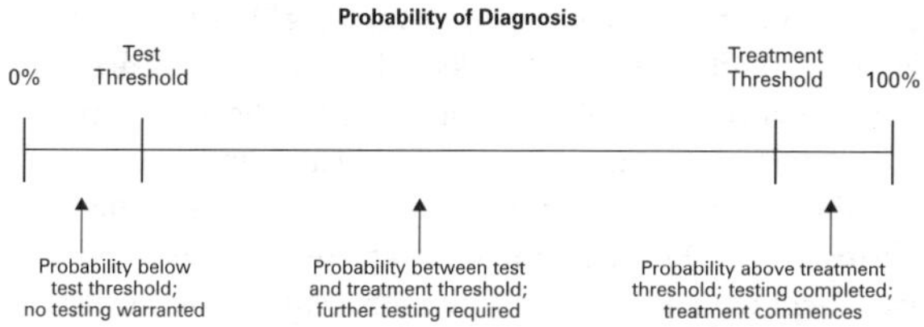

Probability of Diagnosis

| 0% | Test Threshold | | | | Treatment Threshold | 100% |

Probability below test threshold; no testing warranted

Probability between test and treatment threshold; further testing required

Probability above treatment threshold; testing completed; treatment commences

The probability below which the clinician decides a diagnosis warrants no further consideration defines the lower threshold. This threshold is termed the no test-test threshold or, simply, the *test threshold*. In the case of posttraumatic torso pain described above, the diagnosis of rib fracture fell above the test threshold and the diagnosis of myocardial infarction fell below it. In our opening scenario, heart failure dropped below the diagnostic threshold when we received the results of the chest radiograph; we did not, for instance, order an echocardiogram. Immune-mediated pulmonary hemorrhage remained below the test threshold throughout the entire investigation.

For a disorder with a pretest probability above the treatment threshold, a confirming test that raises the probability further would not assist diagnostically. On the other end of the scale, for a disorder with a pretest probability below the test threshold, an exclusionary test that lowers the probability further would not help diagnostically. When the clinician believes the pretest probability is high enough to test for and not high enough to warrant beginning treatment (ie, when probability is between the two thresholds), testing will be diagnostically useful, and it will be most valuable if it moves the probability across either threshold.

What determines our treatment threshold? The greater the adverse effects of treating, the more we will be inclined to choose a high treatment threshold. For instance, because a diagnosis of pulmonary embolus involves long-term anticoagulation with appreciable risks of hemorrhage, we are very concerned about falsely labeling patients. The invasiveness of the next test we are considering will also impact our threshold. If results from the next test (such as a ventilation-perfusion scan) are benign, we will be ready to choose a high treatment threshold. We will be more reluctant to institute an invasive test associated with risks to the patient, such as pulmonary angiogram, and this will drive our treatment threshold downward. That is, we will be more inclined to accept a risk of a false-positive diagnosis because a higher treatment threshold implies putting some patients through the test unnecessarily.

Similar considerations bear on the test threshold. The more serious a missed diagnosis, the lower we will set our test threshold. Since a missed diagnosis of a pulmonary embolus could be fatal, we would be inclined to set our diagnostic threshold low. However, this is again counterbalanced by the risks associated with the next test we are considering. If the risks are low, we will be comfortable with our low diagnostic threshold. The higher the risks, the more it will push our threshold upward.

USING SYSTEMATIC RESEARCH TO AID IN THE DIAGNOSTIC PROCESS

How do clinicians generate differential diagnoses and arrive at pretest estimates of disease probability? They remember prior cases with the same clinical problem(s), so that disorders diagnosed frequently have higher probability than diagnoses made less frequently. Remembered cases are easily and quickly available, and they are calibrated to our local practices. Yet our memories are imperfect, and the probabilities that result are subject to bias and error.[6-8]

Two sorts of systematic investigations can inform the process of generating a differential diagnosis. One type of study addresses the manifestations with which a disease or condition presents. The second—and more important—type of study directly addresses the underlying causes of a presenting symptom, sign, or constellation of symptoms and signs (see Part 1C1, "Differential Diagnosis"). In our opening scenario, the question would be: When patients present with acute cough and shortness of breath, what are the ultimate diagnoses and the relative frequency of these diagnoses?

Having generated an initial differential diagnosis with associated pretest probabilities, how can you incorporate additional information to arrive at an ultimate diagnosis? For each finding, you must implicitly ask: How frequently will this result be seen in patients with one particular diagnostic possibility (or target condition) in relation to the frequency with which it is seen in the competing diagnostic conditions? Once again, you may intuitively refer to your own past experience. Alternatively, you may use data from research studies focusing on test properties. For instance, in our scenario, the Prospective Investigation of Pulmonary Embolism Diagnosis (PIOPED) study of ventilation-perfusion scanning in the diagnosis of pulmonary embolism[1] provided the likelihood ratio that allowed calculation of the posttest probability of 90% (see Part 1C2, "Diagnostic Tests").

Some articles provide evidence about differential diagnosis as well as diagnostic test properties. For example, in a study of diagnostic tests for anemia in aged persons, investigators compared blood tests with bone marrow results in 259 elderly persons, finding iron deficiency in 94 (36%).[9] The investigators also reported a diagnosis of anemia in the remaining 165 patients. Thus, although this study focused on evaluating tests for iron deficiency, it also provides information about disease frequency.

In the following sections of the book, we provide guidelines for you to assess the validity of both types of formal investigations related to diagnosis: studies that focus on a constellation of presenting symptoms or signs and determine patients' ultimate diagnoses, and studies that explore the properties of a diagnostic test. In each case, we suggest that validity will depend on the answers to questions regarding two key design features: Did the investigators enroll the right group of patients; and did they undertake the appropriate investigations to determine the true diagnosis? As we deal in sequence with each of the three types of study, we will explain how you can use the results to improve the accuracy of diagnosis in your clinical practice. As for therapy, prognosis, and harm, the systematic reviews of all diagnostic test articles addressing a particular issue will provide the strongest inferences (see Part 1E, "Summarizing the Evidence"). To understand and interpret such reviews, we must use the principles of assessing primary diagnostic studies.

References

1. The PIOPED Investigators. Value of the ventilation/perfusion scan in acute pulmonary embolism. Results of the Prospective Investigation of Pulmonary Embolism Diagnosis (PIOPED). *JAMA*. 1990;263:2753-2759.

2. Sox HC, Blatt MA, Higgins MC, Marton KI. *Medical Decision Making*. Boston: Butterworths; 1988.

3. Glass RD. *Diagnosis: A Brief Introduction*. Melbourne: Oxford University Press; 1996.

4. Barondess JA, Carpenter CCJ, eds. *Differential Diagnosis*. Philadelphia: Lea & Febiger; 1994.

5. Pauker SG, Kassirer JP. The threshold approach to clinical decision making. *N Engl J Med*. 1980;302:1109-1117.

6. Schmidt HG, Norman GR, Boshuizen HP. A cognitive perspective on medical expertise: theory and implication. *Acad Med*. 1990;65:611-621.

7. Bordage G. Elaborated knowledge: a key to successful diagnostic thinking. *Acad Med*. 1994;69:883-885.

8. Regehr G, Norman GR. Issues in cognitive psychology: implications for professional education. *Acad Med*. 1996;71:988-1001.

9. Guyatt GH, Patterson C, Ali M, et al. Diagnosis of iron-deficiency anemia in the elderly. *Am J Med*. 1990;88:205-209.

DIFFERENTIAL DIAGNOSIS

W. Scott Richardson, Mark Wilson, Jeroen Lijmer, Gordon Guyatt, and Deborah Cook

The following EBM Working Group members also made substantive contributions to this section: Peter Wyer, C. David Naylor, Jonathan Craig, Luz Maria Letelier, and Virginia Moyer

IN THIS SECTION

CLINICAL SCENARIO

A 33-Year-Old Man With Palpitations: What Is the Cause?

You are a primary care physician seeing a patient from your practice, a 33-year-old man who presents with heart palpitations. He describes the new onset as episodes of fast, regular chest pounding that come on gradually, last from 1 to 2 minutes, and occur several times per day. He reports no relationship of symptoms to activities and no change in exercise tolerance. You have previously noted that this patient tends to suffer from anxiety, and he now tells you that he fears heart disease. He has no other symptoms, no personal or family history of heart disease, and he takes no medications. You find his heart rate is 90 bpm and regular, and physical examinations of his eyes, thyroid gland, and lungs are normal. His heart sounds also are normal, without click, murmur, or gallop. His 12-lead ECG is normal, without arrhythmia or signs of preexcitation.

You suspect that anxiety explains this patient's palpitations, that they are mediated by hyperventilation, and that they may be part of a panic attack. Also, although there are no findings to suggest cardiac arrhythmia or hyperthyroidism, you wonder if these disorders are common enough in this sort of patient to warrant serious consideration. You reject pheochromocytoma as too unlikely to consider further. Thus, you can list causes of palpitations, but you want more information about the frequency of these causes to choose a diagnostic workup. You ask the question, "In patients presenting with heart palpitations, what is the frequency of underlying disorders?"

FINDING THE EVIDENCE

Your office computer networks with the medical library, where MEDLINE is on CD-ROM. In the MEDLINE file for current years, you enter three text words: "palpitations" (89 citations), "differential diagnosis" (7039 citations), and "cause or causes" (71,848 citations). You combine these sets, yielding 17 citations. Reviewing the titles and abstracts onscreen, you see a paper by Weber and Kapoor that explicitly addresses the differential diagnosis in patients presenting with palpitations.[1] With a keystroke and a mouse click, you review this article's full text.

ARE THE RESULTS VALID?

Table 1C-1 summarizes the guides for an article about the diagnostic possibilities.

TABLE 1C–1

Users' Guide for an Article About Differential Diagnosis

Are the results valid?

- Did the investigators enroll the right patients? Was the patient sample representative of those with the clinical problem?

- Was the definitive diagnostic standard appropriate? Was the diagnostic process credible?

- For initially undiagnosed patients, was follow-up sufficiently long and complete?

What are the results?

- What were the diagnoses and their probabilities?

- How precise are the estimates of disease probability?

How can I apply the results to patient care?

- Are the study patients similar to the one being considered in my own practice?

- Is it unlikely that the disease possibilities or probabilities have changed since this evidence was gathered?

Did the Investigators Enroll the Right Patients? Was the Patient Sample Representative of Those With the Clinical Problem?

This question asks about two related issues: defining the clinical problem and ensuring a representative population.

First, how do the investigators define the clinical problem under study? The definition of the clinical problem determines the population from which the study patients should be drawn. Thus, investigators studying hematuria might include patients with microscopic and gross hematuria, with or without symptoms. On the other hand, investigators studying asymptomatic, microscopic hematuria would exclude those with symptoms or with gross hematuria.

Differing definitions of the clinical problem will yield different frequencies of underlying diseases. Including patients with gross hematuria or urinary symptoms will raise the frequency of acute infection as the underlying cause relative to those without symptoms. Assessing the validity of an article about differential diagnosis begins with a search for a clear definition of the clinical problem.

Having defined the target population by clinical problem statement, investigators next assemble a patient sample. Ideally, the sample mirrors the target population in all important ways, so that the frequency of underlying diseases in the sample approximates that of the target population. We call a patient sample that mirrors the underlying target population *representative.* The more representative the sample, the more accurate the resulting disease probabilities.

Investigators seldom use the strongest method of ensuring representativeness, which is to obtain a random sample of the entire population of patients with the clinical problem. The next strongest methods are either (1) to include all patients with the clinical problem from a defined geographic area or (2) to include a consecutive series of all patients with the clinical problem who receive care at the investigators' institution(s). To the extent that a nonconsecutive case series opens the study to the differential inclusion of patients with different underlying disorders, it compromises study validity.

You can judge the representativeness of the sample by examining the setting from which patients come. Patients with ostensibly the same clinical problem can present to different clinical settings, resulting in different services seeing different types of patients. Typically, patients in secondary or tertiary care settings have higher proportions of more serious or more uncommon diseases than patients seen in primary care settings. For instance, in a study of patients presenting with chest pain, a higher proportion of referral practice patients had coronary artery disease than the primary care practice patients, even in patients with similar clinical histories.[2]

To further evaluate representativeness, you can note investigators' methods of identifying patients, how carefully they avoided missing patients, and whom they included and excluded. The wider the spectrum of patients in the sample, the more representative the sample should be of the whole population and, therefore, the more valid the results will be. For example, in a study of *Clostridium difficile* colitis in 609 patients with diarrhea, the patient sample consisted of adult inpatients whose diarrheal stools were tested for cytotoxin, thereby excluding any patients whose clinicians chose not to test.[3] Including only those tested is likely to raise the probability of *C difficile* in relation to the entire population of patients with diarrhea.

Weber and Kapoor[1] defined palpitations broadly as any one of several patient complaints (eg, fast heartbeats, skipped heartbeats, etc) and included patients with new and recurring palpitations. They obtained patients from three clinical settings (emergency department, inpatient floors, and a medical clinic) in one university medical center in a middle-sized North American city. Of the 229 adult patients presenting consecutively for care of palpitations at their center during the study period, 39 refused participation; the investigators included the remaining 190 patients, including 62 from the emergency department. No important subgroups appear to have been excluded, so these 190 patients probably represent the full spectrum of patients presenting with palpitations.

Was the Definitive Diagnostic Standard Appropriate? Was the Diagnostic Process Credible?

Articles about differential diagnosis will provide valid evidence only if the investigators arrive at a correct final diagnosis. To do so, they must develop and apply explicit criteria when assigning each patient a final diagnosis. Their criteria should include not only the findings needed to confirm each diagnosis, but also those findings useful for rejecting each diagnosis. For example, published diagnostic criteria for infective endocarditis include both criteria for verifying the infection and criteria for rejecting it.[4,5] Investigators can then classify study patients into diagnostic groups that are mutually exclusive, with the exception of patients whose symptoms stem from more than one etiologic factor. This allows clinicians to understand which diagnoses remain possible for any undiagnosed patients.

Diagnostic criteria should include a search that is sufficiently comprehensive to ensure detection of all important causes of the clinical problem. The more comprehensive the investigation, the smaller the chance that investigators will reach invalid conclusions about disease frequency. For example, a retrospective study of stroke in 127 patients with mental status changes failed to include a comprehensive search for all causes of delirium, and 118 cases remained unexplained.[6] Since the investigators did not describe a complete and systematic search for causes of delirium, the disease probabilities appear less credible.

The goal of developing and applying explicit, credible criteria is to ensure a reproducible diagnosis, and the ultimate test of reproducibility is a formal agreement evaluation. Your confidence in investigators will increase if, as in a study of causes of dizziness,[7] investigators formally demonstrate the extent to which they achieved agreement in diagnosis.

While reviewing the diagnostic criteria, keep in mind that "lesion finding" is not necessarily the same thing as "illness explaining." In other words, using explicit and credible criteria, investigators may find that patients have two or more disorders that might explain the clinical problem, causing some doubt as to which disorder is the culprit. Better studies of disease probability will include some assurance that the disorders found actually did account for the patients' illnesses. For example, in a sequence of studies of syncope, investigators required that the symptoms occur simultaneously with an arrhythmia before that arrhythmia was judged to be the cause.[8] In a study of chronic cough, investigators gave cause-specific therapy and used positive responses to this to strengthen the case for these disorders actually causing the chronic cough.[9]

Explicit diagnostic criteria are of little use unless they are applied consistently. This does not mean that every patient must undergo every test. Instead, for many clinical problems, the clinician takes a detailed yet focused history and performs a problem-oriented physical examination of the involved organ systems, along with a few initial tests. Then, depending on the diagnostic clues from this information, further inquiry proceeds down one of multiple branching pathways. Ideally, investigators would evaluate all patients with the same initial workup and then follow the clues, using prespecified testing sequences. Once a definitive test result confirms a final diagnosis, then further confirmatory testing is unnecessary and unethical.

You may find it easy to decide whether patients' illnesses have been well investigated if they were evaluated prospectively using a predetermined diagnostic approach. When clinicians do not standardize their investigation, this becomes harder to judge. For example, in a study of precipitating factors in 101 patients with decompensated heart failure, although all patients underwent a history and physical examination, the lack of standardization of subsequent testing makes it difficult to judge the accuracy of the disease probabilities.[10]

In the Weber and Kapoor study,[1] the investigators developed a priori explicit and credible criteria for confirming each possible disorder causing palpitations and listed their criteria in an appendix, along with supporting citations. They evaluated study patients prospectively and assigned final diagnoses using two principal means: a structured interview completed by one of the investigators and the combined diagnostic evaluation (ie, history, examination, and testing) chosen by the individual physician seeing the patient at the index visit. In addition, all patients completed self-administered questionnaires designed to assist in detecting various psychiatric disorders. Electrocardiograms were obtained in a majority of patients (166 of 190), and a large number underwent other testing for cardiac disease as well. Whenever relevant, the investigators required that the palpitations occurred at the same time as the arrhythmias before they would attribute the symptoms to that arrhythmia. However, they did not report on agreement for the ultimate decisions about the diagnoses attributed to each patient.

Thus, the diagnostic workup was reasonably comprehensive—although not exhaustive—for common disease categories. Since the subsequent testing ordered by the individual physicians was not fully standardized, some inconsistency may have been introduced, although it does not appear likely to have distorted the probabilities of common disease categories, such as psychiatric or cardiac causes.

For Initially Undiagnosed Patients, Was Follow-up Sufficiently Long and Complete?

Even when investigators consistently apply explicit and comprehensive diagnostic criteria, some patients' clinical problems may remain unexplained. The higher the number of undiagnosed patients, the greater the chance of error in the estimates of disease probability. For example, in a retrospective study of various causes of dizziness in 1194 patients in an otolaryngology clinic, about 27% remained undiagnosed.[11] With more than a quarter of patients' illnesses unexplained, the disease probabilities for the overall sample might be inaccurate.

If the study evaluation leaves patients undiagnosed, investigators can follow these patients over time, searching for additional clues leading to eventual diagnoses and observing the prognosis. The longer and more complete this follow-up is, the greater will be our confidence in the benign nature of the condition in patients who remain undiagnosed yet unharmed at the end of the study. How long is long enough? No single answer would correctly fit all clinical problems, but we would suggest 1 to 6 months for symptoms that are acute and self-limited and 1 to 5 years for chronically recurring or progressive symptoms.

USING THE GUIDE

Returning to our earlier discussion, Weber and Kapoor[1] identified a diagnosable etiology of palpitations in all but 31 (16.3%) of 190 patients included in their study. The investigators followed nearly all of the study patients (96%) for at least a year, during which time one additional diagnosis (symptomatic correlation with ventricular premature beats) was made in those initially undiagnosed. None of the 31 undiagnosed patients had a stroke or died.

WHAT ARE THE RESULTS?

What Were the Diagnoses and Their Probabilities?

In many studies of disease probability, the authors display the main results in a table listing the diagnoses made, along with the numbers and percentages of patients found with those diagnoses. For some symptoms, patients may have more than one underlying disease coexisting with and, presumably, contributing to the clinical problem. In these situations, authors often identify the major diagnosis for such patients and separately tabulate contributing causes. Alternatively, authors sometimes identify a separate, multiple-etiology group.

Weber and Kapoor[1] present a table that tells us that 58 patients (31%) were diagnosed with psychiatric causes and 82 (43%) had cardiac disorders, while thyrotoxicosis was found in five (2.6%), and none had pheochromocytoma. This distribution differed across clinical settings. For instance, cardiac disorders were more than twice as likely to occur in patients presenting to the emergency department, compared to patients presenting to the outpatient clinic.

How Precise Are the Estimates of Disease Probability?

Even when valid, these disease probabilities are only estimates of the true frequencies. You can examine the precision of these estimates using the confidence intervals (CIs) presented by the authors. If the authors do not provide them for you, you can calculate them yourself using the following formula:

$$95\% \ CI = P + 1.96 \ \sqrt{[P \ (1 - P)]/n,}$$

where P is the proportion of patients with the etiology of interest and n is the number of patients in the sample. This formula becomes inaccurate when the number of cases is 5 or fewer, and approximations are available for this situation.

For instance, consider the category of psychiatric causes of palpitations in the Weber and Kapoor[1] study. Using the above formula, we would start with $P = 0.31$, $(1 - P) = 0.69$, and $n = 190$. Working through the arithmetic, we find the CI to be 0.31 ± 0.066. Thus, although the most likely true proportion is 31%, it may range between 24.4% and 37.6%.

Whether you will deem the confidence intervals sufficiently precise depends on where the estimated proportion and confidence intervals fall in relation to your test or treatment thresholds. If both the estimated proportion and the entire 95% confidence interval are on the same side of your threshold, then the result is precise enough to permit firm conclusions about disease probability for use in planning tests or treatments. Conversely, if the confidence limit around the estimate crosses your threshold, the result may not be precise enough for definitive conclusions about disease probability. You might still use a valid but imprecise probability result, while keeping in mind the uncertainty and what it might mean for testing or treatment.

USING THE GUIDE

Weber and Kapoor do not provide the 95% CIs for the probabilities they found. However, as we just illustrated, if you were concerned about how close the probabilities were to your thresholds, you could calculate the 95% CIs yourself.

HOW CAN I APPLY THE RESULTS TO PATIENT CARE?

Are the Study Patients Similar to Those in My Own Practice?

As mentioned previously, we suggest you ask yourself whether the setting or patients are so different from those in your practice that you should disregard the results.[12] For instance, consider whether the patients in your practice come from areas where one or more of the underlying disorders are endemic, which could make the occurrence of these disorders much more likely in your situation than was found in the study.

USING THE GUIDE

Weber and Kapoor[1] recruited the 190 patients with palpitation from those presenting to the outpatient clinics, the inpatient medical and surgical services, and the emergency department (62 of the 190) in one university medical center in a middle-sized North American city. Thus, these patients are likely to be similar to the patients seen in your hospital emergency department, and you can use the study results to help inform the pretest probabilities for the patient in the scenario.

Is It Unlikely That the Disease Possibilities or Probabilities Have Changed Since This Evidence Was Gathered?

As time passes, evidence about disease frequency can become obsolete. Old diseases can be controlled or, as in the case of smallpox, eliminated.[13] New diseases or, at least, new epidemics of disease can arise. Such events can so alter the spectrum of possible diseases or their likelihood that previously valid and applicable studies may lose their relevance. For example, consider how dramatically the arrival of human immunodeficiency virus (HIV) transformed the list of diagnostic possibilities for such clinical problems as generalized lymphadenopathy, chronic diarrhea, and unexplained weight loss.

Similar changes can occur as the result of progress in medical science or public health. For instance, in studies of fever of unknown origin, new diagnostic technologies have substantially altered the proportions of patients who are found to have malignancy or whose fevers remain unexplained.[14-16] Treatment advances that improve survival, such as chemotherapy for childhood leukemia, can bring about shifts in disease likelihood because the treatment might cause complications, such as secondary malignancy years after cure of the disease. Public health measures that control such diseases as cholera can alter the likelihood of occurrence of the remaining etiologies of the clinical problems that the prevented disease would have caused—in this example, acute diarrhea.

USING THE GUIDE

The palpitations study was published in 1996 and the text states that the study period was 8 months during 1991. In this instance, you know of no new developments likely to cause a change in the spectrum or probabilities of disease in patients with palpitations.

CLINICAL RESOLUTION

Let us return to the patient in your practice. Considering the possible causes of his palpitations, your leading hypothesis is that acute anxiety is the cause of your patient's palpitations. You do not believe that the diagnosis of anxiety is so certain that you can rule out other disorders (ie, the pretest probability is below your threshold for treatment without testing). After reviewing the Weber and Kapoor[1] palpitations study, you decide to include in your list of "active alternatives" some cardiac arrhythmias (as common, serious, and treatable) and hyperthyroidism (as less common but serious and treatable) and you arrange testing to exclude these disorders (ie, these alternatives are above your threshold for treatment without testing). Finally, given that none of the 190 study patients had pheochromocytoma, and since your patient has none of the other clinical features of this disorder, you place it into your "other hypotheses" category (ie, below your test threshold) and decide to delay testing for this condition.

References

1. Weber BE, Kapoor WN. Evaluation and outcomes of patients with palpitations. *Am J Med*. 1996;100:138–148.

2. Sox HC, Hickam DH, Marton KI, et al. Using the patient's history to estimate the probability of coronary artery disease: a comparison of primary care and referral practices. *Am J Med*. 1990;89:7–14.

3. Katz DA, Bates DW, Rittenberg E, et al. Predicting *Clostridium difficile* stool cytotoxin results in hospitalized patients with diarrhea. *J Gen Intern Med*. 1997;12:57–62.

4. von Reyn CF, Levy BS, Arbeit RD, Friedland G, Crumpacker CS. Infective endocarditis: an analysis based on strict case definitions. *Ann Intern Med*. 1981;94:505–517.

5. Durack DT, Lukes AS, Bright DK, and the Duke Endocarditis Service. New criteria for diagnosis of infective endocarditis: utilization of specific echocardiographic findings. *Am J Med*. 1994;96:200–209.

6. Benbadis SR, Sila CA, Cristea RL. Mental status changes and stroke. *J Gen Intern Med*. 1994;9:485–487.

7. Kroenke K, Lucas CA, Rosenberg ML, et al. Causes of persistent dizziness: a prospective study of 100 patients in ambulatory care. *Ann Intern Med*. 1992;117:898-904.

8. Kapoor WN. Evaluation and outcome of patients with syncope. *Medicine*. 1990;69:160–175.

9. Pratter MR, Bartter T, Akers S, et al. An algorithmic approach to chronic cough. *Ann Intern Med*. 1993;119:977–983.

10. Ghali JK, Kadakia S, Cooper R, Ferlinz J. Precipitating factors leading to decompensation of heart failure: traits among urban blacks. *Arch Intern Med*. 1988;148:2013–2016.

11. Katsarkas A. Dizziness in aging—a retrospective study of 1194 cases. *Otolaryngol Head Neck Surg*. 1994;110:296–301.

12. Glasziou P, Guyatt GH, Dans AL, Dans LF, Straus SE, Sackett DL. Applying the results of trials and systematic reviews to individual patients [editorial]. *ACP Journal Club*. 1998;129:A15–A16.

13. Barquet N, Domingo P. Smallpox: the triumph over the most terrible of the ministers of death. *Ann Intern Med*. 1997;127:635–642.

14. Petersdorf RG, Beeson PB. Fever of unexplained origin: report on 100 cases. *Medicine*. 1961;40:1–30.

15. Larson EB, Featherstone HJ, Petersdorf RG. Fever of undetermined origin: diagnosis and follow up of 105 cases, 1970–1980. *Medicine*. 1982;61:269–292.

16. Knockaert DC, Vanneste LJ, Vanneste SB, Bobbaers HJ. Fever of unknown origin in the 1980s: an update of the diagnostic spectrum. *Arch Intern Med*. 1992;152:51–55.

Diagnostic Tests

Roman Jaeschke, Gordon Guyatt, and Jeroen Lijmer

The following EBM Working Group members also made
substantive contributions to this section: Peter Wyer,
Virginia Moyer, Deborah Cook, Jonathan Craig, Luz Maria Letelier,
John Williams, C. David Naylor, W. Scott Richardson, Mark Wilson,
and James Nishikawa

IN THIS SECTION

CLINICAL SCENARIO

How Accurate is CT Scanning in Suspected Appendicitis?

A 32-year-old woman enters the emergency department presenting with right lower quadrant pain. She is single and is employed by a company that sells Internet-related products. She is sexually active, having had three sexual partners during the past year, and her last menstrual period ended 3 weeks ago. Yesterday, she began to feel unwell and lost her appetite. During the past few hours the pain became much worse and she felt febrile, but she did not take her temperature. She has not experienced any vaginal discharge. She came to the emergency department when the pain became so severe that she started to worry whether something serious might be wrong.

On examination, you see a moderately ill woman with a temperature of 38.2° C and otherwise normal vital signs, who displays tenderness and guarding in the right lower quadrant and questionable rebound tenderness. You find no cervical motion tenderness, nor do you see cervical discharge. Laboratory examination findings include a white blood cell count of 11,000/mm³. Your differential diagnosis includes appendicitis, pelvic inflammatory disease, and ectopic pregancy; as you are debating whether to refer directly to surgery or to begin by obtaining a gynecologist's opinion, your colleague, an interventional radiologist, stops by on his way back from performing an emergency pulmonary angiogram. You describe the patient you are attending to and he mentions that up to 15% of needless laparotomies and up to 20% of admissions can be avoided if a computed tomographic (CT) scan is performed in patients like this one. He mentions "a very good paper that you must read, since it was published in the *New England Journal of Medicine*" although the citation and the details of the investigators' methods and study results currently escape him.

The patient is stable and currently comfortable, and the emergency department has quieted down since the morning rush. A colleague is ready to allow you a break and you decide you can afford to invest 30 minutes to look for and examine the paper recommended by the radiologist.

FINDING THE EVIDENCE

Upstairs in the library, you use the computer to search the PubMed database. You select "diagnosis" and "specificity" from the clinical queries page (www.ncbi.nlm.nih.gov/entrez/query/static/clinical.html) to have a preformatted search for diagnostic test studies. With the key words "CT" and "appendicitis," the search yields 39 citations. When you limit the search to English-language papers with abstracts that were published during the past 5 years, you find that 18 recent articles remain. The 18 abstracts include two narrative reviews, four retrospective studies, two studies focusing on specific imaging signs, and two studies focusing on a selected group of patients. Two of the abstracts provide no quantitative information about the test's performance and one is from a journal your library does not carry. The remaining five abstracts report a high level of accuracy of the test. The title of the most recent article best fits the patient with right lower quadrant tenderness in that it refers to the value of helical CT scanning for differentiating between appendicitis and acute gynecologic conditions.[1] Furthermore, the *New England Journal of Medicine* article is older and seems less relevant in that it analyzes issues related to cost and patient impact, rather than focusing on diagnostic test accuracy. You decide to retrieve the more recent paper.

In the ensuing discussion of the validity, results, and applicability of studies examining the properties of diagnostic tests, we will focus both on the scenario that included the diagnosis of pulmonary embolism using ventilation-perfusion scanning (see Part 1C, "The Process of Diagnosis") and on the article about the value of CT scanning in the diagnosis of appendicitis. Table 1C-2 summarizes our Users' Guide for a study of interpreting test results.

TABLE 1C–2

Users' Guide for an Article About Interpreting Diagnostic Test Results

Are the results valid?

- Did clinicians face diagnostic uncertainty?

- Was there a blind comparison with an independent gold standard applied similarly to the treatment group and to the control group?

- Did the results of the test being evaluated influence the decision to perform the gold standard?

What are the results?

- What likelihood ratios were associated with the range of possible test results?

How can I apply the results to patient care?

- Will the reproducibility of the test result and its interpretation be satisfactory in my clinical setting?

- Are the results applicable to the patient in my practice?

- Will the results change my management strategy?

- Will patients be better off as a result of the test?

ARE THE RESULTS VALID?

Did Clinicians Face Diagnostic Uncertainty?

A diagnostic test is useful only to the extent that it distinguishes between conditions or disorders that might otherwise be confused. Almost any test can differentiate healthy persons from severely affected ones; this ability, however, tells us nothing about the clinical utility of a test. The true, pragmatic value of a test is therefore established only in a study that closely resembles clinical practice. Another way to understand this point is to refer back to Figure 1C-1 in Part 1C, "The Process of Diagnosis." Note that the population of interest comprises patients whose predicament falls between the test and treatment thresholds.

A vivid example of how choosing the right population can dash the hopes raised with the introduction of a diagnostic test comes from the story of carcinoembryonic antigen (CEA) testing in patients with colorectal cancer. When measured in 36 people with known advanced cancer of the colon or rectum, CEA was elevated in 35 of them. At the same time, much lower levels were found in people without cancer who suffered from a variety of other conditions.[2] The results suggested that CEA might be useful in diagnosing colorectal cancer—or even in screening for the disease. In subsequent studies of patients with less advanced stages of colorectal cancer (and, therefore, lower disease severity) and patients with other cancers or other gastrointestinal disorders (and, therefore, different but potentially confused disorders), the accuracy of CEA testing as a diagnostic tool plummeted and clinicians abandoned CEA measurement for cancer diagnosis and screening. Carcinoembryonic antigen testing has proved useful only as one element in the follow-up of patients with known colorectal cancer.[3]

In an empiric study of design-related bias in studies of diagnostic tests, Lijmer and colleagues related features of the design to the power of tests.[4] Their findings included a large overestimate of the power of the test to distinguish between target-positive and target-negative patients when the investigators enrolled separate test and normal control populations (relative diagnostic odds ratio, [OR] 3.0; 95% confidence interval [CI], 2.0-4.5).

This example contrasts with the PIOPED study that demonstrated the utility of ventilation-perfusion scanning in the diagnosis of pulmonary embolism.[5] Here, investigators recruited the whole spectrum of patients suspected of having pulmonary embolism, including those who entered the study with high, medium, and low clinical suspicion of the condition. The patient sample in the helical CT study from the scenario related to scanning and appendicitis mentioned earlier in this section was appropriate because it comprised consecutive, nonpregnant women presenting to the emergency department of a large general hospital—ones in whom acute appendicitis or an acute gynecologic condition was suspected.

Was There a Blind Comparison With an Independent Gold Standard Applied Similarly to the Treatment Group and the Control Group?

The accuracy of a diagnostic test is best determined by comparing it to the "truth." Accordingly, readers must assure themselves that an appropriate *reference standard* (such as biopsy, surgery, autopsy, or long-term follow-up) has been applied to every patient, along with the test under investigation.[6] In the PIOPED study, the investigators used the pulmonary angiogram as the reference standard, and this was as "gold" as could be achieved without sacrificing the patients.

One way a *gold standard* can go wrong is if the test is part of the gold standard. For instance, one study evaluated the utility of measuring both serum and urinary amylase in making the diagnosis of pancreatitis.[7] The investigators constructed a gold standard that relied on a number of tests, including ones for serum and urinary amylase. This incorporation of the test into the gold standard is likely to inflate the estimate of the test's diagnostic power. Thus, clinicians should insist on the independence of the test and gold standard.

In reading articles about diagnostic tests, if you cannot accept the reference standard (within reason, that is—after all, nothing is perfect), then the article is unlikely to provide valid results for your purposes. If you do accept the reference standard, the next question to ask is whether the test results and the reference standard were assessed blindly (that is, by interpreters who were unaware of the results of the other investigation). Clinical experience demonstrates the importance of this independence or *blinding*. Once clinicians see a pulmonary nodule on a CT scan, they can see the previously undetected lesion on the chest radiograph; once they learn the results of an echocardiogram, they hear the previously inaudible cardiac murmur. The Lijmer et al empiric study of diagnostic test bias to which we have referred demonstrated the bias associated with unblinding even though the magnitude was small (relative diagnostic OR, 1.3; 95% CI, 1.0-1.9).[4]

The more likely that knowledge of the reference standard result could influence the interpretation of a new test, the greater is the importance of the blinded interpretation. Similarly, the more susceptible the gold standard is to changes in interpretation as a result of knowledge of the test, the more important is the blinding of the gold standard interpreter. In their study, the PIOPED investigators did not state explicitly that the tests were interpreted blindly. However, one could deduce from the effort they put into ensuring reproducible, independent readings that the interpreters were, in fact, blind; through correspondence with one of the authors, we have confirmed that this was indeed the case.

In the study of the use of CT in the diagnosis of suspected appendicitis, the investigators used surgical and pathologic findings as the reference standard for patients who went to surgery. For patients who did not go to surgery, the findings at clinical follow-up—including outpatient clinic visits and telephone calls during at least a 2-month period after the CT scan—provided the gold standard. The researchers did not report blinding of the physicians for the results of the helical CT scan. Particularly for patients in whom the diagnosis was made by long-term follow-up, knowledge of the CT result could have created a bias toward making the test look better than it really was.

Did the Results of the Test Being Evaluated Influence the Decision to Perform the Reference Standard?

The properties of a diagnostic test will be distorted if its results influence whether patients undergo confirmation by the reference standard. This situation, sometimes called *verification bias*[8,9] or *workup bias*,[10,11] applies when, for example, patients with suspected coronary artery disease whose exercise test results are positive are more likely to undergo coronary angiography (the gold standard) than those whose exercise test results are negative. The Lijmer et al study showed a large magnitude of bias associated with use of different reference tests for positive and negative results.[4]

Verification bias proved a problem for the PIOPED study as well. Patients whose ventilation-perfusion scans were interpreted as "normal/near normal" and "low probability" were less likely to undergo pulmonary angiography (69%) than those with more positive ventilation-perfusion scans (92%). This is not surprising, since clinicians might be reluctant to subject patients with a low probability of pulmonary embolism to the risks of angiography.

Most articles would stop here, and readers would have to conclude that the magnitude of the bias resulting from different proportions of patients with high- and low-probability ventilation-perfusion scans undergoing adequate angiography is uncertain but perhaps large. However, the PIOPED investigators applied a second reference standard to the 150 patients with low-probability or normal/near normal scans who failed to undergo angiography (136 patients) or in whom angiogram interpretation was uncertain (14 patients): they would be judged to be free of pulmonary embolism if they did well without treatment. Accordingly, the PIOPED investigators followed each of these patients for 1 year without treating them with anticoagulant drugs. Clinically evident pulmonary embolism developed in none of these patients during this time, from which we can conclude that clinically important pulmonary embolism (if we define clinically important pulmonary embolism as requiring anticoagulation therapy to prevent subsequent adverse events) was not present at the time they underwent ventilation-perfusion scanning.

In the helical CT study, the investigators established the reference standard in all patients. However, the test results probably influenced which reference standard—surgery or follow-up—was chosen. As we have mentioned previously, to the extent that CT results influenced the decision regarding the final diagnosis, the study provides an excessively optimistic picture of the test properties.

WHAT ARE THE RESULTS?

What Likelihood Ratios Were Associated With the Range of Possible Test Results?

The starting point of any diagnostic process is the patient presenting with a constellation of symptoms and signs. Consider two patients with nonspecific chest pain and shortness of breath without findings suggesting diagnoses such as pneumonia, airflow obstruction, or heart failure, in whom the clinician suspects pulmonary embolism. One is a 78-year-old woman 10 days after surgery and the other is a 28-year-old man experiencing a high level of anxiety. Our clinical hunches about the probability of pulmonary embolism as the explanation for these two patients' complaints—that is, their pretest probabilities—are very different. In the older woman, the probability is high; in the young man, it is low. As a result, even if both patients have intermediate-probability ventilation-perfusion scans, subsequent management is likely to differ in each. One might well treat the elderly woman immediately with heparin but order additional investigations in the young man.

Two conclusions emerge from this line of reasoning. First, regardless of the results of the ventilation-perfusion scan, they do not tell us whether pulmonary embolism is present. What they do accomplish is to modify the pretest probability of that condition, yielding a new posttest probability. The direction and magnitude of this change from pretest to posttest probability are determined by the test's properties, and the property of most value is the likelihood ratio.

As depicted in Table 1C-3, constructed from the results of the PIOPED study, there were 251 people with angiographically proven pulmonary embolism and 630 people whose angiograms or follow-up excluded that diagnosis. For all patients, ventilation-perfusion scans were classified into four levels: high probability, intermediate probability, low probability, and normal or near-normal. How likely is a high-probability scan among people who do have pulmonary embolism? Table 1C-3 shows that 102 of 251 (or 0.406) people with the condition had high-probability scans. How often is the same test result, a high-probability scan, found among people in whom pulmonary embolism was suspected but has been ruled out? The answer is 14 of 630 (or 0.022) of them.

The ratio of these two likelihoods is called the *likelihood ratio* (LR); for a high probability scan, it equals 0.406 ÷ 0.022 (or 18.3). In other words, a high-probability ventilation-perfusion scan is 18.3 times as likely to occur in a patient with—as opposed to without—a pulmonary embolism.

TABLE 1C–3

Test Properties of Ventilation Perfusion (V/Q) Scanning

	Pulmonary Embolism				
	Present		**Absent**		
Scan Results	**Number**	**Proportion**	**Likelihood Number**	**Proportion**	**Ratio**
High probability	102	102/251 = 0.406	14	14/630 = 0.022	18.3
Intermediate probability	105	105/251 = 0.418	217	217/630 = 0.344	1.20
Low probability	39	39/251 = 0.155	273	273/630 = 0.433	0.36
Normal/near normal	5	5/251 = 0.020	126	126/630 = 0.200	0.10
Total	251		630		

In a similar fashion, we can calculate the likelihood ratio for each level of the diagnostic test results. Each calculation involves answering two questions: First, how likely it is to obtain a given test result (say, a low-probability ventilation-perfusion scan) among people with the target disorder (pulmonary embolism)? Second, how likely is it to obtain the same test result (again, a low-probability scan) among people without the target disorder? For a low-probability ventilation-perfusion scan, these likelihoods are 39/251 (0.155) and 273/630 (0.433), respectively, and their ratio (the likelihood ratio for low-probability scan) is 0.36. Table 1C–3 provides the results of the calculations for the other scan results.

What do all these numbers mean? The Likelihood ratios indicate by how much a given diagnostic test result will raise or lower the pretest probability of the target disorder. A likelihood ratio of 1.0 means that the posttest probability is exactly the same as the pretest probability. Likelihood ratios >1.0 increase the probability that the target disorder is present, and the higher the likelihood ratio, the greater is this increase. Conversely, likelihood ratios <1.0 decrease the probability of the target disorder, and the smaller the likelihood ratio, the greater is the decrease in probability and the smaller is its final value.

How big is a "big" likelihood ratio, and how small is a "small" one? Using likelihood ratios in your day-to-day practice will lead to your own sense of their interpretation, but consider the following a rough guide:

- Likelihood ratios of >10 or < 0.1 generate large and often conclusive changes from pre- to posttest probability;

- Likelihood ratios of 5–10 and 0.1–0.2 generate moderate shifts in pre- to posttest probability;

- Likelihood ratios of 2–5 and 0.5–0.2 generate small (but sometimes important) changes in probability; and

- Likelihood ratios of 1–2 and 0.5–1 alter probability to a small (and rarely important) degree.

Having determined the magnitude and significance of the likelihood ratios, how do we use them to go from pretest to posttest probability? We cannot combine likelihoods directly, the way we can combine probabilities or percentages; their formal use requires converting pretest probability to odds, multiplying the result by the Likelihood ratio, and converting the consequent posttest odds into a posttest probability. Although it is not too difficult (see Part 2D, "Therapy and Understanding the Results, Measures of Association"), this calculation can be tedious and off-putting; fortunately, there is an easier way.

A *nomogram* proposed by Fagan[12] (Figure 1C-2) does all the conversions and allows an easy transition from pretest to posttest probability. The left-hand column of this nomogram represents the pretest probability, the middle column represents the likelihood ratio, and the right-hand column shows the posttest probability. You obtain the posttest probability by anchoring a ruler at the pretest probability and rotating it until it lines up with the likelihood ratio for the observed test result.

FIGURE 1C–2

Likelihood Ratio Nomogram

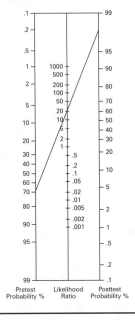

Recall the elderly woman mentioned earlier with suspected pulmonary embolism after abdominal surgery. Most clinicians would agree that the probability of this patient having the condition is quite high—about 70%. This value then represents the pretest probability. Suppose that her ventilation-perfusion scan was reported as being within the realm of high probability. Figure 1C-2 shows how you can anchor a ruler at her pretest probability of 70% and align it with the Likelihood ratio of 18.3 associated with a high-probability scan. The results: her posttest probability is >97%. If, by contrast, her ventilation-perfusion scan result is reported as intermediate (Likelihood ratio, 1.2), the probability of pulmonary embolism hardly changes (it increases to 74%), whereas a near-normal result yields a posttest probability of 19%.

The pretest probability is an estimate. We have already pointed out that the literature dealing with differential diagnosis can help us in establishing the pretest probability (see Part 1C, "The Process of Diagnosis"). Clinicians can deal with residual uncertainty by examining the implications of a plausible range of pretest probabilities. Let us assume the pretest probability in this case is as low as 60%, or as high as 80%. The posttest probabilities that would follow from these different pretest probabilities appear in Table 1C-4.

We can repeat this exercise for our second patient, the 28-year-old man. Let us consider that his presentation is compatible with a 20% probability of pulmonary embolism. Using our nomogram (see Figure 1C-2), the posttest probability with a high-probability scan result is 82%; with an intermediate-probability result, it is 23%; and with a near-normal result, it is 2%. The pretest probability (with a range of possible pretest probabilities from 10% to 30%), likelihood ratios, and posttest probabilities associated with each of the four possible scan results also appear in Table 1C-4.

TABLE 1C–4

Pretest Probabilities, Likelihood Ratios of Ventilation-Perfusion Scan Results, and Posttest Probabilities in Two Patients With Suspected Pulmonary Embolism

Pretest Probability %/(Range)*	Scan Result (LR)	Posttest Probability %/(Range)*
78-Year-Old Woman With Sudden Onset of Dyspnea Following Abdominal Surgery		
70 (60-80)	High Probability (18.3)	97 (96-99)
70 (60-80)	Intermediate Probability (1.2)	74 (64-83)
70 (60-80)	Low Probability (0.36)	46 (35-59)
70 (60-80)	Normal/Near Normal (0.1)	19 (13-29)
28-Year-Old Man With Dyspnea and Atypical Chest Pain		
20 (10-30)	High Probability (18.3)	82 (67-89)
20 (10-30)	Intermediate Probability (1.2)	23 (12-34)
20 (10-30)	Low Probability (0.36)	8 (4-6)
20 (10-30)	Normal/Near Normal (0.1)	2 (1-4)

* The values in parentheses represent a plausible range of pretest probabilities. That is, although the best guess as to the pretest probability is 70%, values of 60% to 80% would also be reasonable estimates.

LR indicates Likelihood ratio.

The investigation of women with possible appendicitis showed that the CT scan was positive in all 32 in whom that diagnosis was ultimately confirmed. Of the 68 who did not have appendicitis, 66 had negative scan results. These data translate into a Likelihood ratio of 0 associated with a negative test and a Likelihood ratio of 34 for a positive test. These numbers effectively mean that the test is extremely powerful. A negative result excludes appendicitis, and a positive test makes appendicitis highly likely.

Having learned to use likelihood ratios, you may be curious about where to find easy access to the Likelihood ratios of the tests you use regularly in your own practice. The Rational Clinical Examination[13] is a series of systematic reviews of the diagnostic properties of the history and physical examination that have been published in *JAMA*. Black and colleagues have summarized much of the available information about diagnostic test properties in the form of a medical text.[14]

Sensitivity and Specificity. Readers who have followed the discussion to this point will understand the essentials of interpretation of diagnostic tests. In part because they remain in wide use, it is also helpful to understand two other terms in the lexicon of diagnostic testing: sensitivity and specificity.

You may have noted that our discussion of likelihood ratios omitted any talk of "normal" and "abnormal" tests. Instead, we presented four different ventilation-perfusion scan interpretations, each with its own Likelihood ratio. However, this is not the way the PIOPED investigators presented their results. They relied on the older (but less useful) concepts of sensitivity and specificity.

Sensitivity is the proportion of people with the target disorder in whom a test result is positive and *specificity* is the proportion of people without the target disorder in whom a test result is negative. To use these concepts, we have to divide test results into normal and abnormal categories; in other words, we must create a two-column x two-column table. Table 1C-5 presents the general form of a 2 x 2 table that we use to understand sensitivity and specificity. Look again at Table 1C-5 and observe that we could transform a 4 x 2 table such as Table 1C-4 into any of three such 2 x 2 tables, depending on what we call normal or abnormal (or depending on what we call negative and positive test results). Let us assume that we call only high-probability scans abnormal (or positive).

TABLE 1C-5

Comparison of the Results of a Diagnostic Test With the Results of Reference Standard Using a 2 x 2 Table*

	Reference Standard	
Test Results	**Disease Present**	**Disease Absent**
Disease present	True Positive (*a*)	False Positive (*b*)
Disease absent	False Negative (*c*)	True Negative (*d*)

* Sensitivity (Sens)	$= \dfrac{a}{a+c}$	
Specificity (Spec)	$= \dfrac{d}{b+d}$	
Likelihood ratio for positive test (LR+)	$= \dfrac{sens}{1-spec}$	$= \dfrac{a/(a+c)}{b/(b+d)}$
Likelihood ratio for negative test (LR−)	$= \dfrac{1-sens}{spec}$	$= \dfrac{c/(a+c)}{d/(b+d)}$

Table 1C-6 presents a 2 x 2 table comparing the results of a ventilation perfusion scan with the results of pulmonary angiogram as a reference standard.

TABLE 1C–6

Comparison of the Results of Diagnostic Test (Ventilation-Perfusion Scan) With the Results of Reference Standard (Pulmonary Angiogram) Assuming Only High-Probability Scans Are Positive (Truly Abnormal)*

| | Angiogram | |
Scan Category	Pulmonary Embolism Present	Pulmonary Embolism Absent
High probability	102	14
Others	149	616
Total	251	630

* Sensitivity, 41%; specificity, 98%; Likelihood ratio of a high-probability test result, 18.3; Likelihood ratio of other results, 0.61.

   To calculate sensitivity from the data in Table 1C-6, we look at the number of people with proven pulmonary embolism (251) who were diagnosed as having the target disorder on ventilation-perfusion scan (102) characterized by a sensitivity of 102/251, or approximately 41% (a/a+c). To calculate specificity, we look at the number of people without the target disorder (630) whose ventilation-perfusion scan results were classified as normal (616), yielding a specificity of 616/630, or 98% (d/b+d). We can also calculate likelihood ratios for the positive and negative test results using this cutpoint: 18.3 and 0.61, respectively.

   Let us see how the test performs if we decide to put the threshold of positive vs negative in a different place in the table. For example, let us call only the normal/near-normal ventilation perfusion scan result negative. As shown in the 2 x 2 table depicted in Table 1C-7, the sensitivity is now 246/251, or 98% (among 251 people with pulmonary embolism, 246 are diagnosed on ventilation-perfusion scan), but what has happened to specificity? Among 630 people without pulmonary embolism, test results in only 126 are negative (specificity, 20%). The corresponding likelihood ratios are 1.23 and 0.1. Note that with this cut we not only lose the diagnostic information associated with the high-probability scan result, but we also interpret intermediate- and low-probability results as if they increase the likelihood of pulmonary embolism, when in fact they decrease the likelihood. You can generate the third 2 x 2 table by setting the cutpoint in the middle. If your sensitivity and specificity values are 82% and 63%, respectively, and associated Likelihood ratios of a positive and a negative test are 2.25 and 0.28, you have it right.

TABLE 1C-7

Comparison of the Results of Diagnostic Test (Ventilation-Perfusion Scan) With the Results of Reference Standard (Pulmonary Angiogram) Assuming Only Normal/Near-Normal Scans Are Negative (Truly Normal)*

	Angiogram	
Scan Category	Pulmonary Embolism Present	Pulmonary Embolism Absent
High, intermediate, and low probability	246	504
Near normal/normal	5	126
Total	**251**	**630**

* Sensitivity, 98%; specificity, 20%; Likelihood ratio of high, intermediate, and low probability, 1.23; Likelihood ratio of near normal/normal, 0.1.

In using sensitivity and specificity you must either discard important information or recalculate sensitivity and specificity for every cutpoint. We recommend the Likelihood ratio approach because it is much simpler and much more efficient.

USING THE GUIDE

Thus far, we have established that the results are likely true for the people who were included in the PIOPED study, and we have ascertained the Likelihood ratio associated with different results of the test. We have concluded that the helical CT scanning study may have overestimated the power of the test, but not so seriously as to completely invalidate the results. How useful are the tests likely to be in our clinical practice?

HOW CAN I APPLY THE RESULTS TO PATIENT CARE?

Will the Reproducibility of the Test Result and Its Interpretation Be Satisfactory in My Clinical Setting?

The value of any test depends on its ability to yield the same result when reapplied to stable patients. Poor reproducibility can result from problems with the test itself (eg, variations in reagents in radioimmunoassay kits for determining hormone levels). A second cause of different test results in stable patients arises whenever a test requires interpretation (eg, the extent of ST-segment elevation on an electrocardiogram). Ideally, an article about a diagnostic test will address the reproducibility of the test results using a measure that corrects for agreement by chance. This is especially important when expertise is required in performing or interpreting the test. You can confirm this by recalling the clinical disagreements that arise when you and one or more colleagues examine the same ECG, ultrasound, or CT scan, even when all of you are experts.

If the reproducibility of a test in the study setting is mediocre and disagreement between observers is common, and yet the test still discriminates well between those with and without the target condition, it is very useful. Under these circumstances, the likelihood is good that the test can be readily applied to your clinical setting. If reproducibility of a diagnostic test is very high and observer variation is very low, either the test is simple and unambiguous or those interpreting it are highly skilled. If the latter applies, less skilled interpreters in your own clinical setting may not do as well.

USING THE GUIDE

The helical CT study made no reference to reproducibility, other than to say that the residents initially interpreted the scans and the consultants agreed in all but one case. The authors did not describe the degree of experience of the radiologists, but the residents' involvement suggests that unusual expertise is not mandatory for accurate interpretation of the images.

Are the Results Applicable to the Patient in My Practice?

Test properties may change with a different mix of disease severity or with a different distribution of competing conditions. When patients with the target disorder all have severe disease, likelihood ratios will move away from a value of 1.0 (sensitivity increases). If patients are all mildly affected, likelihood ratios move toward a value of 1.0 (sensitivity decreases). If patients without the target disorder have competing conditions that mimic the test results seen in patients who do have the target disorder, the likelihood ratios will move closer to 1.0 and the test will appear less useful (specificity decreases). In a different clinical setting in which fewer of the disease-free patients have these competing conditions, the likelihood ratios will move away from 1.0 and the test will appear more useful (sensitivity increases).

The phenomenon of differing test properties in different subpopulations has been demonstrated most strikingly for exercise electrocardiography in the diagnosis of coronary artery disease. For instance, the more extensive the severity of coronary artery disease, the larger are the likelihood ratios of abnormal exercise electrocardiography for angiographic narrowing of the coronary arteries.[15] Another example comes from the diagnosis of venous thromboembolism, where compression ultrasound for proximal-vein thrombosis has proved more accurate in symptomatic outpatients than in asymptomatic postoperative patients.[16]

Sometimes, a test fails in just the patients one hopes it will best serve. The likelihood ratio of a negative dipstick test for the rapid diagnosis of urinary tract infection is approximately 0.2 in patients with clear symptoms and thus a high probability of urinary tract infection, but is over 0.5 in those with low probability,[17] rendering it of little help in ruling out infection in the latter. If you practice in a setting similar to that of the investigation and if the patient under consideration meets all the study inclusion criteria and does not violate any of the exclusion criteria, you can be confident that the results are applicable. If not, a judgment is required. As with therapeutic interventions, you should ask whether there are compelling reasons why the results should not be applied to the patients in your practice, either because of the severity of disease in those patients or because the mix of competing conditions is so different that generalization is unwarranted. The issue of generalizability may be resolved if you can find an overview that pools the results of a number of studies.[18]

USING THE GUIDE

The participants in the PIOPED study were a representative sample of patients with suspected pulmonary embolism from a number of large general hospitals. Therefore, the results are readily applicable to most clinical practices in North America. There are groups such as critically ill patients to whom we might be reluctant to generalize the results; such patients were excluded from the study and are likely to have had a different spectrum of competing conditions than other patients.

The patients enrolled in the study of CT scanning in acute appendicitis constitute a representative sample of women presenting to the emergency department with right lower quadrant pain. The patient before you, in whom the differential diagnosis includes appendicitis and pelvic inflammatory disease, meets study eligibility criteria. Thus, you can be confident that the results will apply in her case.

Will the Results Change My Management Strategy?

It is useful, when making, learning, teaching, and communicating management decisions, to link them explicitly to the probability of the target disorder. As we have described, for any target disorder there are probabilities below which a clinician would dismiss a diagnosis and order no further tests—the test threshold. Similarly, there are probabilities above which a clinician would consider the diagnosis confirmed and would stop testing and initiate treatment—the treatment threshold. When the probability of the target disorder lies between the test and treatment thresholds, further testing is mandated[19] (see Part 1C, "The Process of Diagnosis").

Once we decide what our test and treatment thresholds are, posttest probabilities have direct treatment implications. Let us suppose that we are willing to treat those patients with a probability of pulmonary embolism of 80% or higher (knowing that we will be treating 20% of them unnecessarily). Furthermore, let us suppose we are willing to dismiss the diagnosis of pulmonary embolism in those with a posttest probability of 10% or less. You may wish to apply different numbers here; the treatment and test thresholds are a matter of judgment and they differ for different conditions depending on the risks of therapy (if risky, you want to be more certain of your diagnosis) and the danger of the disease if left untreated (if the danger of missing the disease is high—such as in pulmonary embolism—you want your posttest probability to be very low before abandoning the diagnostic search). In the 28-year-old man discussed earlier in this section, a high-probability scan results in a posttest probability of 82% and may dictate treatment (or, at least, further investigation) and an intermediate probability scan (23% posttest probability) will dictate further testing (perhaps bilateral leg venography, ultrasound, or pulmonary angiography), whereas a low-probability or normal scan (probabilities of less than 10%) will exclude the diagnosis of pulmonary embolism. In the elderly woman, a high-probability scan dictates treatment (97% posttest probability of pulmonary embolism) and an intermediate result (74% posttest probability) may be compatible with either treatment or further testing (likely a pulmonary angiogram), whereas any other result mandates further testing.

If most patients have test results with Likelihood ratios near 1.0, the test will not be very useful. Thus, the usefulness of a diagnostic test is strongly influenced by the proportion of patients suspected of having the target disorder whose test results have very high or very low Likelihood ratios. In the patients suspected of having pulmonary embolism in our ventilation-perfusion scan example, a review of Table 1C-3 allows us to determine the proportion of patients with extreme results (either high probability with an Likelihood ratio of over 10, or normal/ near-normal scans with an Likelihood ratio of 0.1). The proportion can be calculated as (102+14+5+126)/881, or 247/881 = 28%. Clinicians who have been frustrated by frequent intermediate- or low-probability results in patients with suspected pulmonary embolism will already know that this proportion (28%) is far from optimal. Thus, despite the high Likelihood ratio associated with a high-probability scan and the low Likelihood ratio associated with a normal/near-normal result, ventilation perfusion scanning is of limited usefulness in patients with suspected pulmonary embolism.

A final comment has to do with the use of sequential tests. We have demonstrated how each item of history—or each finding on physical examination—represents a diagnostic test. We generate pretest probabilities that we modify with each new finding. In general, we can also use laboratory tests or imaging procedures in the same way. However, if two tests are very closely related, application of the second test may provide little or no information, and the sequential application of likelihood ratios will yield misleading results. For example, once one has the results of the most powerful laboratory test for iron deficiency, serum ferritin, additional tests such as serum iron or transferrin saturation add no further useful information.[20] *Clinical prediction rules* deal with the lack of independence of a series of tests that can be applied to a diagnostic dilemma and provide the clinician with a way of combining their results. For instance, the clinician in the scenario that opened this section could have used a rule that incorporates respiratory symptoms, heart rate, leg symptoms, oxygen saturation, electrocardiographic findings, and other aspects of history and physical examination to accurately classify patients with suspected pulmonary embolism as being characterized by high, medium, and low probability.[21]

USING THE GUIDE

Given the extreme likelihood ratios of helical CT scanning in women with abdominal pain, CT results are very likely to change management. For any patient with an intermediate likelihood of appendicitis, a positive scan will suggest immediate surgery, and a negative scan will mandate continued observation with treatment of alternative diagnostic possibilities (in this case, pelvic inflammatory disease).

Will Patients Be Better Off as a Result of the Test?

The ultimate criterion for the usefulness of a diagnostic test is whether the benefits that accrue to patients are greater than the associated risks.[22] How can we establish the benefits and risks of applying a diagnostic test? The answer lies in thinking of a diagnostic test as a therapeutic maneuver (see Part 1B1, "Therapy"). Establishing whether a test does more good than harm will involve (1) randomizing patients to a diagnostic strategy that includes the test under investigation or to one in which the test is not available and (2) following patients in both groups forward in time to determine the frequency of patient-important target outcomes.

When is demonstrating accuracy sufficient to mandate the use of a test, and when does one require a randomized controlled trial? The value of an accurate test will be undisputed when the target disorder is dangerous if left undiagnosed, if the test has acceptable risks, and if effective treatment exists. This is the case for both of the tests we have considered in detail in this section. A high probability or normal/near-normal results of a ventilation-perfusion scan may well eliminate the need for further investigation and may result in anticoagulant agents being appropriately given or appropriately withheld (with either course of action having a substantial positive influence on patient outcome).

The researchers who conducted the investigation of helical CT scanning in women with abdominal pain asked clinicians to formulate management plans before CT results were available and compared the plan to the one that clinicians followed after receiving the CT result. Of 100 patients, clinicians sent home 43 patients whom they would otherwise have admitted for observation, and they sent 13 others, whom they would otherwise have observed, to the operating room for immediate appendectomy. The evident benefits for patients and for the health care system—patients prefer to be at home than in a hospital, along with the fact that delayed appendectomy risks additional complications—eliminate the need for a randomized trial of CT scanning vs standard diagnostic approaches in women presenting to the emergency department with abdominal pain.

In other clinical situations, tests may be accurate and management may even change as a result of their application, but their impact on patient outcome may be far less certain. Consider one of the issues we raised in our discussion of framing clinical questions (see Part 1A1, "Finding the Evidence"). We presented a patient with apparently resectable non-small-cell carcinoma of the lung and wondered whether the clinician should order a CT scan and base further management on the results, or whether an immediate mediastinoscopy should be undertaken. For this question, knowledge of the accuracy of CT scanning is insufficient. A randomized trial of CT-directed management or mediastinoscopy for all patients is warranted—and indeed, investigators have conducted such a trial.[23] Other examples include catheterization of the right side of the heart for critically ill patients with uncertain hemodynamic status, bronchoalveolar lavage for critically ill patients with possible pulmonary sepsis, bronchial provocation testing for patients with asthma, and the incremental value of magnetic resonance imaging over CT for a wide variety of problems. For these and many other tests, confidence in the right management strategy must await the conduct of well-designed and adequately powered randomized trials.

CLINICAL RESOLUTION

You are sufficiently impressed by the information in the article about helical CT scanning that you decide to bypass the gynecologic consultation. Your radiologist colleague facilitates an emergent scan and soon calls you back, triumphantly announcing that the results are characteristic of appendicitis. The surgeons are soon having the patient whisked to the operating room, and you later hear that the patient is recovering uneventfully after the removal of her inflamed appendix.

References

1. Rao PM, Feltmate CM, Rhea JT, Schulick AH, Novelline RA. Helical computed tomography in differentiating appendicitis and acute gynecologic conditions. *Obstet Gynecol*. 1999;93:417-421.

2. Thomson DM, Krupey J, Freedman SO, Gold P. The radioimmunoassay of circulating carcinoembryonic antigen of the human digestive system. *Proc Natl Acad Sci U S A*. 1969;64:161-167.

3. Bates SE. Clinical applications of serum tumor markers. *Ann Intern Med*. 1991;115:623-638.

4. Lijmer JG, Mol BW, Heisterkamp S, et al. Empirical evidence of design-related bias in studies of diangostic tests. *JAMA*. 1999;282:1061-1066.

5. The PIOPED investigators. Value of ventilation/perfusion scan in acute pulmonary embolism. Results of the prospective investigation of pulmonary embolism diagnosis (PIOPED). *JAMA*. 1990;263:2753-2759.

6. Sackett DL, Haynes RB, Guyatt GH, Tugwell P. *Clinical Epidemiology, A Basic Science for Clinical Medicine*. 2nd ed. Boston: Little, Brown and Company; 1991:53-57.

7. Kemppainen EA, Hedstrom JI, Puolakkainen PA, et al. Rapid measurement of urinary trypsinogen-2 as a screening test for acute pancreatitis. *N Engl J Med*. 1997;336:1788-1793.

8. Begg CB, Greenes RA. Assessment of diagnostic tests when disease verification is subject to selection bias. *Biometrics*. 1983;39:207-215.

9. Gray R, Begg CB, Greenes RA. Construction of receiver operating characteristic curves when disease verification is subject to selection bias. *Med Decis Making*. 1984;4:151-164.

10. Ransohoff DF, Feinstein AR. Problems of spectrum and bias in evaluating the efficacy of diagnostic tests. *N Engl J Med*. 1978;299:926-930.

11. Choi BC. Sensitivity and specificity of a single diagnostic test in the presence of work-up bias. *J Clin Epidemiol*. 1992;45:581-586.

12. Fagan TJ. Nomogram for Bayes's theorem. *N Engl J Med*. 1975;293:257.

13. Sackett DL, Rennie D. The science and art of the clinical examination. *JAMA*. 1992;267:2650-2652.

14. Black ER, Bordley DR, Tape TG, Panzer RJ. *Diagnostic Strategies for Common Medical Problems*. 2nd ed. Philadelphia: American College of Physicians; 1999.

15. Hlatky MA, Pryor DB, Harrell FE. Factors affecting sensitivity and specificity of exercise electrocardiography. *Am J Med*. 1984;77:64-71.

16. Ginsberg JS, Caco CC, Brill-Edwards PA, et al. Venous thrombosis in patients who have undergone major hip or knee surgery: detection with compression US and impedance plethysmography. *Radiology*. 1991;181:651-654.

17. Lachs MS, Nachamkin I, Edelstein PH, et al. Spectrum bias in the evaluation of diagnostic tests: lessons from the repid dipstick test for urinary tract infection. *Ann Intern Med*. 1992;117:135-140.

18. Irwig L, Tosteson AN, Gatsonis C, et al. Guidelines for meta-analyses evaluating diagnostic tests. *Ann Intern Med*. 1994;120:667-676.

19. Sackett DL, Haynes RB, Guyatt GH, Tugwell P. *Clinical Epidemiology, a Basic Science for Clinical Medicine*. 2nd ed. Boston: Little, Brown and Company; 1991:145-148.

20. Guyatt GH, Oxman A, Ali M, et al. Laboratory diagnosis of iron-deficiency anemia: an overview. *J Gen Intern Med*. 1992;7:145-153.

21. Wells PS, Ginsberg JS, Anderson DR, et al. Use of a clinical model for safe management of patients with suspected pulmonary embolism. *Ann Intern Med*. 1998;129:997-1005.

22. Guyatt GH, Tugwell PX, Feeny DH, Haynes RB, Drummond M. A framework for clinical evaluation of diagnostic technologies. *CMAJ*. 1986;134:587-594.

23. Canadian Lung Oncology Group. Investigation for mediastinal disease in patients with apparently operable lung cancer. *Ann Thorac Surg*. 1995;60:1382-1389.

PROGNOSIS

Adrienne Randolph, Heiner Bucher, W. Scott Richardson, George Wells, Peter Tugwell, and Gordon Guyatt

The following EBM Working Group members also made substantive contributions to this section: Deborah Cook, Jonathan Craig, and Jeremy Wyatt

IN THIS SECTION

CLINICAL SCENARIO

Age 71, a Prior Stroke: What Is the Prognosis?

You are a Swiss internist seeing a 71-year-old man recovering from a right lower lobe pneumonia. The patient, who suffered a right hemispheric stroke 1 year ago, has little function of his left arm but is able to walk with a crutch. He is in sinus rhythm. For at least 15 years, he had hypertension that probably was poorly controlled. His echocardiogram has revealed left ventricular hypertrophy and mild left ventricular dysfunction. A Doppler examination of his carotid arteries shows nonsignificant stenosis of less than 50% bilaterally. He takes aspirin 300 mg per day, an angiotensin-converting enzyme (ACE) inhibitor, and a thiazide diuretic now control his hypertension.

From a lively discussion with the patient, you learn that he is a connoisseur of French wines and that since his early retirement he spends several months each year in Southern France, where he owns a little cottage. The patient grumbles that since the stroke, "things are not going the way they should" and you try to console him. Later on, speaking to the patient's wife, you find she is concerned about her husband's difficulty accepting his disability. She feels that owning two residences, with all of the commuting between them, is too much for both of them. The back-and-forth driving and the care for the two houses has completely become her burden, and she states that the pneumonia was the "proof for her husband's exhaustion." She feels that information about his risks of a recurrent stroke and

> death could help him and his family to "settle
> things." Because your knowledge about the progno-
> sis of survivors of stroke is vague, you tell the
> patient's wife that you will obtain specific informa-
> tion to address her concerns, and you promise to
> report back to her and to the patient.

FINDING THE EVIDENCE

Your hospital does not offer access to Best Evidence or the
Cochrane Library, but at least you have an Internet connection. During a break, you connect to the Internet and to
MEDLINE at the US National Library of Medicine Web site
via PubMed. You enter the term "stroke" and, using the the-
saurus, you find the correct Medical Subject Heading
(MeSH) term, "cerebral infarction." Combining the search
with the terms "epidemiology," "recurrence," and "prognosis"
yields a number of relevant results. You identify one interest-
ing article, "Long-Term Risk of Recurrent Stroke After a
First-ever Stroke," from the Oxfordshire Community Project
and obtain a copy from the library.[1]

Clinicians help patients in three broad ways: by diagnosing what is wrong with them, by administering treatment
that does more good than harm, and by giving them an indication of what the future is likely to hold. Clinicians require
studies of patient *prognosis*—those examining the possible
outcomes of a disease and the probability with which they
can be expected to occur—to achieve the second and third
goals. Although they strive to restore health, sometimes clinicians can only offer relief of discomfort and preparation
for death or long-term disability by means of presenting the
expected future course of the patient's illness.

To estimate a patient's prognosis, we examine outcomes in groups of patients with a similar clinical presentation—patients in the first year after stroke, for example. We may then refine our prognosis by looking at subgroups and deciding into which subgroup the patient falls. We may define these subgroups by such demographic variables as age (younger patients may fare better than older ones), by disease-specific variables (patients' outcome may differ depending on whether the stroke was hemorrhagic or thrombotic), or by comorbid factors (those with underlying hypertension, even if treated, may have worse outcomes). When these variables or factors really do predict which patients do better or worse, we call them *prognostic factors.*

Authors often distinguish between prognostic factors and *risk factors,* which are those patient characteristics associated with the development of the disease in the first place. For example, smoking is an important risk factor for the development of lung cancer, but it is not as important a prognostic factor as tumor stage in someone who has lung cancer. The issues in studies of prognostic factors and risk factors are identical, both for assessing validity and for using the results in patient care.

Knowledge of a patient's prognosis can help clinicians make the right diagnostic and treatment decisions. If a patient will get well anyway, clinicians should not recommend high-risk invasive procedures or waste money on expensive or potentially toxic treatments. If a patient is at low risk of adverse outcomes, even beneficial treatments may not be worthwhile. For example, stress ulcer prophylaxis to prevent gastrointestinal bleeding may not be worthwhile in nonintubated patients without a coagulopathy who are at extremely low risk of clinically important hemorrhage.[2] In another example, young nonsmoking patients with mild hypercholesterolemia without hypertension or a family history of coronary disease may conclude that their risk of adverse cardiovascular outcomes during the coming decade or two is so low that they will not take lipid-lowering medication. On the other hand, patients may be destined to have poor outcomes despite whatever treatment we offer. Aggressive therapy in such individuals may only prolong suffering and waste resources.

Knowledge of prognosis is also useful for resolution of issues broader than the care of the individual patient. Organizations may attempt to compare the quality of care across clinicians, or institutions, by measuring the outcomes of care. However, differences in outcome may be caused by the variability in the underlying severity of illness rather than by the treatments, clinicians, or health care institutions under study. If we know patients' prognoses, we may be able to compare populations and adjust for differences in prognosis to obtain a more accurate indication of how management is affecting outcome.

Certain issues are common to all these reasons for determining prognosis—communicating to patients their likely fate, guiding our treatment decisions, and comparing outcomes in populations to make inferences about quality of care—and some differ. In this section of the book, we focus on how to use articles that may contain valid prognostic information that will be useful in counseling patients (Table 1D-1).

TABLE 1D-1

Users' Guides to an Article About Prognosis

Are the results valid?

- Was the sample of patients representative?
- Were the patients sufficiently homogeneous with respect to prognostic risk?
- Was follow-up sufficiently complete?
- Were objective and unbiased outcome criteria used?

What are the results?

- How likely are the outcomes over time?
- How precise are the estimates of likelihood?

How can I apply the results to patient care?

- Were the study patients and their management similar to those in my practice?
- Was the follow-up sufficiently long?
- Can I use the results in the management of patients in my practice?

Using the same methodology as investigators addressing issues of harm (see Part 1B2, "Harm"), investigators addressing issues of prognosis use cohort and case-control designs in their studies to explore the determinants of outcome. Implicitly, randomized controlled trials also address issues of prognosis. The results reported for both the treatment group and the control group provide prognostic information: the control group results tell us about the prognosis in patients who did not receive treatment, and the treatment group results tell us about the prognosis in patients receiving the intervention. In this sense, each arm of a randomized trial represents a cohort study. If the randomized trial meets criteria we will describe later in this section, it can provide extremely useful information about patients' likely fate.

For issues of harm, the choice of appropriate treatment and control groups is crucial. For issues of prognosis, if there is a control group at all (and for populations in which patients all have more or less the same prognosis, this need not be the case), the controls are patients with different prognostic factors. In the same way that articles addressing issues of diagnosis evaluate tests that distinguish between those with and without a target condition or disease, prognostic studies may suggest factors that differentiate between those at low and high risk for a target outcome or adverse event. Issues in evaluating prognostic studies, however, are sufficiently different from those related to harm or diagnosis that clinicians may find the following guides helpful.

ARE THE RESULTS VALID?

Was the Sample of Patients Representative?

Bias has to do with systematic differences from the truth. A prognostic study is biased if it yields a systematic overestimate or underestimate of the likelihood of adverse outcomes in the patients under study. When a sample is systematically different from the underlying population—and is therefore likely to be biased because patients will have a better or worse prognosis than those in that population—that sample as "unrepresentative."

How can you recognize an unrepresentative sample? First, look to see if patients pass through some sort of filter before entering the study. If they do, the result is likely to be from a sample that is systematically different from the underlying population of interest (such as patients who have suffered a myocardial infarction or stroke, or with new-onset diabetes). One such filter is the sequence of referrals that leads patients from primary to tertiary centers. Tertiary centers often care

for patients with rare and unusual disorders or increased illness severity. Research describing the outcomes of patients in
tertiary centers may not be applicable to the general patient
suffering from the disorder in the community.

For example, when children are admitted to the hospital
with febrile seizures, parents want to know the risk that their
child will have more seizures in the future. This risk is much
lower in population-based studies (reported risks range
from 1.5% to 4.6%) than in clinic-based studies (reported
risks are 2.6% to 76.9%).[3] Those in clinic-based studies may
have other neurologic problems predisposing them to have
higher rates of recurrence. For you to adequately counsel
parents, you need to know how similar your patient is to the
patients in the various samples.

Failure to clearly define the patients who entered the
study increases the risk that the sample is unrepresentative.
To help you decide about the representativeness of the sample, look for a clear description of which patients were
included and excluded from a study. The way the sample was
selected should be clearly specified, along with the objective
criteria used to diagnose the patients with the disorder.

Were the Patients Sufficiently Homogeneous With Respect to Prognostic Risk?

Prognostic studies are most useful if individual members of
the entire group of patients being considered are similar
enough that the outcome of the group is applicable to each
group member. This will be true only if patients are at a similar well-described point in their disease process. The point
in the clinical course need not be early, but it does need to be
consistent. For instance, in a study of the prognosis of children with acquired brain injury, researchers looked not at
the entire population, but at a subpopulation who remained
unconscious after 90 days.[4]

After ensuring that the stage of the disease process is not a variable influencing outcome (because investigators held it constant), it is important to consider other factors that might influence patient outcome. For instance, consider the example of acquired brain injury. A study examining neurologic outcome that pooled patients with and without head trauma without distinguishing between them may not be very useful if these two groups have different prognoses. If the overall mortality rate reported in a study is 50% but the patient population is made up of identifiable subgroups, one of which has a mortality rate near zero and the other of which has a mortality rate near 100%, the 50% estimate will be valid for the whole group but not valid for any individual in that group. If the patients are heterogeneous with respect to risk of adverse outcome, the study will be much more

useful if the investigators define subgroups that are at lower and higher risk than the overall group.

For example, Pincus and colleagues followed a cohort of patients with rheumatoid arthritis for 15 years.[5] They separated the patients into a number of cohorts depending on their demographic characteristics, disease variables, and functional status. They found that older patients and those with greater impairment of functional status (eg, modified walking time and activities of daily living) died earlier than others. In another example, the authors of the study of children with acquired brain injury found that patients with posttraumatic injuries did much better than those with anoxic injuries. Of 36 patients with closed head trauma, 23 (64%) regained enough social function to be able to express their wants and needs and nine (25%) eventually regained the capacity to walk independently. Of 13 children with anoxic injuries, none regained important social or cognitive function.[4]

Not only must investigators consider all important prognostic factors, but they must also consider them in relation to one another. Consider the Framingham study, in which investigators examined (among many other things) risk factors for stroke.[6] They reported that the rate of stroke in patients with atrial fibrillation and rheumatic heart disease was 41 per 1000 person-years, which was very similar to the rate for patients with atrial fibrillation but without rheumatic heart disease. However, patients with rheumatic heart disease were, on average, much younger than those who did not have rheumatic heart disease. To properly understand the impact of rheumatic heart disease, investigators in these circumstances must consider separately (1) the relative risk of stroke in young people with and without rheumatic disease, and (2) the risk of stroke in elderly people with and without rheumatic disease. We call this separate consideration an *adjusted analysis*. Once adjustments were made for age (and also for gender and hypertensive status of the patients), the investigators found that the rate of stroke was sixfold greater in patients with rheumatic heart disease and atrial fibrillation than in patients with atrial fibrillation who did not have rheumatic heart disease. If a large number of variables have a major impact on prognosis, investigators should use sophisticated statistical techniques to determine the most powerful predictors. Such an analysis may lead to a clinical decision rule that guides clinicians in simultaneously considering all the important prognostic factors.

How can you decide if the groups are sufficiently homogeneous with respect to their risk? On the basis of your clinical experience—and your understanding of the biology of the condition being studied—can you think of factors that the investigators have neglected that are likely to define subgroups with very different prognoses? To the extent that the answer is "yes," the validity of the study is compromised.

Was Follow-up Sufficiently Complete?

A high patient dropout rate threatens the validity of a study of prognosis. As the number of patients who do not return for follow-up increases, the likelihood of bias also increases (eg, those who are followed may be at systematically higher or lower risk than those not being followed). How many patients lost to follow-up is too many? The answer depends on the relationship between the proportion of patients who are lost and the proportion of patients who have suffered the adverse outcome of interest. The larger the number of patients whose fate is unknown relative to the number who have suffered an event, the greater is the threat to the study's *validity*.

For instance, let us assume that 30% of a particularly high-risk group (such as elderly patients with diabetes) have suffered an adverse outcome (such as cardiovascular death) during long-term follow-up. If 10% of the patients have been lost to follow up, the true rate of patients who had died may be as low as approximately 27% or as high as 40%. Across this range, the clinical implications would not change appreciably, and the loss to follow-up does not threaten the validity of the study. However, in a much lower-risk patient sample (otherwise healthy middle-aged men, for instance) the observed event rate may be 1%. In this case, if we assumed that all 10% of the patients lost to follow up had died, the event rate of 11% might have very different implications.

A large loss to follow-up constitutes a more serious threat to validity when the patients who are lost may be different from those who are easier to find. In one study, for example, after much effort, 180 of 186 patients treated for neurosis were followed.[7] The death rate was 3% among the 60% who were easily traced. Among those who were more difficult to find, however, the death rate was 27%. If a differential fate for those followed and those lost is plausible (and in most prognostic studies, it will be), loss to follow-up that is large in relation to the proportion of patients suffering the adverse outcome of interest constitutes an important threat to validity.

Were Objective and Unbiased Outcome Criteria Used?

Outcome events can vary from those that are objective and easily measured (eg, death), to those requiring some judgment (eg, myocardial infarction), to those that may require considerable judgment and are challenging to measure (eg, disability or quality of life). Investigators should clearly specify and define their target outcomes before the study and, whenever possible, they should base their criteria on objective measures. In addition, they should specify the intensity and frequency of monitoring. As the subjectivity of the outcome definition increases, it becomes more important that individuals determining the outcomes are blinded to the presence of prognostic factors.

The study of children with acquired brain injury mentioned earlier in this section provides a good example of the issues involved in measuring outcome.[4] The examiners found that patients' families frequently optimistically interpreted interactions with the patients. The investigators therefore required that development of a social response in the affected children needed verification by study personnel, and they made the date that consciousness returned dependent on the date of the next outpatient visit. For instance, for a child who remained unconscious 1 year after injury and who was conscious on the next clinic visit 16 months after the original injury, the duration of unconsciousness would be recorded as being 1 year.

Returning to the patient scenerio, and the article describing the prognosis of stroke patients, the Oxfordshire Community Stroke Project prospectively registered all 675 patients with a first-ever stroke at the time they entered one of the participating hospitals.[1] Thus, patients were recruited at a common, early starting point. Since the study was community based, the population may be representative for a unselected cohort of British first-ever stroke patients. Their mean age was 72 years and 47% were male. In 81% of the patients, cerebral infarction was the cause of stroke; 10% had primary intracerebral hemorrhage; and 5% had subarachnoid hemorrhage—a pattern common to other stroke natural history studies.

One might speculate that a number of risk factors could influence the risk of subsequent stroke, including initial stroke severity, the patient's age, type of stroke, and presence of diabetes, heart failure, or blood pressure. The investigators analyzed all but the first of these factors and found no difference in prognosis across subgroups.

The investigators succeeded in achieving 100% follow-up by a study nurse who evaluated patients at 1 month, 6 months, 1 year after their event, and annually thereafter. The authors provided a detailed definition of what they meant by a stroke (for instance, they excluded asymptomatic new lesions on CT scans). However, they made no attempt to blind the nurse to possible prognostic factors.

WHAT ARE THE RESULTS?

How Likely Are the Outcomes Over Time?

The quantitative results from studies of prognosis or risk are the number of events that occur over time. We will use the example of a man asking a physician about the prognosis of his elderly mother who has dementia to illustrate common expressions of this relationship that provide complementary information about prognosis.

The patient's son asks, "What are the chances that my mother will still be alive in 5 years?" A high-validity study of the prognosis of patients with dementia provides a simple and direct answer in absolute terms.[8] Five years after presentation to the clinic, about one half of the patients (50%) had died. Thus, there is about a 50:50 chance that his mother will be alive in 5 years.

The patient's son might then indicate that the only person he knows with Alzheimer disease is a 65-year-old uncle who was diagnosed 10 years ago and is still living. He is surprised that his mother's chance of dying in the next 5 years is so high. This gives the clinician the opportunity to discuss some of the prognostic factors for death in patients with Alzheimer disease. The high-validity study examining the prognosis of demented patients suggested that older patients, those with more severe dementia, those with behavioral problems, and those with hearing loss died earlier.

The son might then ask whether his mother's chance of survival is expected to change over time. That is, although she may be at low risk for the next 2 years, will the risk jump sharply after that? Neither the absolute nor relative expressions of results address this question. For this answer we should turn to a *survival curve*, a graph of the number of events over time (or conversely, the chance of being free of these events over time) (see Part 2D, "Therapy and Understanding the Results, Measures of Association"). The events must be discrete (eg, death, stroke, or recurrence of cancer) and the time at which they occur must be precisely known.

Figure 1D-1 shows two survival curves—one of survival after a myocardial infarction[9] and the other depicting the results of hip replacement surgery in terms of when patients needed a revision because something had gone wrong after the initial surgery.[10] Note that the chance of dying after a myocardial infarction is highest shortly after the event (reflected by an initially steep downward slope of the curve, which then becomes flat), whereas very few hip replacements require revision until much later (this curve, by contrast, starts out flat and then steepens). The study of patients with dementia provided a survival curve that suggests that the chance of dying is more or less constant during the first 7 years after referral to the clinic for dementia (Figure ID-2)[8].

FIGURE 1D–1

Survival Curves

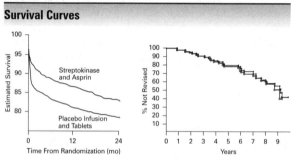

Left, survival after myocardial infarction. **Right,** results of hip replacement surgery, proportion of patients who survived without needing a new procedure (revision) after their initial hip replacement.

Reproduced with permission from The Lancet Publishing Group (left) and *The Journal of Bone and Joint Surgery* (right).

How Precise Are the Estimates of Likelihood?

The more precise the estimate of prognosis a study provides, the less we need be uncertain around the estimated prognosis and the more useful it is to us. Usually, risks of adverse outcomes are reported with their associated 95% confidence intervals (CIs). If the study is valid, the 95% CI defines the range of risks within which it is highly likely that the true risk lies (see Part 2C, "Therapy and Understanding the Results, Confidence Intervals"). For example, the study of the prognosis of patients with dementia provides the 95% CI around the 49% estimate of survival at 5 years after presentation, ie, 39% to 58%. Note that in most survival curves, the earlier follow-up periods usually include results from more patients than do the later periods (owing to losses to follow-up and because patients are not enrolled in the study at the same time). This means that the survival curves are more precise in the earlier periods, which should be indicated by narrower confidence bands around the left-hand parts of the curve.

FIGURE 1D–2

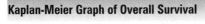

Kaplan-Meier Graph of Overall Survival

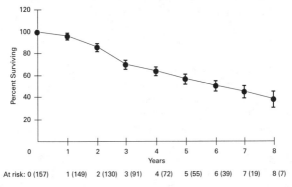

Note standard errors of the entire cohort and the number of patients at risk each year.

Reproduced with permission from Wiley-Liss, Inc, a subsidiary of John Wiley & Sons, Inc.

USING THE GUIDE

The Oxfordshire study found that the absolute risk of death during the first year after a stroke was 31% (95% CI, 27%-34%) and the absolute risk of dying over the next 4 years averaged approximately 4% per year. For patients who survived, the risk of a recurrent stroke was 8.6% (95% CI, 6.5%-10.7%) in the first 6 months, 4.6% (95% CI, 2.6%-6.6%) in the next 6 months, and 6.7% (95% CI, 2.7%-7.3%), 5.0% (95% CI, 1.0%-5.6%), 3.3%, and 1.3%, respectively, in the second, third, fourth, and fifth years (the authors do not accurately report the confidence intervals for the fourth and fifth years). In patients with recurrent strokes, 61% were sufficiently severe that they led to disability in activities of daily living that continued for more than 7 days while 24% led to symptoms that resolved within a week.

The investigators examined whether certain factors—sex, age, smoking, or the presence of diabetes, atrial fibrillation, cardiac failure, a transient ischemic attack, angina or myocardial infarction, intermittent claudication, or hypertension—influenced the risk of recurrent stroke. Of these factors, only smoking influenced the risk—smokers had an increased risk (OR, 1.66; 95% CI, 1.10 -2.51).

HOW CAN I APPLY THE RESULTS TO PATIENT CARE?

Were the Study Patients and Their Management Similar to Those in My Practice?

The authors should describe the study patients in enough detail that you can make a comparison with patients in your practice. The patients' characteristics and the way they are defined should be described explicitly. One factor rarely reported in prognostic studies that could strongly influence outcome is therapy. Therapeutic strategies often vary markedly among institutions and change over time as new treatments become available or old treatments regain popularity. To the extent that our interventions are therapeutic or detrimental, overall patient outcome could improve or become worse.

Was Follow-up Sufficiently Long?

Since the presence of illness often precedes the development of an outcome event by a long period, investigators must follow patients for long enough to detect the outcomes of interest. For example, recurrence in some women with early breast cancer can occur many years after initial diagnosis and treatment.[11] A prognostic study may provide an unbiased assessment of outcome over a short period of time if it meets the validity criteria in Table 1D-1, but it may be of little use if a patient is interested in prognosis over a long period of time.

Can I Use the Results in the Management of Patients in My Practice?

Prognostic data often provide the basis for sensible decisions about therapy. Knowing the expected clinical course of a patient's condition can help you judge whether treatment should be offered at all. For example, warfarin markedly decreases the risk of stroke, in patients with nonrheumatic atrial fibrillation and is indicated for many patients with this disorder.[12] However, in one study, the frequency of stroke in patients with "lone" atrial fibrillation (patients 60 years of age or younger with no associated cardiopulmonary disorders) was 1.3% over a 15-year period.[13] Most patients with a prognosis this good are likely to feel that, for them, the risks of anticoagulant therapy outweigh the benefits.

Even if the prognostic result does not help with selection of appropriate therapy, it can help you in counseling a concerned patient or relative. Some conditions, such as asymptomatic hiatal hernia or asymptomatic colonic diverticulae, have such a good overall prognosis that they have been termed "nondisease."[14] On the other hand, a prognostic result of uniformly bad prognosis provides the clinician with a starting place for a discussion with the patient and family, leading to counseling about end-of-life concerns.

CLINICAL RESOLUTION

Returning to the opening scenario, our review of the validity criteria suggests that the investigators obtained an unbiased assessment of recurrent stroke risk in their cohort study.[1] The 71-year-old patient introduced at the beginning of this section resembles the majority of those in the cohort study in terms of age and type of stroke, and we can readily generalize the results to his care. The minimum follow-up in the study was 2 years and certain patients were followed up to 6.5 years, allowing investigators to provide estimates for patients up to 5 years.

Given that he has survived the first year after his stoke, the patient's risk of dying within the next 4 years is approximately

16%, and there is another 16% risk of recurrent stroke. Given their relatively narrow confidence intervals, we can be reasonably secure using these estimates. Since aspirin administration likely reduces the risk of recurrent stroke by approximately 25%, we would need to treat 25 patients like the man under consideration for 4 years to prevent a single stroke; the number needed to treat (NNT) = 100 / (16% – 12%). Given the low toxicity of low-dose daily aspirin, we can confidently recommend that therapy to our patient.

Despite his complaints about his state of health, the patient tends to take an optimistic view of life. He is pleased to know that in 4 years his chance of being alive and no more disabled than he is at present is almost 70%. He uses this fact to help persuade his wife to maintain the dual residences, at least for the time being.

References

1. Burn J, Dennis M, Bamford J, Sandercock P, Wade D, Warlow C. Long-term risk of recurrent stroke after a first-ever stroke: the Oxfordshire Community Project. *Stroke*. 1994;25:333-337.

2. Cook DJ, Fuller HD, Guyatt GH, et al. Risk factors for gastrointestinal bleeding in critically ill patients. *N Engl J Med*. 1994;330:377-381.

3. Ellenberg JH, Nelson KB. Sample selection and the natural history of disease: studies of febrile seizures. *JAMA*. 1980;243:1337-1340.

4. Kriel RL, Krach LE, Jones-Saete C. Outcome of children with prolonged unconsciousness and vegetative states. *Pediatr Neurol*. 1993;9:362-368.

5. Pincus T, Brooks RH, Callahan LF. Prediction of long-term mortality in patients with rheumatoid arthritis according to simple questionnaire and joint count measures. *Ann Intern Med*. 1994;120:26-34.

6. Dawber TR, Kannel WB, Lyell LP. An approach to longitudinal studies in a community: The Framingham study. *Ann NY Acad Sci*. 1963;107:539.

7. Sims AC. Importance of high tracing-rate in long-term medical follow up studies. *Lancet*. 1973;2:433.

8. Walsh JS, Welch G, Larson EB. Survival of outpatients with Alzheimer-type dementia. *Ann Intern Med*. 1990;113:429-434.

9. ISIS-2 (Second International Study of Infarct Survival) Collaborative Group. Randomised trial of intravenous streptokinase, oral aspirin, both, or neither among 17,187 cases of suspected acute myocardial infarction: ISIS-2. *Lancet*. 1988;2:349-360.

10. Dorey F, Amstutz H. The validity of survivorship analysis in total joint arthroplasty. *J Bone J Surg AM*. 1989;71A(4):544-548.

11. Early Breast Cancer Trialists' Collaborative Group. Systemic treatment of early breast cancer by hormonal, cytotoxic, or immune therapy: 133 randomised trials involving 31000 recurrences and 24000 deaths among 75000 women. *Lancet*. 1992;339:1-15.

12. Segal JB, McNamara RL, Miller MR, et al. Prevention of thromboembolism in atrial fibrillation: a meta-analysis of trials of anticoagulants and antiplatelet drugs. *J Gen Intern Med*. 2000;15:56-67.

13. Kopecky SL. The natural history of lone atrial fibrillation: a population-based study over three decades. *N Engl J Med*. 1987;317:669-674.

14. Meador CK. The art and science of nondisease. *N Engl J Med*. 1965;272:92.

SUMMARIZING THE EVIDENCE

Andrew Oxman, Gordon Guyatt, Deborah Cook, and Victor Montori

The following EBM Working Group members also made substantive contributions to this section: Rose Hatala, Ann McKibbon, Trisha Greenhalgh, Jonathan Craig, and Roman Jaeschke

IN THIS SECTION

CLINICAL SCENARIO

Should We Offer Thrombolytic Drugs to Patients Presenting With Acute Thrombotic Stroke?

You are one of a group of neurologists working at an academic medical center. Your institution is not currently administering thrombolytic therapy to patients who present with acute thrombotic stroke. Some of your colleagues, convinced that thrombolysis will reduce ultimate mortality and morbidity in patients with acute thrombotic stroke, are enthusiastic about offering these patients tissue plasminogen activator (tPA) if they present within a few hours of symptom onset. Other members of your group are much more reluctant to initiate a policy of offering thrombolysis. You are undecided.

Your group has decided to address the issue formally. You join a subcommittee charged with collecting the evidence and generating an initial summary. The subcommittee decides to begin by looking for a systematic review.

FINDING THE EVIDENCE

You start by looking in the Cochrane Library 2000, Issue 1. You enter the terms "stroke" and "tissue plasminogen activator," locate a relevant review in the Cochrane Database of Systematic Reviews, and find that the latest update was in July 1999.[1]

For most of their questions, clinicians can find more than one relevant study. In the same way that it is important to use rigorous methods in primary research to protect against bias and random error, it is also important to use rigorous methods when summarizing the results of several studies. Traditional literature reviews, commonly found in journals and textbooks, typically provide an overview of a disease or condition. This overview may include a discussion of one or more aspects of disease etiology, diagnosis, prognosis, or management and will address a number of clinical, background, and theoretical questions.

For example, a review article or a chapter from a textbook on asthma might include sections on etiology, diagnosis, and prognosis and examine a wide variety of options for the treatment and prevention of asthma. Typically, authors of traditional reviews make little or no attempt to be systematic in the formulation of the questions they are addressing, the search for relevant evidence, or the summary of the evidence they consider. Medical students and clinicians looking for background information nevertheless often find these reviews very useful in obtaining a broad picture of a clinical condition or area of inquiry (see Part 1A1, "Finding the Evidence").

Unfortunately, expert reviewers often make conflicting recommendations and their advice frequently lags behind or is inconsistent with the best available evidence.[2] One important reason for this phenomenon is the use of unsystematic approaches to collecting and summarizing the evidence. Indeed, in one study, self-rated expertise was inversely related to the methodologic rigor of the review.[3]

In this section of the book, we focus on reviews that address specific clinical questions (eg, foreground information). Clinicians seeking to address focused management issues in providing patient care will find such reviews particularly useful (see Part 1A1, "Finding the Evidence").

Authors sometimes use the terms overview, systematic review, and meta-analysis interchangeably. We use the term *overview* for any summary that attempts to address a focused clinical question, *systematic review* for any summary that attempts to address a focused clinical question using methods designed to reduce the likelihood of bias; and *meta-analysis* describes reviews that use quantitative methods to summarize the results. Investigators must make a host of decisions in preparing a systematic review, including determining the focus; identifying, selecting, and critically appraising the relevant studies (which we will call the *primary studies*); collecting and synthesizing (either quantitatively or nonquantitatively) the relevant information; and drawing conclusions. To avoid errors in systematic reviews requires an organized approach; enabling users to assess the validity of the results requires explicit reporting of the methods.

During the past decade, rapid expansion has occurred in the literature in terms of describing the methods used in systematic reviews, including studies that provide an empiric basis for guiding decisions about the methods used in summarizing evidence.[4-6] Here, we emphasize key points from the perspective of a clinician needing to make a decision about patient care.

In applying the Users' Guides, you will find it useful to have a clear understanding of the process of conducting a systematic review. Figure 1E-1 demonstrates how the process begins with the definition of the question, which is synonymous with specifying selection criteria for deciding which studies to include in a review. These criteria define the population, the exposures or interventions, and the outcomes of interest (see Part 1A1, "Finding the Evidence"). A systematic review will also restrict the included studies to those that meet minimal methodologic standards. For example, systematic reviews that address a question of therapy will often include only randomized controlled trials.

FIGURE 1E–1

The Process of Conducting a Systematic Review

Define the Question

- Specify inclusion and exclusion criteria
    Population
    Intervention or exposure
    Outcome
    Methodology
- Establish a priori hypotheses to explain heterogeneity

Conduct Literature Search

- Decide on information sources: databases, experts, funding agencies, pharmaceutical companies, hand-searching, personal files, registries, citation lists of retrieved articles
- Determine restrictions: time frame, unpublished data, language
- Identify titles and abstracts

Apply Inclusion and Exclusion Criteria

- Apply inclusion and exclusion criteria to titles and abstracts
- Obtain full articles for eligible titles and abstracts
- Apply inclusion and exclusion criteria to full articles
- Select final eligible articles
- Assess agreement on study selection

Create Data Abstraction

- Data abstraction: participants, interventions, comparison interventions, study design
- Results
- Methodologic quality
- Assess agreement on validity assessment

Conduct Analysis

- Determine method for pooling of results
- Pool results (if appropriate)
- Decide on handling missing data
- Explore heterogeneity
    Sensitivity and subgroup analysis
- Explore possibility of publications bias

Having specified their selection criteria, reviewers must conduct a comprehensive search that yields a large number of potentially relevant titles and abstracts. They then apply the selection criteria to the titles and abstracts, arriving at a smaller number of articles that they can retrieve. Once again, the reviewers apply the selection criteria, this time to the complete reports. Having completed the culling process, they assess the methodologic quality of the articles and abstract data from each study. Finally, they summarize the data, including, if appropriate, a quantitative synthesis or meta-analysis. The analysis includes an examination of differences among the included studies, an attempt to explain differences in results (exploring heterogeneity), a summary of the overall results, and an assessment of their precision and validity. Guidelines for assessing the validity of reviews and using the results correspond to this process (Table 1E-1).

TABLE 1E-1

Users' Guides for How to Use Review Articles

Are the results valid?

- Did the review explicitly address a sensible clinical question?
- Was the search for relevant studies detailed and exhaustive?
- Were the primary studies of high methodologic quality?
- Were assessments of studies reproducible?

What are the results?

- Were the results similar from study to study?
- What are the overall results of the review?
- How precise were the results?

How can I apply the results to patient care?

- How can I best interpret the results to apply them to the care of patients in my practice?
- Were all clinically important outcomes considered?
- Are the benefits worth the costs and potential risks?

ARE THE RESULTS VALID?

Did the Review Explicitly Address a Sensible Clinical Question?

Consider a systematic review that pooled results from all cancer therapeutic modalities for all types of cancer to generate a single estimate of the impact on mortality. Next, consider a review that pooled results of the effects in patients suffering from clinically manifest atherosclerosis (whether in the heart, head, or lower extremities) of all doses of all antiplatelet agents (including aspirin, sulfinpyrazone, and dipyridamole) on major thrombotic events (including myocardial infarctions, strokes, and acute arterial insufficiency in the leg) and mortality. Finally, reflect on a review that addressed the impact of a wide range of aspirin doses to prevent thrombotic stroke in patients who had experienced a transient ischemic attack (TIA) in the carotid circulation.

Clinicians would not find the first of these reviews useful; they would conclude it is too broad. Most clinicians are uncomfortable with the second question, still considering it excessively broad. For this second question, however, a highly credible and experienced group of investigators found the question reasonable and published the results of their meta-analysis in a leading journal.[7-9] Most clinicians are comfortable with the third question, although some express concerns about pooling across a wide range of aspirin doses.

What makes a systematic review too broad or too narrow? Elsewhere in this book, we have argued that identifying the population, the interventions or exposures, and the outcomes of interest is a useful way of structuring a clinical question (see Part 1A1, "Finding the Evidence"). When deciding if the question posed in the review is sensible, clinicians need to ask themselves whether the underlying biology is such that they would expect; that is, the same treatment effect across the range of patients. They should ask the parallel question about the other components of the study question. For example, is the underlying biology such that, across the range of interventions and outcomes included, they expect more or less the same treatment effect? Clinicians can also construct a similar set of questions for other areas of clinical inquiry. For example, across the range of patients, ways of testing, and criterion or gold standard for diagnosis, does one expect more or less the same likelihood ratios associated with studies examining a diagnostic test (see Part 1C2, "Diagnostic Tests")?[10]

The reason that clinicians reject a systematic review that pools across all modes of cancer therapy for all types of cancer is that they know that some cancer treatments are effective in certain cancers, whereas others are harmful. Combining the results of these studies would yield a meaningless estimate of effect that would not be applicable to any of the interventions.

Clinicians who reject the second review might also argue that the biologic variation in antiplatelet agents is likely to lead to important differences in treatment effect. Further, they may contend that there are important differences in the biology of atherosclerosis in the vessels of the heart, head, and legs. Moreover, because clinicians need to make specific decisions about specific patients, they may be inclined to seek a summary of the evidence for the intervention they are considering in patients who most resemble the patient before them.

Those who would endorse the second review would argue the similar underlying biology of antiplatelet agents— and atherosclerosis in different parts of the body—and thus anticipate a similar magnitude of treatment effects. Moreover, they would point out that the best estimate of effect for an individual patient will often come from a broader review rather than a narrower one. There are three reasons for this.

First, focusing on a narrow group of patients (eg, the most severe, or least severe), interventions (such as a single aspirin dose in our cerebrovascular disease example), or studies (eg, those only in the English language)—in each case, a subgroup of those one might have chosen—increases the risk of chance producing a spurious result.[11, 12] Second, focusing on a subgroup introduces a risk of false conclusions owing to bias, if the criterion used to select the subgroup is confounded with another determinant of treatment effect. For example, a reviewer may select studies based on the type of patient even though the quality of studies of those patients is methodologically weaker than other studies, resulting in a spurious overestimate of treatment effect. Third, review of all potentially relevant data facilitates exploration of the possible explanations for variability in study results—the patients, the interventions, and the ways of measuring outcome. Thus, a broadly focused review provides a better basis for estimating the effect of a specific agent for a specific manifestation; it also provides a better basis for determining whether to believe a subgroup analysis, rather than a narrowly focused review that risks an inappropriate subgroup analysis.

Turning to the third question, most clinicians would accept that the biology of aspirin action is likely to be similar in patients whose TIA reflected right-sided or left-sided brain ischemia, in patients older than 75 years and in younger patients; in men and women, across doses, over periods of follow-up ranging from 1 to 5 years, and in patients with stroke who have been identified by the attending physician and those identified by a team of expert reviewers. The similar biology is likely to result in a similar magnitude of treatment effect. Nonetheless, even within this more narrowly focused question, there is still variation in the types of patients and the types of interventions, as well as possible differences in the types of outcome measures and methods of the included studies. Thus, there will still be a need to examine possible sources of variation in the results. As a result, the question about whether it is sensible to pool across studies cannot, in general, be resolved until one has looked at the results. If the effect was similar across studies, the results support pooling; if not, they raise questions about any inferences one can make from the pooled results.

The task of the clinician, then, is to decide whether, across the range of patients, interventions or exposures, and outcomes, it is plausible that the intervention will have a similar impact. Doing so requires a precise statement of what range of patients, exposures, and outcomes the reviewer has decided to consider; in other words, explicit selection criteria for studies included in the review are necessary. In addition, criteria are necessary that specify what types of studies were considered relevant. Generally these should be similar to the primary validity criteria we have described for original reports of research in other parts of this book (see Table 1E-2). Explicit eligibility criteria not only facilitate the user's decision regarding whether the question was sensible, but also make it less likely that the authors will preferentially include studies that support their own prior conclusions.

TABLE 1E-2

Guides for Selecting Articles That Are Most Likely to Provide Valid Results[3]

Therapy	• Were patients randomized? • Was follow-up complete?
Diagnosis	• Was the patient sample representative of those with the disorder? • Was the diagnosis verified using credible criteria that were independent of the clinical manifestations under study?
Harm	• Did the investigators demonstrate similarity in all known determinants of outcome, or adjust for differences in the analysis? • Was follow-up sufficiently complete?
Prognosis	• Was there a representative and well-defined sample of patients at a similar point in the course of disease? • Was follow-up sufficiently complete?

Bias in choosing articles to cite is a problem for both systematic reviews and original reports of research (in which the discussion section often includes comparisons with the results of other studies). Gøtzsche, for example, reviewed citations in reports of trials of new nonsteroidal anti-inflammatory drugs in rheumatoid arthritis.[13] Among 77 articles in which the authors could have referenced other trials with and without outcomes favoring the new drug, nearly 60% (44) cited a higher proportion of the trials with favorable outcomes. In 22 reports of controlled trials of cholesterol lowering, Ravnskov found a similar bias toward citing positive studies.[14] In 26 reports of RCTs in general medical journals, Clarke and Chalmers found only two articles in which the results were discussed in the context of an updated systematic review.[15] Users should exercise caution when interpreting the results of a study outside of the context of a systematic review.

Was the Search for Relevant Studies Detailed and Exhaustive?

Authors of a systematic review should conduct a thorough search for studies that meet their inclusion criteria. Their search should include the use of bibliographic databases, such as MEDLINE and EMBASE, the Cochrane Controlled Trials Register (containing more than 250,000 RCTs), and databases of current research.[16] They should check the reference lists of the articles they retrieve, and they should seek personal contact with experts in the area. It may also be important to examine recently published abstracts presented at scientific meetings and to look at less frequently used databases, including those that summarize doctoral theses and databases of ongoing trials held by pharmaceutical companies. Listing these sources, it becomes evident that a MEDLINE search alone will not be satisfactory. Unless the authors tell us what they did to locate relevant studies, it is difficult to know how likely it is that relevant studies were missed.

There are two reasons that reviewers should contact experts in the area under consideration. The first is to identify published studies that may have been missed (including studies that are labeled "in press" and those that have not yet been indexed or referenced). The second is to identify unpublished studies and to include them to avoid publication bias.

Publication bias occurs when the publication of research depends on the direction of the study results and whether they are statistically significant. Studies in which an intervention is not found to be effective sometimes are not published. Because of this, systematic reviews that fail to include unpublished studies may overestimate the true effect of an intervention.[17-21]

If investigators include unpublished studies in a review, they should obtain full written reports and they should appraise the validity of both published and unpublished studies. Reviewers may also use statistical techniques to explore the possibility of publication bias and other reporting biases, although the power of these techniques to detect bias is limited.[22] Systematic reviews based on a small number of studies with small sample sizes are the most susceptible to *publication bias,* and users should be cautious about drawing conclusions in such cases. Results that seem too good to be true may well not be true.

Reviewers may go even farther than simply contacting the authors of primary studies. They may recruit these investigators as collaborators in their review, and in the process they may obtain individual patient records. Access to individual patient records facilitates powerful analysis and strengthens the inferences from a systematic review.

Were the Primary Studies of High Methodologic Quality?

Even if a review article includes only RCTs, knowing whether they were of good quality is important. Unfortunately, peer review does not guarantee the validity of published research (see Part 1B1, "Therapy").[23] For exactly the same reason that the guides for using original reports of research begin by asking if the results are valid, it is essential to consider the validity of primary articles in systematic reviews.

Differences in study methods might explain important differences among the results.[24-26] For example, less rigorous studies tend to overestimate the effectiveness of therapeutic and preventive interventions.[27] Even if the results of different studies are consistent, determining their validity still is important. Consistent results are less compelling if they come from weak studies than if they come from strong studies.

Consistent results from observational studies are particularly suspect. Physicians may systematically select patients with a good prognosis to receive therapy, and this pattern of practice may be consistent over time and geographic setting. Observational studies summarized in a systematic review,[28] for instance, have consistently shown average relative risk reductions in major cardiovascular events of about 50% with hormone replacement therapy. The only large RCT addressing this issue found no effect of hormone replacement therapy on cardiovascular risk.[29]

There is no one correct way to assess the quality of studies, although in the context of a systematic review the focus should be on validity and users should be cautious about the use of scales to assess the quality of studies.[30, 31] Some investigators use long checklists to evaluate methodologic quality, whereas others focus on three or four key aspects of the study. When considering whether to trust the results of a review, check to see whether the authors examined criteria similar to those we have presented in other sections of this book (see Part 1B1, "Therapy"; Part 1C, "The Process of Diagnosis"; Part 1B2, "Harm"; and Part 1D, "Prognosis"). Reviewers should apply these criteria both in selecting studies for inclusion and in assessing the validity of the included studies (see Figure 1E-1 and Table 1E-2).

Were Assessments of Studies Reproducible?

As we have seen, authors of systematic review articles must decide which studies to include, how valid they are, and what data to extract. These decisions require judgment by the reviewers and are subject to both mistakes (ie, random errors) and bias (ie, systematic errors). Having two or more people participate in each decision guards against errors; if there is good agreement beyond chance between the reviewers, the clinician can have more confidence in the results of the systematic review.

USING THE GUIDE

Returning to our opening scenario, the Cochrane review you located included trials enrolling patients with acute ischemic stroke in whom CT excluded hemorrhage.[1] These patients were randomized to receive or not receive thrombolytic therapy, and an intention-to-treat analysis had been or could be conducted. (An intention-to-treat analysis examines outcomes for study participants based on the treatment arm to which they were originally randomized rather than the treatment they actually received.) You are concerned that the impact of treatment might differ substantially in patients who present early or late, in those with major or minor deficits, in those who received different thrombolytic agents, and in studies with different ways of measuring functional status or different durations of follow-up. Nevertheless, you are uncertain about the extent to which these variables might affect outcome, and you suspect that combining results across all patients, interventions, and outcomes might prove informative.

The reviewers searched the Cochrane Registry of Controlled Trials and EMBASE. In addition, they hand-searched a number of Japanese-language journals; contacted 321 pharmaceutical companies; contacted principal investigators in Europe, the United States, Japan, and China; attended a number of international stroke treatment symposia; and searched references quoted in the articles they found. It is likely they obtained all the relevant trials.

Of the 17 trials included, seven used centralized randomization of patients to treatment or control groups to ensure concealment. In 13 studies, participants and health care personnel were then blinded to allocation by using sealed, prepacked, and identical-looking thrombolytic and placebo infusions. Because of bleeding complications of thrombolytic therapy, blinding of participants and health care personnel may be difficult to ensure, underscoring the importance of blinding the outcome assessors; long-term outcome assessors were blinded to allocation in only four of the studies. The reviewers do not report on the proportion of patients lost to follow-up in any trial.

One of the review's authors decided whether potentially eligible trials met inclusion criteria. A different author extracted the data but then verified them with the principal investigators and corrected any errors. In 10 trials, the authors of the systematic review were able to obtain scores on a measure of functional status, the Rankin instrument, on individual patients. Scores of up to two out of five on this functional status measurement instrument indicate that patients are still able to look after themselves,[32] so the investigators classified scores of three to five on this instrument as characterizing a poor outcome. In another two trials for which they could not obtain individual data, scores of two or greater represented a poor outcome.

Overall, the methods of the systematic review—and the methodologic quality of the trials included in the systematic review—were strong.

WHAT ARE THE RESULTS?

Were the Results Similar From Study to Study?

Most systematic reviews document important differences in patients, exposures, outcome measures, and research methods from study to study. As a result, the most common answer to the initial question about whether we can expect similar results across the range of patients, interventions, and outcomes is "perhaps."

Fortunately, one can resolve this unsatisfactory situation. Having completed the review, investigators should present the results in a way that allows clinicians to check the validity of the initial assumption. That is, did results prove similar from study to study?

There are two things to consider when deciding whether the results are sufficiently similar to warrant making a single estimate of treatment effects that applies across the populations, interventions, and outcomes studied. First, how similar are the best estimates of the treatment effect (that is, the *point estimates*) from the individual studies? The more different they are, the more clinicians should question the decision to pool results across studies.

Second, to what extent are differences among the results of individual studies greater than you would expect by chance? Users can make an initial assessment by examining the extent to which the confidence intervals overlap. The greater the overlap, the more comfortable one is with pooling results. Widely separated confidence intervals flag the presence of important variability in results that requires explanation.

Clinicians can also look to formal statistical analyses called tests of heterogeneity, which assess the degree of difference or variance among samples, groups, or populations. When the P value associated with the test of heterogeneity is small (eg, < .05), chance becomes an unlikely explanation for the observed differences in the size of the effect (see Part 2B, "Therapy and Understanding the Results, Hypothesis Testing"). Unfortunately, a higher *P* value (.1, or even .3) does not necessarily rule out important heterogeneity. The reason is that, when the number of studies and their sample sizes are both small, the test of heterogeneity is not very powerful. Hence, large differences between the apparent magnitude of the treatment effect between studies—that is, the point estimates—dictates caution in interpreting the overall findings, even in the face of a nonsignificant test of homogeneity. Conversely, if the differences in results across studies are not clinically important, then heterogeneity is of little concern, even if it is statistically significant.

Reviewers should try to explain between-study variability in findings. Possible explanations include differences between patients (eg, thrombolytic therapy in acute myocardial infarction may be much more effective in patients who present shortly after the onset of chest pain than those who present much later), between interventions (eg, tPA may have a larger treatment effect than streptokinase), between outcome measurement (eg, the effect may differ if the outcome is measured at 30 days rather than at 1 year after myocardial infarction), or methodology (eg, the effect may be smaller in blinded trials or in those with more complete follow-up). Although appropriate and, indeed, necessary, this search for explanations of heterogeneity in study results may be misleading. Furthermore, how is the clinician to deal with residual heterogeneity in study results that remains unexplained? We will deal with this issue in our discussion of the applicability of the study results.

What Are the Overall Results of the Review?

In clinical research, investigators collect data from individual patients. Because of the limited capacity of the human mind to handle large amounts of data, investigators use statistical methods to summarize and analyze them. In systematic reviews, investigators collect data from individual studies. Investigators must also summarize these data and, increasingly, they are relying on quantitative methods to do so.

Simply comparing the number of positive studies to the number of negative studies is not an adequate way to summarize the results. With this sort of "vote counting," large and small studies are given equal weight, and (unlikely as it may seem) one investigator may interpret a study as positive, whereas another investigator may interpret the same study as negative.[33] For example, a clinically important effect that is not statistically significant could be interpreted as positive in light of clinical importance and negative in light of statistical significance. There is a tendency to overlook small but important effects if studies with statistically nonsignificant (but potentially clinically important) results are counted as negative.[34] Moreover, a reader cannot tell anything about the magnitude of an effect from a vote count even when studies are appropriately classified using additional categories for studies with a positive or negative trend.

Typically, meta-analysts weight studies according to their size, with larger studies receiving more weight. Thus, the overall results represent a weighted average of the results of the individual studies. Occasionally studies are also given more or less weight depending on their quality, or poorer-quality studies might be given a weight of zero (excluded) either in the primary analysis or in a secondary analysis that tests the extent to which different assumptions lead to different results (a sensitivity analysis).

You should look to the overall results of a systematic review the same way you look to the results of primary studies. In a systematic review of a therapeutic question, you should look for the relative risk and relative risk reduction or the odds ratio (see Part 2D, "Therapy and Understanding the

Results, Measures of Association"). In systematic reviews regarding diagnosis, you should look for summary estimates of the likelihood ratios (see Part 1C2, "Diagnostic Tests").

Sometimes the outcome measures that investigators have used in different studies are similar but not identical. For example, different trials might measure functional status using different instruments. If the patients and the interventions are reasonably similar, estimating the average effect of the intervention on functional status still might be worthwhile. One way of doing this is to summarize the results of each study as an effect size.[35] The *effect size* is the difference in outcomes between the intervention and control groups divided by the standard deviation. The effect size summarizes the results of each study in terms of the number of standard deviations of difference between the intervention and control groups. Investigators can then calculate a weighted average of effect sizes from studies that measured a given outcome in different ways.

You may find it difficult to interpret the clinical importance of an effect size. For example, if the weighted average effect is one half of a standard deviation, is this effect clinically trivial or is it large? Once again, you should look for a presentation of the results that conveys their practical importance (eg, by translating the summary effect size back into natural units[36]). For instance, clinicians may have become familiar with the significance of differences in walk test scores in patients with chronic lung disease. Investigators can then convert the effect size of a treatment on a number of measures of functional status (eg, the walk test and stair climbing) back into differences in walk test scores.[37]

Although it is generally desirable to have a quantitative summary of the results of a review, it is not always appropriate. When quantitative summaries are inappropriate, investigators should still present tables or graphs that summarize the results of the primary studies.

How Precise Were the Results?

In the same way that it is possible to estimate the average effect across studies, it is possible to estimate a confidence interval around that estimate, that is, a range of values with a specified probability (typically 95%) of including the true effect (see Part 2C, "Therapy and Understanding the Results, Confidence Intervals").

USING THE GUIDE

Returning to our opening scenario, four trials used streptokinase, three trials used urokinase, two used Pro-Urokinase, and eight used tPA. Data from six trials for death during the first 7 to 10 days showed that 16.6% of those receiving thrombolytic agents and 9.8% of the control patients died (OR, 1.85; 95% CI, 1.48-2.32). The P value for the test of heterogeneity showed borderline significance with the value for the tPA trials being lower and nonsignificant (OR, 1.24; 95% CI, 0.85-1.81). Considering data from 11 trials, investigators found that thrombolytic therapy increased fatal intracranial hemorrhage from 1.0% to 5.4% (OR, 4.15; 95% CI, 2.96-5.84), and the results were consistent across studies.

The final assessment of outcome (at 1 month in six trials, 3 months in nine trials, and 6 months in two trials) showed an increase in deaths from 15.9% to 19% (OR, 1.31; 95% CI, 1.13-1.52). The results showed considerable heterogeneity ($P < .01$).

Thrombolysis reduced the combined endpoint of death and dependency (55.2% in patients receiving thrombolysis and 59.7% in those allocated to the control group (OR, 0.83; 95% CI, 0.73-0.94). The results were consistent across the trials.

The authors explored possible sources of heterogeneity for differences in death rate. Despite large differences in point estimates (urokinase OR, 0.71; streptokinase OR, 1.43; tPA OR, 1.16), differences among drugs failed to reach statistical significance. Death rate was increased when streptokinase and aspirin were given together in comparison to streptokinase alone. The authors failed to find a relationship between control event rate and mortality, though they note that individual data would be required to properly explore the relationship between stroke severity and thrombolytic benefit and harm. Trials in which some patients were randomized within 3 hours and some were randomized after 3 hours showed no difference in deaths between the two groups.

HOW CAN I APPLY THE RESULTS TO PATIENT CARE?

How Can I Best Interpret the Results to Apply Them to the Care of Patients in My Practice?

Even if the true underlying effect is identical in each of a set of studies, chance will ensure that the observed results differ (see Part 2A, "Therapy and Harm, Why Study Results Mislead—Bias and Random Error"). As a result, systematic reviews risk capitalizing on the play of chance. Perhaps the studies with older patients happened, by chance, to be those with the smaller treatment effects. The reviewer may erroneously conclude that the treatment is less effective in elderly patients. The more subgroup analyses the reviewer undertakes, the greater is the risk of a spurious conclusion.

The clinician can apply a number of criteria to distinguish subgroup analyses that are credible from those that are not. Criteria that make a hypothesized difference in subgroups more credible include the following: conclusions drawn on the basis of within-study rather than between-study comparisons; a large difference in treatment effect across subgroups; a highly statistically significant difference in treatment effect (eg, the lower the P value on the comparison of the different effect sizes in the subgroups, the more credible the difference); a hypothesis that was made before the study began and that was one of only a few that were tested; consistency across studies; and indirect evidence in support of the difference (eg, "biologic plausibility"). If these criteria are not met, the results of a subgroup analysis are less likely to be trustworthy and you should assume that the overall effect across all patients and all treatments, rather than the subgroup effect, applies to the patient at hand and to the treatment under consideration.

What are clinicians to do if subgroup analyses fail to provide an adequate explanation for unexplained heterogeneity in study results? Although a number of reasonable possibilities exist, including not to pool findings at all, we suggest that, pending further trials that may explain the differences, clinicians should look to a summary measure from all of the best available studies for the best estimate of the impact of the intervention or exposure.[38-40]

Were All Clinically Important Outcomes Considered?

Although it is a good idea to look for focused review articles because they are more likely to provide valid results, this does not mean that you should ignore outcomes that are not included in a review. For example, the potential benefits of hormone replacement therapy include a reduced risk of fractures and a reduced risk of coronary heart disease, and potential downsides include an increased risk of breast cancer and endometrial cancer. Focused reviews of the evidence are more likely to provide valid results of the impact of hormone replacement therapy on each one of these four outcomes, but a clinical decision requires considering all of them.

Systematic reviews frequently do not report the adverse effects of therapy. One reason is that the individual studies often measure these adverse effects either in different ways or not at all, making pooling, or even effective summarization, difficult. Costs are an additional outcome that you will often find absent from systematic reviews.

Are the Benefits Worth the Costs and Potential Risks?

Finally, either explicitly or implicitly, the clinician and patient must weigh the expected benefits against the costs and potential risks (see Part 1F, "Moving From Evidence to Action"). Although this is most obvious for deciding whether to use a therapeutic intervention or a preventive one, providing patients with information about causes of disease or prognosis also can have both benefits and risks. For example, informing city dwellers about the health risks of air pollution exposures might result in their reducing their risk of exposure, with potential benefits; however, it might also cause anxiety or make their lives less convenient. Informing an asymptomatic woman with newly detected cancer about her prognosis might help her to plan better, but it might also label her, cause anxiety, or increase the period during which she is "sick."

A valid review article provides the best possible basis for quantifying the expected outcomes, but these outcomes still must be considered in the context of your patient's values and concerns about the expected outcomes of a decision.

Ultimately, trading off benefits and risks will involve value judgments (see Part 1F, "Moving From Evidence to Action"), and in individual decision making, these values should come from the patient.

CLINICAL RESOLUTION

Returning to the opening scenario, the committee decides it can confidently reach two conclusions on the basis of the systematic review. First, thrombolytic therapy increases the odds of intracranial hemorrhage by a factor of between approximately 3 and 6, with the best estimate being approximately 4. In absolute terms, thrombolytic therapy will cause one intracranial hemorrhage for every 23 patients who are treated. Second, thrombolytic therapy reduces the odds of the combined outcome of death and dependency after approximately 3 months by approximately 5% to 30%, the best estimate being an OR of 0.83 (17%). In absolute terms, 22 patients need to be treated to prevent one patient from dying or becoming seriously dependent after 3 months. A third conclusion also seems likely: the concomitant administration of aspirin increases the risk of intracranial hemorrhage.

The committee concludes that many areas of uncertainty remain. They include questions about whether the risk of death during the 3-month period after stroke is lower for tPA than the combined estimate suggests, as well as the relative effect on both hemorrhage and death and disability, according to the severity and nature of symptoms at initial presentation. Given the extent and nature of the uncertainties, the committee agrees that administration of thrombolytic therapy should be restricted to highly selected patients who are ready to risk an increase in the likelihood of early death to achieve a subsequent reduction in morbidity.

References

1. Wardlaw JM, del Zoppo G, Yamaguchi T. Thrombolysis for acute ischaemic stroke. *Cochrane Database Syst Rev.* 2000;2:CD000213.

2. Antman EM, Lau J, Kupelnick B, Mosteller F, Chalmers TC. A comparison of results of meta-analyses of randomized control trials and recommendations of clinical experts: treatments for myocardial infarction. *JAMA.* 1992;268:240-248.

3. Oxman AD, Guyatt GH. The science of reviewing research. *Ann N Y Acad Sci.* 1993;703:125-133; discussion 133-134.

4. Clarke M, Olsen KL, Oxman AD, eds. The Cochrane Review Methodology Database. In: *The Cochrane Library.* Oxford: Update Software; 2000, issue 1.

5. Clarke M, Oxman AD, eds. Cochrane Reviewers' Handbook 4.0 [updated July 1999]. In: *The Cochrane Library.* Oxford: Update Software; 2000, issue 1.

6. Egger M, Davey Smith G, Altman DG, eds. *Systematic Reviews in Health Care: Meta-Analysis in Context.* 2nd ed. London: BMJ Books; 2000.

7. Antiplatelet Trialists' Collaboration. Collaborative overview of randomised trials of antiplatelet therapy, I: prevention of death, myocardial infarction, and stroke by prolonged antiplatelet therapy in various categories of patients. *BMJ.* 1994;308:81-106.

8. Antiplatelet Trialists' Collaboration. Collaborative overview of randomised trials of antiplatelet therapy, II: maintenance of vascular graft or arterial patency by antiplatelet therapy. *BMJ.* 1994;308:159-168.

9. Antiplatelet Trialists' Collaboration. Collaborative overview of randomised trials of antiplatelet therapy, III: reduction in venous thrombosis and pulmonary embolism by antiplatelet prophylaxis among surgical and medical patients. *BMJ.* 1994;308:235-246.

10. Irwig L, Tosteson AN, Gatsonis C, et al. Guidelines for meta-analyses evaluating diagnostic tests. *Ann Intern Med.* 1994;120:667-676.

11. Counsell CE, Clarke MJ, Slattery J, Sandercock PA. The miracle of DICE therapy for acute stroke: fact or fictional product of subgroup analysis? *BMJ.* 1994;309:1677-1681.

12. Clarke MJ, Halsey J. D.I.C.E. 3: the need for cautious interpretation of meta-analyses. Paper presented at: First Symposium on Systematic Reviews: Beyond the Basics; January 1998; Oxford.

13. Gøtzsche PC. Reference bias in reports of drug trials. *Br Med J (Clin Res Ed)*. 1987;295:654-656.

14. Ravnskov U. Cholesterol lowering trials in coronary heart disease: frequency of citation and outcome. *BMJ*. 1992;305:15-19.

15. Clarke M, Chalmers I. Discussion sections in reports of controlled trials published in general medical journals: islands in search of continents? *JAMA*. 1998;280:280-282.

16. The *meta*Register of Controlled Trials (*m*RCT). Current Controlled Trials. Available at: *www.controlled-trials.com/*. Accessed January 31, 2001.

17. Dickersin K. The existence of publication bias and risk factors for its occurrence. *JAMA*. 1990;263:1385-1389.

18. Dickersin K, Min Y, Meinert CL. Factors influencing publication of research results. *JAMA*. 1992;267:374-378.

19. Dickersin K. How important is publication bias? A synthesis of available data. *AIDS Educ Prev*. 1997;9(suppl 1):15-21.

20. Stern JM, Simes RJ. Publication bias: evidence of delayed publication in a cohort study of clinical research projects. *BMJ*. 1997;315:640-645.

21. Ioannidis JP. Effect of the statistical significance of results on the time to completion and publication of randomized efficacy trials. *JAMA*. 1998;279:281-286.

22. Egger M, Davey Smith G, Schneider M, Minder C. Bias in meta-analysis detected by a simple, graphical test. *BMJ*. 1997;315:629-634.

23. Williamson JW, Goldschmidt PG, Colton T. The quality of medical literature: analysis of validation assessments. In: Bailar JC, Mosteller F, eds. *Medical Uses of Statistics.* 2nd ed. Waltham: NEJM Books; 1992:370-391.

24. Horwitz RI. Complexity and contradiction in clinical trial research. *Am J Med*. 1987;82:498-510.

25. Detsky AS, Naylor CD, O'Rourke K, McGeer AJ, L'Abbe KA. Incorporating variations in the quality of individual randomized trials into meta-analysis. *J Clin Epidemiol*. 1992;45:255-265.

26. Moher D, Pham B, Jones A, et al. Does quality of reports of randomised trials affect estimates of intervention efficacy reported in meta-analyses? *Lancet*. 1998;352:609-613.

27. Kunz R, Oxman AD. The unpredictability paradox: review of empirical comparisons of randomised and non-randomised clinical trials. *BMJ*. 1998;317:1185-1190.

28. Stampfer MJ, Colditz GA. Estrogen replacement therapy and coronary heart disease: a quantitative assessment of the epidemiologic evidence. *Prev Med*. 1991;20:47-63.

29. Hulley S, Grady D, Bush T, et al. Randomized trial of estrogen plus progestin for secondary prevention of coronary heart disease in postmenopausal women. Heart and Estrogen/progestin Replacement Study (HERS) Research Group. *JAMA*. 1998;280:605-613.

30. Moher D, Jadad AR, Nichol G, Penman M, Tugwell P, Walsh S. Assessing the quality of randomized controlled trials: an annotated bibliography of scales and checklists. *Control Clin Trials*. 1995;16:62-73.

31. Juni P, Witschi A, Bloch R, Egger M. The hazards of scoring the quality of clinical trials for meta-analysis. *JAMA*. 1999;282: 1054-1060.

32. de Haan R, Limburg M, Bossuyt P, van der Meulen J, Aaronson N. The clinical meaning of Rankin 'handicap' grades after stroke. *Stroke*. 1995;26:2027-2030.

33. Glass GV, McGaw B, Smith ML. *Meta-analysis in Social Research*. Beverly Hills: Sage Publications; 1981:18-20.

34. Cooper HM, Rosenthal R. Statistical versus traditional procedures for summarizing research findings. *Psychol Bull*. 1980;87:442-449.

35. Rosenthal R. *Meta-analytic Procedures for Social Research.* 2nd ed. Newbury Park: Sage Publications; 1991.

36. Smith K, Cook D, Guyatt GH, Madhavan J, Oxman AD. Respiratory muscle training in chronic airflow limitation: a meta-analysis. *Am Rev Respir Dis*. 1992;145:533-539.

37. Lacasse Y, Wong E, Guyatt GH, King D, Cook DJ, Goldstein RS. Meta-analysis of respiratory rehabilitation in chronic obstructive pulmonary disease. *Lancet*. 1996;348:1115-1119.

38. Peto R. Why do we need systematic overviews of randomized trials? *Stat Med*. 1987;6:233-244.

39. Oxman AD, Guyatt GH. A consumer's guide to subgroup analyses. *Ann Intern Med*. 1992;116:78-84.

40. Yusuf S, Wittes J, Probstfield J, Tyroler HA. Analysis and interpretation of treatment effects in subgroups of patients in randomized clinical trials. *JAMA*. 1991;266:93-98.

Moving From Evidence to Action

Gordon Guyatt, Robert Hayward, W. Scott Richardson,
Lee Green, Mark Wilson, Jack Sinclair, Deborah Cook,
Paul Glasziou, Alan Detsky, and Eric Bass

PJ Devereaux also made substantive contributions to this section

IN THIS SECTION

CLINICAL SCENARIO

Warfarin in Atrial Fibrillation: Is It the Best Choice for This Patient?

You are a primary care practitioner considering the possibility of warfarin therapy in a 76-year-old woman with congestive heart failure and chronic atrial fibrillation who has just entered your practice. Aspirin is the only antithrombotic agent that the patient has received during the 10 years she has had atrial fibrillation. Her other medical problems include stage I hypertension, which she has had since sometime in her fifth decade, and for which she has been taking hydrochlorothiazide and benazepril. Her previous physicians' records suggest that in recent years her systolic blood pressure was 130 to 140 mm Hg and her diastolic pressure was 80 to 90 mm Hg. Current blood pressure is 136/84 mm Hg, with a heart rate of 76 beats per minute, suggesting effective rate control. The patient does not have valvular disease, diabetes, or other comorbidity, and she does not smoke.

The duration of the patient's atrial fibrillation dissuades you from considering cardioversion or antiarrhythmic therapy. The patient lives alone. Although she has never had a significant fall, you are concerned that warfarin would present a risk of intracranial hemorrhage that may prove to be greater than its benefit in terms of stroke prevention. You find she places a high value on avoiding a stroke and a somewhat lower value on avoiding a major bleeding episode. Although she is not fond of medical care, she would accept the inconvenience associated with monitoring anticoagulant therapy.

The question of whether and when to offer anti-coagulant therapy to patients with nonvalvular atrial fibrillation arises often in your practice, but there is little agreement on the topic among you and your partners. You are all convinced that warfarin anticoagulant therapy for nonvalvular atrial fibrillation prevents strokes, but some believe that it causes too many bleeding complications. Several patients in the practice with atrial fibrillation have suffered embolic strokes despite aspirin therapy, but two patients suffered serious gastrointestinal bleeding while taking warfarin. Things became even more confusing recently when one of your colleagues, known as a maverick, declared that clopidogrel is the correct agent to use for patients with nonvalvular atrial fibrillation.

You make no change to the patient's medication regimen today, but you make a note to yourself to reconsider when she returns and to raise the issue at a staff meeting next week.

FINDING THE EVIDENCE

You have little inclination to review the voluminous original literature relating to the benefits of anticoagulant therapy in reducing stroke or its risk of bleeding, but you hope to find an evidence-based recommendation to guide you and your colleagues. You decide to search for two sources of such a recommendation: a practice guideline and a decision analysis.

You bring up your Web browser and go to your favorite search engine, Google.com. Entering the term "practice guidelines," you see that the second item on the results list is "National Guidelines Clearinghouse," at www.guidelines.gov.

This looks promising, as you note that the server appears to reside at the US Agency for Healthcare Research and Quality (AHRQ), formerly known as the Agency for Health Care Policy and Research (AHCPR), which you recall created a series of guidelines using formal evidence-based guidelines methodology.[1]

After linking to the clearinghouse, you see a heading labeled "Guidelines Syntheses." The syntheses area is described as containing

> " . . . syntheses of selected guidelines that cover similar topic areas. Key elements of each synthesis include the scope of the guidelines, the interventions and practices considered, the major recommendations and the corresponding rating schemes and strength of the evidence, the areas of agreement, and the areas of disagreement."

This description seems a close fit for the criteria you have for evidence-based guidelines, but unfortunately, atrial fibrillation is not listed among the syntheses completed thus far. Returning to the main page, you enter the term "atrial fibrillation" in the search box, which yields 22 guidelines. The first one on the list seems promising: "Fifth ACCP Consensus Conference on Antithrombotic Therapy," from the American College of Chest Physicians, completed in 1998. The guideline is summarized on the Clearinghouse site and has been published in the peer-reviewed literature.[2] You click on "Complete summary" and then print the text that appears. You also send an e-mail message to the hospital librarian asking for a copy of the published article. You look forward with some trepidation to reading the material, as you are aware that many guidelines, even from sources presumably as authoritative as specialty societies, are poorly constructed.[3,4]

Before you leave Google.com you enter the phrase "atrial fibrillation decision analysis" in the search text box and the results include the following link:

www.thelancet.com/newlancet/sub/issues/
vol355no9208/body.article956.html.

The article is a recent decision analysis published in *The Lancet* that appears highly suitable.[5]

TREATMENT RECOMMENDATIONS

Each day, clinicians make dozens of patient management decisions. Some are relatively inconsequential, whereas others are important. Each one involves weighing benefits and risks, gains and losses, and recommending or instituting a course of action judged to be in the patient's best interest. Implicit in each decision is a consideration of the relevant evidence, an intuitive integration of that evidence, and a weighing of the likely benefits and risks in light of the patient's preferences. When making choices, clinicians may benefit from structured summaries of the options and outcomes, systematic reviews of the evidence regarding the relationship between options and outcomes, and recommendations regarding the best choices. This section of the book explores the process of developing recommendations, suggests how the process may be conducted systematically, and introduces a taxonomy for differentiating recommendations that are more rigorous (and, thus, are more likely to be trustworthy) from those that are less rigorous (and, thus, are at greater risk of being misleading).

Traditionally, authors of original, or primary, research into therapeutic interventions include recommendations about the use of these interventions in clinical practice in the discussion section of their papers. Authors of systematic reviews and meta-analyses also tend to provide their impressions of the management implications of their studies. Typically, however, authors of individual trials or overviews do not consider all possible management options, but instead focus on a comparison of two or three alternatives. They may also fail to identify subpopulations in which the impact of treatment may vary considerably. Finally, when the authors of systematic reviews provide recommendations, they typically are not grounded in an explicit presentation of societal or patient preferences.

Failure to consider these issues may lead to variability in recommendations given the same data. For example, various recommendations emerged from different meta-analyses of selective decontamination of the gut using antibiotic prophylaxis for pneumonia in critically ill patients despite very similar results. The recommendations varied from suggesting implementation, to equivocation, to rejecting implementation.[6-9] Varying recommendations reflect the fact that investigators reporting primary studies and meta-analyses often make their recommendations without benefit of an explicit standardized process or set of rules.

When benefits or risks are dramatic and are essentially homogeneous across an entire population, intuition may provide an adequate guide to making treatment recommendations. However, such situations are unusual. In most instances, because of their susceptibility to both bias and random error, intuitive recommendations risk misleading the clinician and the patient.

These considerations suggest that when clinicians examine treatment recommendations, they should critically evaluate the methodologic quality of the recommendations. Our goal in this section is to provide clinicians with the tools to conduct such a critical evaluation.

Although recommendations that impact on health resource allocation may be directed at health policymakers, our focus in this book is to dispense advice for practicing clinicians. We will begin by describing the process of developing a recommendation, and we will introduce two formal processes that clinical investigators, experts, and authoritative bodies use in developing recommendations: decision analysis and clinical practice guidelines. We will then offer criteria for deciding when the process is done well and when it is done poorly, along with a hierarchy of treatment recommendations that clinicians may find useful.

Developing Recommendations

Figure 1F-1 presents the steps involved in developing a recommendation, along with the formal strategies for doing so. The first step in clinical decision making is to define the decision. This involves specifying the alternative courses of action and the possible outcomes. Often, treatments are designed to delay or prevent an adverse outcome such as stroke, death, or myocardial infarction. As usual, we will refer to the outcomes that treatment is designed to prevent as *target outcomes*. Treatments are associated with their own adverse outcomes— side effects, toxicity, and inconvenience. In addition, new treatments may markedly increase—or decrease—costs. Ideally, the definition of the decision will be comprehensive—all reasonable alternatives will be considered and all possible beneficial and adverse outcomes will be identified. In patients like the woman described in the opening scenario with nonvalvular atrial fibrillation, options include not treating the condition, giving aspirin, or administering anticoagulant therapy with warfarin. Outcomes include minor and major embolic stroke, intracranial hemorrhage, gastrointestinal hemorrhage, minor bleeding, the inconvenience associated with taking and monitoring medication, and costs to the patient, the health care system, and society.

FIGURE 1F–1

A Schematic View of the Process of Developing a Treatment Recommendation

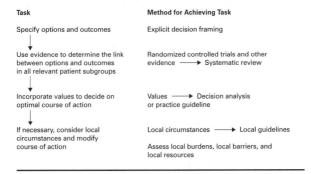

Task	Method for Achieving Task
Specify options and outcomes	Explicit decision framing
Use evidence to determine the link between options and outcomes in all relevant patient subgroups	Randomized controlled trials and other evidence ⟶ Systematic review
Incorporate values to decide on optimal course of action	Values ⟶ Decision analysis or practice guideline
If necessary, consider local circumstances and modify course of action	Local circumstances ⟶ Local guidelines
	Assess local burdens, local barriers, and local resources

Having identified the options and outcomes, decision makers must evaluate the links between the two. What will the alternative management strategies yield in terms of benefit and harm?[10, 11] How are potential benefits and risks likely to vary in different groups of patients?[11, 12] Once these questions are answered, making treatment recommendations involves value judgments about the relative desirability or undesirability of possible outcomes. We will use the term *preferences* synonymously with *values* or *value judgments* in referring to the process of trading off positive and negative consequences of alternative management strategies.

Recently, investigators have applied scientific principles to the identification, selection, and summarization of evidence—and to the valuing of outcomes. We will briefly review the systematic approach to the identification, selection, and summarization of evidence that we have presented in Part 1E, "Summarizing the Evidence," and will then describe the two strategies used to move from evidence to action—that is, decision analysis and practice guidelines.

Systematic Reviews

Unsystematic approaches to identification and collection of evidence risk biased ascertainment. That is, treatment effects may be underestimated or, more commonly, overestimated, and side effects may be exaggerated or ignored. Even if the evidence has been identified and collected in a systematic fashion, if reviewers are then unsystematic in the way they summarize the collected evidence, they run similar risks of bias. One result of these unsystematic approaches may be recommendations advocating harmful treatment; in other cases, there may be a failure to encourage effective therapy. For example, experts advocated routine use of lidocaine for patients with acute myocardial infarction when available data suggested the intervention was ineffective and possibly even harmful, and they failed to recommend thrombolytic agents when data showed patient benefit.[13]

Systematic reviews deal with this problem by explicitly stating inclusion and exclusion criteria for evidence to be considered, conducting a comprehensive search for the evidence, and summarizing the results according to explicit rules that include examining how effects may vary in different patient subgroups (see Part 1E, "Summarizing the Evidence"). When a systematic review pools data across studies to provide a quantitative estimate of overall treatment effect, we call it a *meta-analysis*. Systematic reviews provide strong evidence when the quality of the primary study design is good and sample sizes are large; they provide weaker evidence when study designs are poor and sample sizes are small. Because judgment is involved in many steps in a systematic review (including specifying inclusion and exclusion criteria, applying these criteria to potentially eligible studies, evaluating the methodologic quality of the primary studies, and selecting an approach to data analysis), systematic reviews are not immune from bias. Nevertheless, in their rigorous approach to identifying and summarizing data, systematic reviews reduce the likelihood of bias in estimating the causal links between management options and patient outcomes.

Decision Analysis

Rigorous *decision analysis* provides a formal structure for integrating the evidence about the beneficial and harmful effects of treatment options with the values or preferences associated with those beneficial and harmful effects. Decision analysis applies explicit, quantitative methods to analyzing decisions under conditions of uncertainty; it allows clinicians to compare the expected consequences of pursuing different strategies. The process of decision analysis makes fully explicit all of the elements of the decision, so that they are open for debate and modification.[14-16]

We will use the term *clinical decision analyses* to include studies that use formal, mathematical approaches to analyze decisions faced by clinicians in the course of patient care, such as deciding whether to screen for a condition, choosing a testing strategy, or selecting a type of treatment. Although such analyses can be undertaken to inform a decision for an individual patient ("Should I recommend warfarin to this 76-year-old woman with atrial fibrillation?"), they are undertaken more widely to help inform a decision about clinical policy[17] ("Should I routinely recommend warfarin to patients in my practice with atrial fibrillation?"). The study retrieved by the search in our scenario is an example of the latter, whereas an example of a decision analysis for an individual patient is an analysis of whether to recommend cardiac surgery for an elderly woman with aortic stenosis.[18]

Decision analysis can also be applied to more global questions of health care policy that are viewed from the perspective of society or a national health authority. Examples include analyzing whether or not to screen for prostate cancer[19] and comparing different policies for cholesterol screening and treatment.[20] Decision analyses in health services research share many attributes with clinical analyses[21]; however, a discussion of their differences is beyond the scope of this book.

Most clinical decision analyses are built as decision trees, and the articles usually will include one or more diagrams showing the structure of the decision tree used for the analysis. Reviewing such diagrams will help you understand the model. Figure 1F-2 shows a diagram of a very simplified version of the decision tree for the atrial fibrillation problem mentioned at the beginning of this section. The clinician has three options for patients with atrial fibrillation in whom antiarrhythmic therapy to achieve and maintain sinus rhythm is not a possible management strategy: to offer no prophylaxis, to recommend aspirin, or to recommend warfarin. Regardless of what choice is made, patients may or may not develop embolic events and, in particular, stroke. Prophylaxis lowers the chance of embolism but can cause bleeding in some patients. This simplified model excludes a number of important consequences, including the inconvenience of warfarin monitoring and the unpleasantness of minor bleeding.

As seen in Figure 1F-2, decision trees are displayed graphically, oriented from left to right, with the decision to be analyzed on the left, the compared strategies in the center, and the clinical outcomes on the right. The decision is represented by a square, termed a *decision node.* The lines emanating from the decision node represent the clinical strategies being compared. Chance events are symbolized by circles, called *chance nodes,* and outcome states are shown (in Figure 1F-2) as triangles or (in other decision trees) as rectangles. When a decision analysis includes costs among the outcomes, it becomes an economic analysis and summarizes tradeoffs between health changes and resource expenditure.[22,23]

FIGURE 1F–2

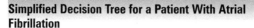

Simplified Decision Tree for a Patient With Atrial Fibrillation

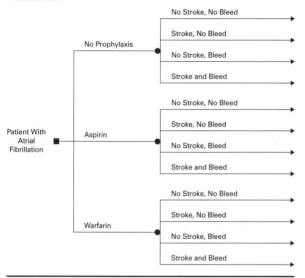

Once a decision analyst has constructed the tree, he or she must generate quantitative estimates of the likelihood of events, or *probabilities*. The scale for probability estimates ranges from 0 (impossible) to 1.0 (absolute certainty). Probabilities must be assigned to each branch emanating from a chance node, and for each chance node, the sum of probabilities must add up to 1.0.

For example, returning to Figure 1F-2, consider the no-prophylaxis strategy (the upper branch emanating from the decision node). This arm has one chance node at which four possible events could occur (the four possible combinations arising from bleeding or not bleeding and from having a stroke or not having a stroke). Figure 1F-3 depicts the probabilities associated with one arm of the decision, the no-prophylaxis strategy (generated by assuming a 1% chance of bleeding and a 10% probability of stroke, with the two events being independent). Patients given no prophylaxis would have a 0.1% chance (a probability of 0.001) of bleeding and having a stroke, a 0.9% chance (a probability of 0.009) of bleeding and not having a stroke, a 9.9% chance (a probability of 0.099) of not bleeding but having a stroke, and an 89.1% chance (a probability of 0.891) of not bleeding and not having a stroke.

FIGURE 1F–3

Decision Tree With Probabilities—No-Prophylaxis Option

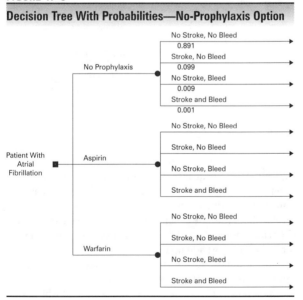

The decision analyst would generate similar probabilities for the other two branches. Presumably, the aspirin branch would have a higher risk of bleeding and a lower risk of stroke. The warfarin branch would have the highest risk of bleeding and the lowest risk of stroke.

These probabilities would not suggest a clear course of action, as the alternative with the lowest risk of bleeding has the highest risk of stroke, and vice versa. Thus, the right choice would depend on the relative value or utility one placed on bleeding and stroke. Decision analysts typically place a utility on each of the final possible outcomes that varies from 0 (death) to 1.0 (full health). Figure 1F-4 presents one possible set of utilities associated with the four outcomes and applied to the no-prophylaxis arm of the decision tree: 1.0 for no stroke or bleeding, 0.8 for no stroke and bleeding, 0.5 for stroke but no bleeding, and 0.4 for stroke and bleeding.

The final step in the decision analysis is to calculate the total value associated with each possible course of action. Given the particular set of probabilities and utilities we have presented, the value of the no-prophylaxis branch would be $(0.891 \times 1.0) + (0.009 \times 0.8) + (0.099 \times 0.5) + (0.001 \times 0.4)$, or 0.948. Depending on the probabilities attached to the aspirin and warfarin branches, they would be judged superior or inferior to the no-prophylaxis branch. If the total value of each of these branches were >0.948, they would be judged preferable to the no-prophylaxis branch; if the total value were <0.948, they would be judged less desirable.

FIGURE 1F–4

Decision Tree With Probabilities and Utilities Included in the No-Prophylaxis Arm of the Tree

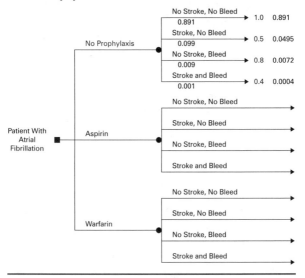

The model presented in Figures 1F-2 to 1F-4 is oversimplified in a number of ways, among which are its omission of the time frame of events and the possibility of a patient suffering multiple events. Decision analysts can make use of software programs that model what might happen to a hypothetical cohort of patients over a series of time cycles (say, periods of 1 year's duration). The model allows for the possibility that patients might move from one health state to another. For instance, one unfortunate patient may suffer a mild stroke in one cycle, continue with minimal functional limitation for a number of cycles, suffer a gastrointestinal bleeding episode in a subsequent cycle and, finally, experience a major stroke. These multistate transition models or Markov models permit more sophisticated and true-to-life depictions—and, presumably, more accurate decision analysis.

Practice Guidelines

Practice guidelines, or "systematically developed statements to assist practitioner and patient decisions about appropriate health care for specific clinical circumstances,"[24] provide an alternative structure for integrating evidence and applying values to reach treatment recommendations.[1, 25-30] Practice guideline methodology places less emphasis on precise quantification than does decision analysis. Instead, it relies on the consensus of a group of decision makers, ideally including experts, front-line clinicians, and patients, who carefully consider the evidence and decide on its implications. The guidelines developers' mandate may be to adduce recommendations for a country, a region, a city, a hospital, or a clinic. Depending on whether the country is the Philippines or the United States, whether the region is urban or rural, whether the institution is a large teaching hospital or a small community hospital, and whether the clinic serves a poor community or an affluent one, guidelines based on the same evidence may differ. For example, clinicians practicing in rural parts of less industrialized countries without resources to monitor its intensity may reject the administration of warfarin to patients with atrial fibrillation.

Both decision analyses and practice guidelines can be methodologically strong or weak and thus may yield either valid or invalid recommendations. In Table 1F-1, we offer four guidelines to assess the validity of a treatment recommendation—one for each step depicted in Table 1F-1—and describe these in detail below.

TABLE 1F-1

Users' Guides for the Validity of Treatment Recommendations

- Did the recommendations consider all relevant patient groups, management options, and possible outcomes?

- Is there a systematic review of evidence linking options to outcomes for each relevant question?

- Is there an appropriate specification of values or preferences associated with outcomes?

- Do the authors indicate the strength of their recommendations?

ASSESSING RECOMMENDATIONS

Did the Recommendations Consider All Relevant Patient Groups, Management Options, and Possible Outcomes?

Recommendations pertain to decisions, and decisions involve particular groups of patients, choices for those patients, and the consequences of the choices. Regardless of whether recommendations apply to diagnosis, prevention, therapy, or rehabilitation, they should specify all relevant patient groups, the interventions of interest, and sensible alternative practices. For example, in a decision analysis of the management of suspected herpes encephalitis, the authors included the three strategies available to clinicians at the time: brain biopsy, empiric vidarabine, or neither option.[31] Although this model represented the decision well at the time of publication, acyclovir has subsequently become available and is now widely used for this disorder. Because the original model did not include an acyclovir strategy, it would no longer accurately portray the decision.

To cite another example, in a guideline based on a careful systematic literature review,[32] the American College of Physicians offers recommendations for medical therapeutic options for preventing strokes.[33] Although the authors mention carotid endarterectomy as an alternative in their practice guidelines, the procedure is not included in the recommendations themselves. These guidelines would have been strengthened if medical management for transient ischemic attacks had been placed in the context of the highly effective surgical procedure.[34]

Treatment recommendations often vary for different subgroups of patients. In particular, those at lower risk of target outcomes that treatment is designed to prevent are less likely to benefit from therapy than those who are at higher risk. For instance, in a guideline concerning hormone replacement therapy in postmenopausal women, the American College of Physicians provided separate recommendations for women who had undergone a hysterectomy and for those at higher risk of cardiovascular disease or breast cancer than for other women.[35]

Recommendations must consider not only all relevant patient groups and management options, but all important consequences of the options as well. Evidence concerning the effects on morbidity, mortality, and quality of life are all relevant to patients, and efficient use of resources dictates attention to costs. If costs are considered, regardless of whether authors use the perspective of patients, insurers, or the health care system or consider broader issues such as the consequences of time lost from work, they can further affect the conclusions. Indeed, a decision analysis that includes economic outcomes is labeled an *economic analysis*.

Making recommendations about screening requires particular attention to identifying all potential outcomes. Attempting to identify disease in asymptomatic individuals may result in a number of negative outcomes that clinicians do not face when diagnosing and treating symptomatic patients. Individuals who screen positive for a disease must live for a longer time with the awareness of their illness and the associated negative psychologic consequences. This is particularly problematic if the condition screened for may remain asymptomatic for long periods of time. For instance, consider a man who screens positive for prostate cancer, but was destined to die of heart disease before the prostate cancer became clinically manifest. Those who screen positive but ultimately prove disease-negative may find the experience traumatic, and people who screen negative but ultimately prove to suffer from the target condition may feel betrayed.

In their guideline on hormone replacement therapy, the American College of Physicians used lifetime probability of developing endometrial cancer, breast cancer, hip fracture, coronary heart disease, and stroke, along with median life expectancy, to estimate risks and benefits for subgroups of women. They acknowledged possible effects of hormone replacement therapy on serum lipoproteins, uterine bleeding, sexual and urinary function, and the need for invasive monitoring, but they did not include these considerations in the model used to synthesize evidence. The effects of hormone replacement therapy on quality of life, which could have a major impact on patient choices, were not explicitly considered.

In a decision analysis concerning anticoagulant therapy for patients suffering from dilated cardiomyopathy,[4] the authors' decision model included all of the clinical events of interest to patients (stroke, other emboli, hemorrhage, and so on). The analysts measured outcomes using quality-adjusted life expectancy, a scale that combines information about both the quantity and the quality of life. This metric fit the clinical decision well, for one can expect that warfarin might affect both the quantity and quality of life.

Is There a Systematic Review of Evidence Linking Options to Outcomes for Each Relevant Question?

Having specified options and outcomes, the next task for decision makers is to estimate the likelihood that each outcome will occur. In effect, they have a series of specific questions. For hormone replacement therapy, the initial question is, "what is the effect of alternative approaches on the incidence of hip fracture, breast cancer, endometrial cancer, myocardial infarction, and sudden coronary death?" Recommendations must consolidate and combine all of the relevant evidence in an appropriate manner. In carrying out this task, decision makers must avoid bias that will distort the results. This requires access to, or conduct of, a systematic review of the evidence bearing on each question. Part 1E, "Summarizing the Evidence," provides guidelines for deciding how likely it is that collection and summarization of the evidence are free from bias.

The best recommendations define admissible evidence, report how it was selected and combined, make key data available for review, and report randomized trials that link interventions with outcomes. However, such randomized trials may be unavailable, and the authors of overviews may reasonably abandon their project if there are no high-quality studies to summarize. Those making recommendations do not have this luxury. For important but ethically, technically, or economically difficult questions, strong scientific evidence may never become available. Because recommendations must deal with the best (often inadequate) evidence available, a variety of studies (published and unpublished) and reports of expert and consumer experience may need to be considered. This means that the strength of the evidence in support of the recommendations can vary widely. Thus, even recommendations that are grounded in rigorous collection and summarization of evidence may yield weak recommendations if the quality of the evidence is poor, an issue to which we will return later in this section (see Table 1F-1).

Is There an Appropriate Specification of Values or Preferences Associated With Outcomes?

Linking treatment options with outcomes is largely a question of fact and a matter of science. Assigning preferences to outcomes, by contrast, is a matter of values. Consider, for example, the relative importance of a possible increased risk of developing breast cancer compared with expectations of decreased risks for fractures in association with hormone replacement therapy. Consequently, it is important that authors report the principal sources of such judgments and the method of seeking consensus.

Clinicians should look for information about who was involved in assigning values to outcomes or who, by influencing recommendations, was implicitly involved in assigning values. Expert panels and consensus groups are often used to determine what a guideline will say. You need to know who the "experts" are, bearing in mind that panels dominated by members of specialty groups may be subject to intellectual, territorial, and even financial biases. Panels that include a balance of experts in research methodology, practicing generalists and specialists, and public representatives are more likely to have considered diverse views in their deliberations than panels restricted to content area experts.

Even with broad representation, the actual process of deliberation can influence recommendations. Therefore, clinicians should look for a report of methods used to synthesize preferences from multiple sources. Informal and unstructured processes may be vulnerable to undue influence by individual panel members, particularly that of the chair of the panel. Explicit strategies for describing and dealing with dissent among judges, or frank reports of the degree of consensus, strengthen the credibility of the recommendations.

Knowing the extent to which patient preferences were considered is particularly important. Many guideline reports, by their silence on the matter of patient preferences, assume that guideline developers adequately represent patients' interests. Although they are reported rarely, it also would be valuable for you to know which principles—such as patient autonomy, nonmaleficence, or distributive justice—were given priority in guiding decisions about the value of alternative interventions. Excellent guidelines will state whether the guideline is intended to optimize values for individual patients, for reimbursement agencies, or for society as a whole. Ideally, guidelines will state the underlying value judgments on which they are based.

For instance, in the guideline on medical therapies to prevent stroke, the American College of Physicians recommended that aspirin be considered the drug of choice in patients with transient ischemic attacks and suggested that ticlopidine be reserved for patients who do not tolerate aspirin.[24] The best estimate of the effect of ticlopidine relative to aspirin in patients with transient ischemic attacks is a 15% reduction in relative risk, a benefit that would translate into the prevention of one stroke for every 70 patients treated in a group of patients with a 10% risk of stroke. The recommendation that aspirin, rather than ticlopidine, be the drug of choice for patients with transient ischemic attack is made, at least in part, on the basis of the increased cost of ticlopidine and the need for checking the white blood cell count in patients receiving ticlopidine. This implicit value judgment could be questioned, and the guideline would be strengthened if the authors had made explicit the values underlying their judgment.

Clinicians using a decision analysis will not face the huge problem of implicit and hidden value judgments that afflict practice guidelines. The reason, as Figure 1F-4 demonstrates, is that decision analysis requires explicit and quantitative specification of values. These values, expressed as utilities, represent measurements of the value to the decision maker of the various outcomes of the decision. Several methods are available to measure these values directly;[5,7,24,25] the issue of which of these methods is best remains controversial.

Regardless of the measurement method used, the authors should report the source of the ratings. In a decision analysis built for an individual patient, the most (and probably only) credible ratings are those measured directly from that patient. For analyses built to inform clinical policy, credible ratings could come from three sources. First, they may come from direct measurements from a large group of patients with the disorder in question and to whom results of the decision analysis could be applied. Second, ratings may come from other published studies of quality-of-life judgments by such patients, as was done in a recent analysis of strategies for chronic atrial fibrillation.[26] Third, they may come from ratings made by an equally large group of people representing the general public. Whoever provides the rating must understand the outcomes they are asked to rate; the more the raters know about the condition, the more credible are their utility ratings.

Do the Authors Indicate the Strength of Their Recommendations?

Multiple considerations should inform the strength or grade of recommendations: the quality of the sources contributing to the systematic review or reviews that bring together the relevant evidence, the magnitude and consistency of the intervention effects in different studies, the magnitude of adverse effects, the burden to the patient and the health care system, the costs, and the relative value placed upon different outcomes. Thus, recommendations may vary from those that rely on evidence from a systematic review of randomized controlled trials that show large treatment effects on patient-important outcomes with minimal side effects, inconvenience, and costs (yielding a very strong recommendation), to those that rely on evidence from observational studies showing a small magnitude of treatment effect with appreciable side effects and costs (yielding a very weak recommendation).

There are two ways that those developing recommendations can indicate their strength. One, most appropriate for practice guidelines, is to formally grade the strength of a recommendation. The other, most appropriate for decision analyses, is to vary the assumptions about the effect of the management options on the outcomes of interest. In this latter approach, a sensitivity analysis, investigators explore the extent to which varying assumptions might impact the ultimate recommendation. We will discuss the two approaches in turn.

Grades of Recommendation

The Canadian Task Force on the Periodic Health Examination proposed the first formal taxonomy of levels of evidence[36-38] focusing on individual studies. We have modified this framework, taking into account that practice guidelines must rest on systemic reviews that bring together evidence from the best available individual studies (Table 1F-2).

The letter grades in Table 1F-2 (A, B, C+, and C) reflect a hierarchy of methodologic strength that ranges from overviews of randomized trials with consistent results to overviews of observational studies with inconsistent results. Randomized trials yield the strongest evidence (grade A). Since inferences about the health effects of interventions are weakened when there are unexplained major differences in effects in different studies, guidelines based on randomized trials are stronger when the results of individual studies are similar, and guidelines are weaker when major differences between studies, or heterogeneity, are present (grade B). Recommendations from observational studies yield weaker evidence (grade C).

We now identify two situations in which evidence from RCTs directly addressing the question of interest is unavailable, but the evidence is nevertheless strong. First, generalization from one group of patients to another may be very secure. For instance, randomized trials show a large reduction of strokes in patients with atrial fibrillation without mitral valve disease. The underlying biology suggests that clinicians are on strong ground generalizing these results to patients with atrial fibrillation who do have mitral valve disease. Second, observational studies may yield a very high level of consistency and a very large magnitude of effect. Insulin therapy for acute diabetic ketoacidosis provides an example of such a situation. We denote the strength of evidence in both these contexts as C+.

If the evidence linking interventions and outcomes comes from systematic reviews of original studies, clinicians can apply the criteria for a valid systematic review and the schema in Table 1F-2 to decide on the strength of evidence supporting recommendations.

The number categories in Table 1F-2 (1 and 2) reflect the balance between benefits and risks of therapy. If the benefits clearly outweigh the risks (or vice versa) and virtually all patients would make the same choice, the recommendation is designated grade 1. When the balance is less certain and different patients may make different choices, we designate the recommendation as grade 2. A number of factors may make for uncertainty in the balance between benefits and risks, including marked variation in patient values and a wide range of confidence intervals around estimates of benefit and risk.

TABLE 1F-2

An Approach to Grading Treatment Recommendations Based on Systematic Reviews of the Relevant Evidence

Grade of Recommendation	Clarity of Risk/Benefit	Methodologic Strength of Supporting Evidence	Implications
1 A	Clear	RCTs without important limitations	Strong recommendation; can apply to most patients in most circumstances without reservation
1 B	Clear	RCTs with important limitations (inconsistent results, methodologic flaws*)	Strong recommendations, likely to apply to most patients
1 C+	Clear	No RCTs directly addressing the question, but results from closely related RCTs can be unequivocally extrapolated, or evidence from observational studies may be overwhelming	Strong recommendation; can apply to most patients in most circumstances
1 C	Clear	Observational studies	Intermediate-strength recommendation; may change when stronger evidence is available
2 A	Unclear	RCTs without important limitations	Intermediate-strength recommendation; best action may differ depending on circumstances or patient's or societal values

Grade of Recommendation	Clarity of Risk/Benefit	Methodologic Strength of Supporting Evidence	Implications
2 B	Unclear	RCTs with important limitations (inconsistent results, methodologic flaws)	Weak recommendation; alternative approaches likely to be better for some patients under some circumstances
2 C	Unclear	Observational studies	Very weak recommendations; other alternatives may be equally reasonable

* These situations include RCTs with both lack of blinding and subjective outcomes where the risk of bias in measurement of outcomes is high, RCTs with large loss to follow-up.

NOTE: Since grade B and C studies are flawed, it is likely that most recommendations in these classes will be level 2.

The following considerations will bear on whether the recommendation is grade 1 or 2: the magnitude and precision of the treatment effect, patients' risk of the target event being prevented, the nature of the benefit and the magnitude of the risk associated with treatment, variability in patient preferences, variability in regional resource availability and health care delivery practices, and cost considerations. Inevitably, weighing these considerations involves subjective judgment.

RCT indicates randomized controlled trial.

If recommendations are developed on the basis of observational studies or if the estimate of the magnitude of the treatment effect is imprecise, clinicians can conclude that the recommendation is relatively weak. Investigators can deal with this weakness in recommendations by testing the effect of the guideline on patient outcomes in a real-world clinical situation. For instance, Weingarten and colleagues examined the impact of implementation of a practice guideline, suggesting that low-risk patients admitted to coronary care units should receive early discharge.[39] On alternate months during a 1-year period, clinicians either received or did not receive a reminder of the guideline recommendations. During the months in which the intervention was in effect, hospital stay for coronary care unit patients was approximately 1 day shorter and the average cost was reduced by more than $1000.00. Mortality and health status at 1 month after discharge were similar in the two groups. Such a study, if methodologically strong, addresses the weakness in the underlying evidence and dramatically raises the grade of the recommendations.

The guideline on hormone replacement therapy described previously demonstrates the limitations of recommendations based on weak evidence.[35] Although the guideline did not grade its recommendations, they are based largely on observational studies and would be characterized as 2C in the schema presented in Table 1F-2. In particular, the guideline relied to a large extent on a meta-analysis of observational studies of the impact of hormone replacement therapy on coronary heart disease, suggesting a relative risk reduction of 0.35. Subsequently, in the first large randomized trial in women with established coronary disease, no reduction in coronary events was found with hormone replacement therapy.[40] Clearly, clinicians should be cautious in their implementation of grade C recommendations.

Sensitivity Analysis

Decision analysts use the systematic exploration of the uncertainty in the data, known as *sensitivity analysis*, to see what effect varying estimates for risks, benefits, and values have on expected clinical outcomes and, therefore, on the choice of clinical strategies. Sensitivity analysis asks the question: is the conclusion generated by the decision analysis affected by the uncertainties in the estimates of the likelihood or value of the outcomes? Estimates can be varied one at a time, termed one-way sensitivity analyses, or can be varied two or more at a time, known as multiway sensitivity analyses. For instance, investigators conducting a decision analysis of the administration of antibiotic agents for prevention of *Mycobacterium avium-intracellulare* in patients with HIV infection found that the cost-effectiveness of prophylaxis decreased if they either assumed a longer life span for patients or made a less sanguine estimate of the drugs' effectiveness.[41] If they simultaneously assumed both a longer life span and decreased drug effectiveness (a two-way sensitivity analysis), the cost-effectiveness decreased substantially. Clinicians should look for a table that lists which variables the analysts included in their sensitivity analyses, what range of values they used for each variable, and which variables, if any, altered the choice of strategies.

Generally, all of the probability estimates should be tested using sensitivity analyses. The range over which they should be tested will depend on the source of the data. If the estimates come from large, high-quality randomized trials with narrow confidence limits, the range of estimates tested can be narrow. The less valid the methods or the less precise the estimates, the wider the range that must be included in the sensitivity analyses.

Decision analysts should also test utility values with sensitivity analyses, with the range of values again determined by the source of the data. If large numbers of patients or knowledgeable and representative members of the general public gave very similar ratings to the outcome states, investigators can use a narrow range of utility values in the sensitivity analyses. If the ratings came from a small group of raters, or if the values for individuals varied widely, then investigators should use a wider range of utility values in the sensitivity analyses. To the extent that the bottom line of the decision analysis does not change with varying probability estimates and varying values, clinicians can consider the recommendation a strong one. When the bottom-line decision shifts with different plausible probabilities or values, the recommendation becomes much weaker.

Table 1F-3 presents a schema for classifying the methodologic quality of treatment recommendations, emphasizing the three key components: consideration of all relevant options and outcomes, a systematic summary of the evidence, and an explicit or quantitative consideration, or both, of societal or patient preferences.

TABLE 1F-3

A Hierarchy of Rigor in Making Treatment Recommendations

Level of Rigor	Systematic Summary of Evidence	Considers All Relevant Options and Outcomes?	Explicit Statement of Values	Sample Methodologies
High	Yes	Yes	Yes	Practice guideline or decision analysis*
Intermediate	Yes	Yes or no	No	Systematic review*
Low	No	Yes or no	No	Traditional review; article reporting primary research

* Sample methodologies may not reflect the level of rigor shown. Exceptions may occur in either direction. For example, if the author of a practice guideline or decision analysis neither systematically collects nor summarizes information and if neither societal nor patients' values are explicitly considered, recommendations will be produced that are of low rigor. Conversely, if the author of a systematic review does consider all relevant options and at least qualitatively considers values, recommendations approaching high rigor can be produced.

Are Treatment Recommendations Desirable at All?

The approaches we have described highlight the view that patient management decisions are always a function of both evidence and preferences. Values are likely to differ substantially among settings. For example, monitoring of anticoagulant therapy might take on a much stronger negative value in a rural setting where travel distances are large, or in a more severely resource-constrained environment where, for example, there is a direct inverse relationship between the resources available for purchase of antibiotic drugs and those allocated to monitoring levels of anticoagulation.

Patient-to-patient differences in values are equally important. The magnitude of the negative value of anticoagulant monitoring, or the relative negative value associated with a stroke vs a gastrointestinal bleeding episode, will vary widely among individual patients, even in the same setting. If decisions are so dependent on preferences, what is the point of recommendations?

This line of argument suggests that investigators should systematically search, accumulate, and summarize information for presentation to clinicians. In addition, investigators may highlight the implications of different sets of values for clinical action. The dependence of the decision on the underlying values—and the variability of values—would suggest that such a presentation would be more useful than a recommendation.

We find this argument compelling. However, its implementation depends on standard methods of summarizing and presenting information that clinicians are comfortable interpreting and using. In addition, it assumes that clinicians will have the time and the methods to ascertain patient values that they can then integrate with the information from systematic reviews of the impact of management decisions on patient outcomes. These requirements are unlikely to be fully met in the immediate future. Moreover, treatment recommendations are likely to remain useful for providing insight, marking progress, highlighting areas where we need more information, and stimulating productive controversy. In any case, clinical decisions are likely to improve if clinicians are aware of the underlying determinants of their actions and are able to be more critical about the recommendations offered to them. Our taxonomy may help to achieve both goals.

CLINICAL RESOLUTION

Let us return to the opening clinical scenario. Addressing the validity of the practice guideline on antithrombotic therapy in atrial fibrillation,[2] you begin by considering whether the guideline developers have addressed all important patient groups, treatment options, and outcomes. You note that they make separate recommendations for patients at varying risk of stroke, but not for patients at different risk of bleeding. The latter omission may occur because studies of prognosis have been inconsistent in the apparent risk factors for bleeding they identified. You have ruled out antiarrhythmic therapy (which another decision analysis of which you are aware suggests as the management option of choice[42]) for the patient before you. The guideline addresses the options you are seriously considering, full- and fixed-dose warfarin and aspirin, but does not mention your eccentric colleague's choice of clopidogrel or a related agent, ticlopidine. The guideline addresses the major outcomes of interest, occlusive (embolic) stroke, hemorrhagic stroke, gastrointestinal bleeding, and other major bleeding events, but does not deal specifically with the need for regular blood testing or the frequent minor bruising associated with warfarin therapy.

Moving to the selection and synthesis of the evidence, you find the guideline's eligibility criteria to be appropriate and the supportive literature search, as documented by the clearinghouse, to be comprehensive. The synthesis method is not stated explicitly, but in reading the text it becomes apparent that it is based on calculation and comparison of absolute and relative event rates for both benefits and risks and that it is tied to the guideline's strength of recommendations.

The authors of the guideline make it clear that they believe patient values are crucial to the decision, although they do not explicitly specify the relative value of stroke and bleeding that underlie their recommendations. The guideline comes down clearly on the side of adjusted-dose warfarin therapy for high-risk patients and aspirin for low-risk patients. Since high-risk patients still bleed with warfarin and low-risk patients experience fewer strokes when they take anticoagulant agents, the recommendations express an implicit relative valuing of strokes vs major and minor bleeding episodes and the inconvenience associated with warfarin therapy.

When, as in this case, guideline developers are implicit, clinicians must examine who the people involved in making recommendations are, and the possible influences on their value judgments. The developers are all expert specialists—the authors do not include patients or primary care physicians. Dupont, the makers of warfarin, funded the production of the guidelines, published as a supplement to the journal *Chest.*[2] This is worth noting, for the funders of any research project may influence its conduct. When, as is often the case in guidelines, investigators are making implicit value judgments, the possible biases that flow from the source of funding are particularly dangerous.

The guideline developers used the predecessor of the grading scheme described earlier in this section, basing all of their recommendations on the results of randomized controlled trials with consistent results, and thus rated them grade A (see Table 1F-2). They classified both of their recommendations that high-risk patients receive warfarin and low-risk patients aspirin as grade 1, meaning they believe that in both cases, the risk-benefit relationship is clear. The patient from the clinical scenario presented earlier in this section falls into the intermediate-risk category. The recommendations suggest that either warfarin or aspirin represents a reasonable option for her. Overall, the guideline meets validity criteria relatively well, and you are inclined to place a high level of trust in the authors' recommendations.

The decision analysis[5] restricts its comparison to warfarin therapy vs no treatment. Its rationale for omitting aspirin is that its efficacy is not proven (although the aspirin effect in other meta-analyses has achieved statistical significance, it has always been on the border). The investigators do not mention any other antiplatelet treatment. They include outcomes of the inconvenience associated with monitoring of anticoagulant therapy, major bleeding episodes, mild stroke, severe stroke, and cost. They omit minor bleeding.

The investigators present their search strategies very clearly. They restrict themselves to the results of computer searches of the published literature but, given this limitation, their searches appear comprehensive. With great clarity, they also describe their rationale for selecting evidence, and their criteria appear rigorous. They note the limitations of one key decision: to choose data from the Framingham study, rather than from randomized controlled trials of therapy for patients with atrial fibrillation, from which to derive their risk estimates.

To generate values, the authors interviewed 57 community-dwelling elderly people with a mean age of 73 years. They used standard gamble methodology to generate utility values. Their key values include utilities, on a 0 to 1.0 scale where 0 is death and 1.0 is full health, of 0.986 for warfarin managed by a general practitioner, 0.880 for a major bleeding episode, 0.675 for a mild stroke, and 0 for a severe stroke.

The investigators conducted a sensitivity analysis that indicated their model was sensitive to variation in patients' utility for being on warfarin. If they assumed utility values for being on warfarin in the upper quartile (1.0; that is, no disutility is suggested for taking warfarin), their analysis suggests that virtually all patients should be receiving warfarin treatment. If they assumed the lower quartile utility, 0.92), the analysis suggests that most patients should not be taking warfarin.

This decision analysis rates high with respect to the validity criteria in Table 1F-1. The utilities in the investigators' core analysis using median patient values and best estimates of risk and risk reduction (their *base case* analysis) match those of the patient in the scenario quite well. The investigators provided tables that suggest the best decision for different patients; when we add the characteristics of the patient being considered in the opening scenario, we find that the verdict is: no benefit from treatment. However, this patient does fit into a cell near the boundary between no benefit and clear benefit, and the investigators' sensitivity analysis suggests that if she places the same value on life taking warfarin as life not taking warfarin, she would benefit from using the drug.

Having reviewed what turns out to be a rigorous guideline and a rigorous decision analysis, you believe that you are in a much stronger position both in your own decision making and in providing guidance to your colleagues. Your residual discomfort stems from the realization that the best decision for many patients, including the patient in the scenario, is critically dependent on the patient's values. You resolve to have a more detailed discussions of the options and the consequences when you see her next.

References

1. Eddy DM. *A Manual for Assessing Health Practices and Designing Practice Policies: The Explicit Approach.* Philadelphia: American College of Physicians; 1992.

2. Laupacis A, Albers G, Dalen J, Dunn MI, Jacobson AK, Singer DE. Antithrombotic therapy in atrial fibrillation. *Chest.* 1998;114:579S-589S.

3. Shaneyfelt TM, Mayo-Smith MF, Rothwangl J. Are guidelines following guidelines? The methodological quality of clinical practice guidelines in the peer-reviewed medical literature. *JAMA.* 1999;281:1900-1905.

4. Grilli R, Magrini N, Penna A, Mura G, Liberati A. Practice guidelines developed by specialty societies: the need for a critical appraisal. *Lancet.* 2000;355:103-106.

5. Thompson R, Parkin D, Eccles M, Sudlow M, Robinson A. Decision analysis and guidelines for anticoagulant therapy to prevent stroke in patients with atrial fibrillation. *Lancet.* 2000;355:956-962.

6. Vandenbroucke-Grauls CMJE, Vendenbroucke JP. Effect of selective decontamination of the digestive tract on respiratory tract infections and mortality in the intensive care unit. *Lancet.* 1991;338:859-862.

7. Selective Decontamination of the Digestive Tract Trialists' Collaborative Group. Meta-analysis of randomised controlled trials of selective decontamination of the digestive tract. *BMJ.* 1993;307:525-532.

8. Heyland DK, Cook DJ, Jaeschke R, Griffith L, Lee HN, Guyatt GH. Selective decontamination of the digestive tract. *Chest.* 1994;105:1221-1229.

9. Kollef MH. The role of selective digestive tract decontamination on mortality and respiratory tract infections. *Chest.* 1994;105:1101-1108.

10. Glasziou PP, Irwig LM. An evidence based approach to individualising treatment. *BMJ.* 1995;311:1356-1358.

11. Sinclair JC, Cook R, Guyatt GH, Pauker SG, Cook DJ. When should an effective treatment be used? Derivation of the threshold number needed to treat and the minimum event rate for treatment. *J Clin Epidemiol.* In press.

12. Smith GD, Egger M. Who benefits from medical interventions? *BMJ.* 1994;308:72-74.

13. Antman EM, Lau J, Kupelnick B, Mosteller F, Chalmers TC. A comparison of results of meta-analyses of randomized control trials and recommendations of clinical experts: treatments for myocardial infarction. *JAMA*. 1992;268:240-248.

14. Keeney RL. Decision analysis: an overview. *Operations Res*. 1982;30:803-838.

15. Eckman MH, Levine HJ, Pauker SG. Decision analytic and cost-effectiveness issues concerning anticoagulant prophylaxis in heart disease. *Chest*. 1992;102:538S-549S.

16. Kassirer JP, Moskowitz AJ, Lau J, Pauker SG. Decision analysis: a progress report. *Ann Intern Med*. 1987;106:275-291.

17. Eddy DM. Clinical decision making: from theory to practice. Designing a practice policy. Standards, guidelines and options. *JAMA*. 1990;263:3077, 3081, 3084.

18. Wong JB, Salem DN, Pauker SG. You're never too old. *N Engl J Med*. 1993;328:971-974.

19. Krahn MD, Mahoney JE, Eckman MH, Trachtenberg J, Pauker SG, Detsky AS. Screening for prostate cancer: a decision analytic view. *JAMA*. 1994;272:773-780.

20. Krahn M, Naylor CD, Basinski AS, Detsky AS. Comparison of an aggressive (U.S.) and a less aggressive (Canadian) policy for cholesterol screening and treatment. *Ann Intern Med*. 1991;115:248-255.

21. Goel V. Decision analysis: applications and limitations. *CMAJ*. 1992;147:413-417.

22. Drummond MF, Richardson WS, O'Brien B, Levine M, Heyland DK, for the Evidence-Based Medicine Working Group. Users' Guides to the Medical Literature XIII. How to use an article on economic analysis of clinical practice. A. Are the results of the study valid? *JAMA*. 1997;277:1552-1557.

23. O'Brien BJ, Heyland DK, Richardson WS, Levine M, Drummond MF, for the Evidence-Based Medicine Working Group. Users' Guides to the Medical Literature XIII. How to use an article on economic analysis of clinical practice. B. What are the results and will they help me in caring for my patients? *JAMA*. 1997;277:1802-1806.

24. Institute of Medicine. *Clinical Practice Guidelines: Directions for a New Program*. Washington, DC: National Academy Press; 1990.

25. AMA/Specialty *Society Practice Parameters Partnership. Attributes to Guide the Development of Practice Parameters.* Chicago: American Medical Association; 1990.

26. American College of Physicians. *Clinical Efficacy Assessment Project: Procedural Manual*. Philadelphia: American College of Physicians; 1986.

27. Gottlieb LK, Margolis CZ, Schoenbaum SC. Clinical practice guidelines at an HMO: development and implementation in a quality improvement model. *QRB*. 1990;16:80-86.

28. Lohr KN, Field MJ. A provisional instrument for assessing clinical practice guidelines. 1991. Unpublished.

29. Woolf SH. Expert Panel on Preventive Services: analytic methodology. 1991. Unpublished.

30. Park RE, Fink A, Brook RH, et al. Physicians' rating of appropriate indications for six medical and surgical procedures. *Am J Public Health*. 1986;76:766-772.

31. Barza M, Pauker SG. The decision to biopsy, treat, or wait in suspected herpes encephalitis. *Ann Intern Med*. 1980;92:641-649.

32. Matchar DB, McCrory DC, Barnett HJM, Feussner JR. Medical treatment for stroke prevention. *Ann Intern Med*. 1994;121:41-53.

33. American College of Physicians. Guidelines for medical treatment for stroke prevention. *Ann Intern Med*. 1994;121:54-55.

34. North American Symptomatic Carotid Endarterectomy Trial Collaborators. Beneficial effect of carotid endarterectomy in symptomatic patients with high-grade carotid stenosis. *N Engl J Med*. 1991;325:445-453.

35. Grady D, Rubin SM, Petitti DB, et al. Hormone therapy to prevent disease and prolong life in postmenopausal women. *Ann Intern Med*. 1992;117:1016-1037.

36. Canadian Task Force on the Periodic Health Examination. The periodic health examination. *CMAJ*. 1979;121:1193-1254.

37. Woolf SH, Battista RN, Anderson GM, Logan AG, Wang E. Assessing the clinical effectiveness of preventive maneuvers: analytic principles and systematic methods in reviewing evidence and developing clinical practice recommendations. *J Clin Epidemiol*. 1990;43:891-905.

38. Sackett DL. Rules of evidence and clinical recommendations on the use of antithrombotic agents. *Arch Intern Med*. 1986;146:464-466.

39. Weingarten SR, Reidinger MS, Conner L, et al. Practice guidelines and reminders to reduce duration of hospital stay for patients with chest pain. *Ann Intern Med*. 1994;120:257-263.

40. Hulley S, Grady D, Bush T, Furberg C, Herrington D, Riggs B, Vittinghoff E. Randomized trial of estrogen plus progestin for secondary prevention of coronary heart disease in post-menopausal women. Heart and Estrogen/progestin Replacement Study (HERS) Research Group. *JAMA*. 1998;280:605-613.

41. Bayoumi AM, Redelmeier DA. Preventing *Mycobacterium avium* complex in patients who are using protease inhibitors: a cost-effectiveness analysis. *AIDS*. 1998;12:1503-1512.

42. Catherwood E, Fitzpatrick WD, Greenberg ML, et al. Cost-effectiveness of cardioversion and antiarrhythmic therapy in non-valvular atrial fibrillation. *Ann Intern Med*. 1999;130:625-636.

Part 2

Beyond the Basics: Using and Teaching the Principles of Evidence-Based Medicine

Part 2 of this printed volume provides detailed, in-depth discussions of the key concepts introduced in Part 1. Directed at those who would like to reach a deeper understanding of statistical concepts, it expands on only a few issues: bias and random error, hypothesis testing, confidence intervals, and measures of association.

In the electronic version of the book, each section of Part 2 is linked to Part 1; and the text of Part 1 highlights the concepts on which Part 2 expands. These expanded discussions include strategies for explaining difficult concepts that instructors of evidence-based medicine (EBM) may find particularly useful.

The CD-ROM Part 2 begins with expansions of issues raised in the "Philosophy of Evidence-Based Medicine," including critics' attacks on EBM. The next section provides a perspective on the fundamental threat to inferences from any primary study: bias and random error. Here, we emphasize the link between addressing issues of therapy and issues of harm. We also include this latter section in the printed volume.

The largest segment of Part 2 addresses issues of delivering the optimal therapy to patients. This segment includes of examples of randomized controlled results that have differed from those predicted by biologic rationale or suggested by observational studies. We also provide examples of numbers needed to treat for a number of therapies, emphasizing how the number needed to treat will vary in patients with differing baseline risks.

This segment expands on a number of statistical issues including intention-to treat analysis, hypothesis testing, confidence intervals, and choosing the best way of expressing the magnitude of a treatment effect ("Measures of Association"), some of which are also included in the paper text. We provide a guide on applying the results of randomized controlled trials to individual patients, and describe how clinicians can definitively determine the best treatment for an individual in "N of 1 Clinical Trials."

Part 2 emphasizes the care clinicians should take when therapy clearly impacts on biologic variables, but may not impact on patient-important outcomes ("Surrogate Outcomes"). On the other hand, we provide a deeper understanding of outcomes that randomized controlled trials have tended to neglect; namely, patients' quality of life. Part 2 provides clinicians with a strategy for deciding whether to generalize results across a class of drugs, or to conclude that a particular drug in a class is superior to others. Finally, we offer insights in to two particular types of studies: those addressing computer decision aids, and qualitative studies focusing on patients' experience of illness and of health care.

Issues related to diagnostic tests on which Part 2 expands include studies related to describing the clinical manifestations of particular diseases and those that generate or test clinical prediction rules. Part 2 provides a guide to help understand how chance can inflate apparent agreement (eg, agreement between physicians assessing an element of physical examination), and chance-corrected measures of agreement that help deal with this problem. Next we provide some examples of likelihood ratios, the ultimate output of studies of diagnostic tests. The related section on prognosis, "Regression and Correlation," deals with concepts of statistical analysis.

Readers of the next segment of Part 2 will deepen their understanding of systematic reviews. What interpretations are possible when studies addressing a similar question yield discrepant results ("Evaluating Differences in Study Results")? When should clinicians believe an analysis that suggests that a drug is effective in one group of patients and not another, or that differing doses have appreciably different effects on outcome ("When to Believe a Subgroup Analysis")? This segment also discusses the difficulties that unpublished studies present for systematic reviews, and the issues involved in choosing the optimal strategy for statistical analysis.

Part 2 concludes with an expanded discussion of how one uses evidence to arrive at a management approach for the individual patient, or for a group of similar patients. Clinicians reading this segment will gain insight into approaches to grade the strength of expert recommendations, and will learn how to make sense of a study that examines the economic implications of alternative treatments. We provide a detailed discussion of studies of screening interventions, and of studies that examine the quality of clinical care. Finally, we address what is perhaps the most important frontier of evidence-based medicine: How can one efficiently and effectively incorporate the values of a specific patient in health care decisions that will influence the subsequent life of that patient?

THERAPY AND HARM
Why Study Results Mislead—Bias and Random Error

Gordon Guyatt

The following EBM Working Group members also made substantive contributions to this section: Sharon Straus, Deborah Cook, and Peter Wyer

IN THIS SECTION

RANDOM ERROR

Our clinical questions have a correct answer that corresponds to an underlying reality or truth. For instance, there is a true underlying magnitude of the impact of beta blockers on mortality in patients with heart failure, of the impact of inhaled steroids on exacerbations in patients with asthma, and of the impact of carotid endarterectomy on incidence of strokes in patients with transient ischemic attacks. Unfortunately, however, we will never know what that true impact really is. Why is this so?

Consider a perfectly balanced coin. Every time we flip the coin, the probability of its landing with head up or tail up is equal—50%. Assume that we, as investigators, do not know that the coin is perfectly balanced—in fact, we have no idea how well balanced it is, and we would like to find out. We can state our question formally: what is the true underlying probability of a resulting head or tail on any given coin flip? Our first experiment addressing this question is a series of 10 coin flips. The result: eight heads and two tails. What are we to conclude? Taking our result at face value, we infer that the coin is very unbalanced (that is, biased in such a way that it yields heads more often than tails) and that the probability of heads on any given flip is 80%.

Few would be happy with this conclusion. The reason for our discomfort is that we know that the world is not constructed so that a perfectly balanced coin will always yield five heads and five tails in any given set of 10 coin flips. Rather, the result is subject to the play of chance—otherwise known as *random error*. Some of the time, 10 flips of a perfectly balanced coin will yield eight heads. On occasion, nine of 10 flips will turn up heads. On rare occasions, we will find heads on all 10 flips.

What if the 10 coin flips yield five heads and five tails? Our awareness of the play of chance makes us very hesitant to conclude that the coin is a true one. We know that not only might we get eight heads and two tails when the real probability of a head is 0.5, but also that a series of 10 coin flips in a very biased coin (a true probability of heads of 0.8, for instance) could yield five heads and five tails.

Let us say that a funding agency, intrigued by the results of our first small experiment, provides us with resources to conduct a larger study. This time, we increase the sample size of our experiment markedly, conducting a series of 1000 coin flips. When we end up with 500 heads and 500 tails, are we ready to conclude that we are dealing with a true coin? Not quite. We know that, were the true underlying probability of heads 51%, we would sometimes see 1000 coin flips yield the very same result we have just observed.

Application. We can apply the above logic to the results of experiments addressing health care issues in human beings. A randomized controlled trial shows that 10 of 100 treated patients die in the course of treatment and that 20 of 100 control patients who do not receive treatment die. Does treatment really reduce the death rate by 50%? Maybe, but awareness of chance will leave us with considerable uncertainty about the magnitude of the treatment effect—and perhaps about whether treatment helps at all. To use a real-world example, in a study of cardiac insufficiency, 228 (17%) of 1320 patients with moderate to severe heart failure allocated to receive placebo died, as did 156 (12%) of 1327 allocated to receive bisoprolol.[1] Although the true underlying reduction in the relative risk of dying is likely to be in the vicinity of the 34% suggested by the study, we must acknowledge that considerable uncertainty remains about the true magnitude of the effect. Let us remember the question with which we started: why is it that, no matter how powerful and well-designed our experiment, we will never be sure of the true treatment effect? The answer is accounted for by chance.

BIAS

What do we mean when we say that a study is valid, believable, or credible? *Validity* is the degree to which a study appropriately answers the question being asked or appropriately measures what it intends to measure. In this book, we use validity as a technical term that relates to the magnitude of *bias*. In contrast to random error, bias leads to systematic deviations (ie, the error has direction) from the underlying truth. In studies of treatment or harm, bias leads to either an underestimate or an overestimate of the underlying beneficial or harmful effect.

Bias may intrude as a result of differences, other than the experimental intervention, between patients in treatment and control groups at the time they enter a study. Alternatively, it may reflect differences that develop after the study begins. At the start of a study each patient, if left untreated, is destined to do well—or poorly. To do poorly means to have an adverse event—say, a stroke—during the course of the study. We often refer to the adverse event that is the focus of a study as the *target outcome* or event.

There are a host of factors that are associated with—or causally related to—the likelihood of a patient suffering the target outcome. Consider a trial in which patients at risk of a cerebrovascular event are studied. If patients' underlying disease (atherosclerosis) is severe, if they have reached advanced age, if their blood pressure is high, or if they are male, they are more likely than others to have a stroke.[2] We call each of these patient characteristics *prognostic factors* or *determinants of outcome*. These prognostic factors determine patients' destiny with respect to whether or not they will suffer the target adverse event.

We can contrast these patient characteristics with such other characteristics as eye color or shoe size. Eye color and shoe size differ from the first set of characteristics in that they are seldom, if ever, related to the likelihood of having a stroke. Patients with blue eyes are no more or less likely to suffer a stroke than those with brown eyes. Those with size 12 shoes are at no greater or lesser risk than those with size 8 shoes.

Prognostic Differences Between Treatment and Control Patients. Bias will intrude if treated and control patients who are not treated differ in substantive outcome-associated ways at the start of the study. Differences in eye color or shoe size will not create bias because they are not associated with the target outcome, but differences in important prognostic factors will lead to bias. For example, if treated patients have more severe atherosclerosis or are older than their control counterparts, their destiny will be to suffer a greater proportion of adverse events than those in the control group, and the results of the study will be biased against the treatment group. That is, the study will yield a systematically lower estimate of the treatment effect than would be obtained were the study groups alike prognostically. Thus, the study results would not reflect the underlying truth.

What if the control group has a higher mean blood pressure, or a greater proportion of men, than the treatment group? In these cases, the bias will be in the opposite direction (ie, it will be against the control group). If control patients begin the study with a greater stroke risk, study results will be biased in favor of the treatment group, and treatment will appear to benefit patients more than it really does. Thus, one source of bias is prognostic differences between treated and control patients at the start of a study.

Placebo Effect. Even if treated and control patients can begin the study with the same fate or destiny, the study may still produce a biased estimate of the treatment effect. For example, patients who believe they are receiving treatment may anticipate that they will do better. As it turns out, such anticipation may have a profound effect on how patients actually do feel and, furthermore, on how they function. This *placebo effect* may bias the results toward suggesting a greater biologic effect of treatment than is really the case.

Differential Administration of Interventions. Another potential source of bias is differential administration of interventions (other than that under study) to patients in the treatment and control groups. For example, in a study of a new treatment for stroke in which a larger proportion of patients in the treatment group receive aspirin or clopidogrel than those in the control group, the results will overestimate the treatment effect. This will not be true if a larger proportion of patients in the treatment group receive saline eye drops or antacid medications. The reason is that saline eye drops and antacids have no impact on the frequency of stroke, whereas aspirin[3] and clopidogrel[4] reduce stroke incidence. *Cointervention* is a technical term used to describe a situation when treatments that do affect the incidence of the target outcome are differentially administered to treatment and control groups.

Note some parallels: we are not concerned about imbalance of eye color or shoe size when patients start the study (which we often call *baseline characteristics*), nor are we concerned about imbalance of saline eye drops or antacid administration once the study starts. What we are concerned about is imbalance in disease severity in the treatment and control patients, and about differential administration of aspirin to the two groups, because they may affect the likelihood of patients having a stroke. Study results will be biased if factors that affect prognosis, either baseline characteristics or subsequent treatment, are unequal in the groups being compared. A *confounding variable* is any prognostic factor or effective treatment that is not equal in the groups being compared. For a study to be unbiased, the groups must start the same (with respect to their likelihood of suffering the target outcome) and stay the same.

Differential Measurement of the Target Outcome. Differential measurement of the target outcome can also introduce bias. For instance, whether a patient has suffered a transient ischemic attack or a small stroke may be a matter of judgment. If all such events are identified and recorded as strokes in the control group and as transient ischemic attacks in the intervention group, the study will overestimate the effect of treatment on stroke reduction.

Loss to Follow-up. Another way that a study may introduce bias related to measurement of outcome is when large numbers of patients are *lost to follow-up*. If rates of adverse outcomes differ in patients lost to follow-up, the necessity of relying on data from patients who were followed will result in findings that differ from the underlying truth.

DIFFERENTIATING DEGREES OF BIAS AND RANDOM ERROR

Students of EBM face conceptual challenges and challenges of nomenclature. When asked to say what makes a study valid, students often respond, "large sample size." Small sample size does not produce bias (and, thus, compromised validity), but it can increase the likelihood of a misleading result through *random error*. You may find the following exercise helpful in clarifying notions of bias and random error.

Consider a set of studies with identical design and sample size that recruit from the same patient pool. Just as an experiment of 10 coin flips will not always yield five heads and five tails, the play of chance will ensure that despite their identical design, each study will have a different result.

Consider four sets of such studies. Within each set, the design and sample size of each individual trial are identical. Two of the four sets of studies have small sample sizes, and two have large sample sizes.

Two sets include only randomized controlled trials (RCTs) in which patients, caregivers, and those assessing outcome are all blinded. Two sets use only an observational design (eg, patients are in treatment or control groups on the basis of their choice, their clinician's choice, or happenstance), which is far more vulnerable to bias. In this exercise we are in the unique position of knowing the true treatment effect. In Figure 2A-1, each of the bull's-eyes in the center of the four components of the figure represents the truth. Each smaller dot represents not a single patient, but the results of one repetition of the study. The farther a smaller dot lies from the central bull's-eye, the larger is the difference between the study result and the underlying true treatment effect.

FIGURE 2A–1

Representation of Four Sets of Identically Conducted Studies Demonstrating Varying Degrees of Bias and Random Error

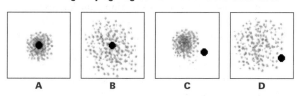

A, A group of randomized controlled trials (large sample size). **B,** A group of randomized controlled trials (small sample size). **C,** A group of observational studies (large sample size). **D,** A group of observational studies (small sample size).

Each set of studies represents the results of RCTs or observational studies and of studies of large or small sample size. Before reading further, examine Figure 2A-1 and draw your own conclusions about the study designs and number of patients in each of the four (A through D) components.

Figure 2A-1(A) represents the results of a series of randomized trials with large sample size. The results are valid and are thus distributed around the true effect, represented by the central bull's-eye, resulting from the strong study design. The results do not fall exactly on target because of chance or random error. However, the large sample size, which minimizes random error, ensures that the result of any individual study is relatively close to the truth.

Contrast this set of results with those depicted in Figure 2A-1(B). Again, the strong study design results in the individual study results being distributed around the truth. However, because the sample size is small and random error is large, the results of individual studies may be far from the truth.

If we think back to our coin flip experiments, this clarifies the difference between the studies in the Figures 2A-1(A) and 2A-1(B). In a series of experiments in which each study involves 10 flips of a true coin, individual results may fall far from the truth, and findings of 70%, or even 80%, heads (or tails) will not be unusual. This situation is analogous to Figure 2A-1(B). If our experiments each involve 1000 coin flips, analogous to Figure 2A-1(A), we will seldom see distributions more extreme than, say 540, or a 54% probability of heads or tails. With the smaller sample size, individual results are far from the truth; with the larger sample size, they are all close to the truth.

Figures 2A-1(A) and 2A-1(B) illustrate the rationale for pooling results of different studies, a process called *meta-analysis*. Assume that the available evidence about therapeutic effectiveness comes from a series of small RCTs. However, there is a problem: Chance will ensure that the study results vary widely, and we will not know which one to believe. Because of a strong study design, the distribution of the results is centered around the truth. As a result of this favorable situation we can, by pooling the results of the studies, decrease random error and increase the strength of our inferences from the uncertainty of Figure 2A-1(B) to the confidence of Figure 2A-1(A).

In Figure 2A-1(C), the center of the set of dots is far from the truth. This is because studies with observational designs, even large ones, are vulnerable to bias. Since the studies share an identical design, each one will be subject to the same magnitude and direction of bias. The results are very precise with minimal random error; however, they are incorrect.

One real-world example of this phenomenon is the apparent benefit of vitamin E on reducing mortality from coronary artery disease suggested by the results of a number of large observational studies.[5] By contrast, a subsequent very large, well-conducted RCT failed to demonstrate any impact of vitamin E on coronary deaths.[6]

A second example comes from the many large observational studies suggesting a reduction in the relative risk of coronary death of about 35% in women taking post-menopausal hormone replacement therapy.[7] Notably, the first RCT comparing hormone replacement therapy to placebo in women at high risk of coronary events showed no benefit.[8] In both of these situations, the likely explanation is that people with a lower underlying risk of coronary artery disease are the ones who tend to take vitamin E and hormone replacement therapy. Their lower initial risk resulted in a consistently biased estimate of effectiveness.

The situation depicted in Figure 2A-1(C) is a particularly dangerous one because the large size of the studies instills confidence in clinicians that their results are accurate. For example, many clinicians, fed by the consistent results of very large observational studies, still believe the prevailing dogma of the beneficial effect of hormone replacement therapy on coronary artery disease mortality.

Like Figure 2A-1(C), Figure 2A-1(D) depicts a series of observational studies leading to biased results that are far from the truth. However, because the sample sizes are all small, the results vary widely from study to study. One might be tempted to conduct a meta-analysis of these data. This is dangerous because we risk converting imprecise estimates with large random error to precise estimates with small random error; both, however, are biased.

STRATEGIES FOR REDUCING BIAS: THERAPY AND HARM

We have noted that bias arises from differences in prognostic factors in treatment and control groups at the start of a study, or from differences in prognosis that arise as a study proceeds. What can investigators do to reduce these biases? Table 2A-1 summarizes the available strategies.

TABLE 2A-1

Ways of Reducing Bias in Studies of Therapy and Harm

Source of Bias	Therapy: Strategy for Reducing Bias	Harm: Strategy for Reducing Bias
Differences noted at the start of the study:		
Treatment and control patients differ in prognosis	Randomization	Statistical adjustment for prognostic factors in the analysis of data
Differences that arise as the study proceeds:		
Placebo effects	Blinding of patients	Choice of outcomes (eg, mortality) less subject to placebo effects
Cointervention	Blinding of caregivers	Documentation of treatment differences and statistical adjustment
Bias in assessment of outcome	Blinding of assessors of outcome	Choice of outcomes (eg, mortality) less subject to observer bias
Loss to follow-up	Ensuring complete follow-up	Ensuring complete follow-up

When studying new treatments, investigators often have a great deal of control. They can reduce the likelihood of differences in the distribution of prognostic features in treated and untreated patients at baseline by randomly allocating patients to the two groups. They can markedly reduce placebo effects by administering placebos that are identical in treatment but biologically inert to control group patients. Blinding clinicians to whether patients are receiving active or placebo therapy can eliminate the risk of important cointervention, and blinding outcome assessors minimizes bias in the assessment of event rates.

In general, investigators studying the impact of potentially harmful exposures have far less control than those investigating the effects of potentially beneficial treatments. They must be content to compare patients whose exposure is determined by their choice or circumstances, and they can address potential differences in patients' fate only by statistical adjustment for known prognostic factors. Blinding is impossible, so their best defense against placebo effects and bias in outcome assessment is to choose endpoints, like death, that are less subject to these biases. Investigators addressing both sets of questions can reduce bias by minimizing loss to follow-up (see Table 2A-1).

These general rules do not always apply. Sometimes, investigators find it difficult or impossible to randomize patients to treatment and control groups. Under such circumstances they choose observational study designs, and clinicians must apply the validity criteria developed for questions of harm to such studies.

Similarly, if the potentially harmful exposure is a drug with beneficial effects, investigators may be able to randomize patients to intervention and control groups. In this case, clinicians can apply the validity criteria designed for therapy questions to the study. Whether for issues of therapy or harm, the strength of inference from RCTs will almost invariably be far greater than the strength of inference from observational studies.

References

1. CIBIS-II Investigators and Committees. The Cardiac Insufficiency Bisoprolol Study II (CIBIS- II): a randomised trial. *Lancet*. 1999;353:9-13.

2. Goldstein LB, Adams R, Becker K, Furberg CD, Gorelick PB, Hademenos G, et al. Primary prevention of ischaemic stroke: a statement for healthcare professionals from the Stroke Council of the American Heart Association. *Stroke.* 2001;32(1):280-299.

3. Gubitz G, Sandercock P, Counsell C. Antiplatelet therapy for acute ischaemic stroke (Cochrane Review). In: *The Cochrane Library*, 1, 2001. Oxford: Update Software.

4. CAPRIE Steering Committee. A randomized, blinded, trial of clopidogrel versus aspirin in patients at risk of ischaemic events (CAPRIE). *Lancet.* 1996;348(9038):1329-1339.

5. Knekt P, Reunanen A, Jarvinen R, Seppanen R, Heliovaara M, Aromaa A. Antioxidant vitamin intake and coronary mortality in a longitudinal population study. *Am J Epidemiol*. 1994;139:1180-1189.

6. Yusuf S, Dagenais G, Pogue J, Bosch J, Sleight P. Vitamin E supplementation and cardiovascular events in high-risk patients. The Heart Outcomes Prevention Evaluation Study Investigators. *N Engl J Med*. 2000;342:154-160.

7. Stampfer MJ, Colditz GA. Estrogen replacement therapy and coronary heart disease: a quantitative assessment of the epidemiologic evidence. *Prev Med*. 1991;20:47-63.

8. Hulley S, Grady D, Bush T, et al. Randomized trial of estrogen plus progestin for secondary prevention of coronary heart disease in postmenopausal women. Heart and Estrogen/progestin Replacement Study (HERS) Research Group. *JAMA*. 1998;280:605-613.

THERAPY AND UNDERSTANDING THE RESULTS

Hypothesis Testing

Gordon Guyatt, Roman Jaeschke, Deborah Cook, and Stephen Walter

Rose Hatala also made substantive contributions to this section

IN THIS SECTION

We have said that there is a true, underlying effect of a treatment that only can be estimated by any individual experiment (see Part 2A, "Therapy and Harm, Why Study Results Mislead—Bias and Random Error"). Investigators use statistical methods to advance their understanding of this true effect. For some time, the essential paradigm for statistical inference in the medical literature has been that of hypothesis testing. The investigator starts with what is called a *null hypothesis* that the statistical test is designed to consider and, possibly, disprove. Typically, the null hypothesis is that there is no difference between treatments being compared. In a randomized trial in which investigators compare an experimental treatment with a placebo control, one can state the null hypothesis as follows: the true difference in effect on the outcome of interest between the experimental and control treatments is zero. For instance, in a comparison of vasodilator treatment in 804 men with heart failure, investigators compared the proportion of enalapril-treated survivors with the proportion of survivors given a combination of hydralazine and nitrates.[1] We start with the assumption that the treatments are equally effective and we adhere to this position unless data make it untenable. In the vasodilator trial, the null hypothesis could be stated more formally as follows: the true difference in the proportion surviving between patients treated with enalapril and those treated with hydralazine and nitrates is zero.

In this hypothesis-testing framework, the statistical analysis addresses the question of whether the observed data are consistent with the null hypothesis. The logic of the approach is as follows: Even if the treatment truly has no positive or negative impact on the outcome (that is, the effect size is zero), the results observed will seldom show exact equivalence; that is, no difference at all will be observed between the experimental and control groups. As the results diverge farther and farther from the finding of "no difference," the null hypothesis that there is no difference between treatment effects becomes less and less credible. If the difference between results of the treatment and control groups becomes large enough, clinicians must abandon belief in the null hypothesis. We will further develop the underlying logic by describing the role of chance in clinical research.

THE ROLE OF CHANCE

In Part 2A, "Therapy and Harm, Why Study Results Mislead—Bias and Random Error," we considered a balanced coin with which the true probability of obtaining either heads or tails in any individual coin toss is 0.5. We noted that if we tossed such a coin 10 times, we would not be surprised if we did not see exactly five heads and five tails. Occasionally, we would get results quite divergent from the 5:5 split, such as 8:2 or even 9:1. Furthermore, very infrequently the 10 coin tosses would result in 10 consecutive heads or tails.

Chance is responsible for this variability in results, and certain recreational games illustrate the way chance operates. On occasion, the roll of two unbiased dice (dice with an equal probability of rolling any number between 1 and 6) will yield two ones or two sixes. On occasion (much to the delight of the recipient), the dealer at a poker game will dispense a hand consisting of five cards of a single suit. Even less frequently, the five cards will not only belong to a single suit, but will also have consecutive face value.

Chance is not restricted to the world of coin tosses, dice, and card games. If we take a sample of patients from a community, chance may result in unusual distributions of chronic disease. Chance also may be responsible for substantial imbalance in event rates in two groups of patients given different treatments that are, in fact, equally effective. Much statistical inquiry is geared to determining the extent to which unbalanced distributions could be attributed to chance and the extent to which one should invoke other explanations (treatment effects, for instance). As we will demonstrate, the conclusions of statistical inquiry are determined to a large extent by the size of the study.

THE *P* VALUE

One way that an investigator can err is to conclude that there is a difference between a treatment group and a control group when, in fact, no such difference exists. In statistical terminology, making the mistake of erroneously concluding there is such a difference is called a *type I error* and the probability of making such an error is referred to as the alpha level. Imagine a situation in which we are uncertain whether a coin is biased. That is, we suspect that a coin toss is more likely to result in either heads or tails. One could construct a null hypothesis that the true proportions of heads and tails are equal (that is, the coin is unbiased). With this scenario, the probability of any given toss landing heads is 50%, as is the probability of any given toss landing tails. We could test this hypothesis by an experiment in which we conducted a series of coin tosses. Statistical analysis of the results of the experiment would address the question of whether the results observed were consistent with chance.

Let us conduct a hypothetical experiment in which the suspected coin is tossed 10 times and on all 10 occasions, the result is heads. How likely is this to have occurred if the coin was indeed unbiased? Most people would conclude that it is highly unlikely that chance could explain this extreme result.

We would therefore be ready to reject the hypothesis that the coin is unbiased (the null hypothesis) and conclude that the coin is biased. Statistical methods allow us to be more precise by ascertaining just how unlikely the result is to have occurred simply as a result of chance if the null hypothesis is true. The law of multiplicative probabilities for independent events (where one event in no way influences the other) tells us that the probability of 10 consecutive heads can be found by multiplying the probability of a single head (1/2) 10 times over; that is, $1/2 \times 1/2 \times 1/2$, and so on. The probability of getting 10 consecutive heads is then slightly less than one in a thousand. In a journal article, one would likely see this probability expressed as a P value, such as $P < .001$. What is the precise meaning of this P value? If the coin were unbiased (that is, if the null hypothesis were true) and one were to repeat the experiment of the 10 coin tosses many times, 10 consecutive heads would be expected to occur by chance less than once in a thousand times. The probability of obtaining either 10 heads or 10 tails is approximately 0.002, or two in a thousand.

In the framework of hypothesis testing, the experiment would not be over, for one has to make a decision. Are we willing to reject the null hypothesis and conclude that the coin is biased? This has to do with how much faith we have in concluding that the coin is biased when, in fact, it is not. In other words, what risk or chance of making a type I error are we willing to accept? The reasoning implies a threshold value that demarcates a boundary. On one side of this boundary we are unwilling to reject the null hypothesis; on the other side we are ready to conclude that chance is no longer a plausible explanation for the results. To return to the example of 10 consecutive heads, most people would be ready to reject the null hypothesis when the results observed would be expected to occur by chance alone less than once in a thousand times.

Let us repeat the thought experiment. This time we obtain nine tails and one head. Once again, it is unlikely that the result is because of the play of chance alone. This time the *P* value is .02. That is, if the coin were unbiased and the null hypothesis were true, results as extreme as—or more extreme than—those observed (that is, 10 heads or 10 tails, nine heads and one tail, or nine tails and one head) would be expected to occur by chance alone two times per hundred repetitions of the experiment.

Given this result, are we willing to reject the null hypothesis? The decision is arbitrary and is a matter of judgment. Statistical convention, however, would suggest that the answer is "yes," because the conventional boundary or threshold that demarcates the plausible from the implausible is five times per hundred, which is represented by a *P* value of .05. This boundary is dignified by long tradition, although other choices of boundary could be equally reasonable. We call results that fall beyond this boundary (that is, *P* value <.05) *statistically significant*. The meaning of statistically significant, therefore, is "sufficiently unlikely to be due to chance alone that we are ready to reject the null hypothesis."

Let us repeat our experiment twice more, both times with a new coin. On the first repetition we obtain eight heads and two tails. Calculation of the *P* value associated with an 8/2 split tells us that, if the coin were unbiased, results as or more extreme than 8/2 (or 2/8) would occur solely as a result of the play of chance 11 times per hundred ($P = .11$). We have crossed to the other side of the conventional boundary between what is plausible and what is implausible. If we accept the convention, the results are not statistically significant and we will not reject the null hypothesis.

On our final repetition of the experiment, we obtain seven tails and three heads. Experience tells us that such a result, although not the most common, would not be unusual even if the coin were unbiased. The *P* value confirms our intuition: results as extreme as or more extreme than this 7/3 split would occur under the null hypothesis 34 times per hundred (*P* = .34). Again, we will not reject the null hypothesis.

Although medical research is concerned with questions other than determining whether coins are unbiased, the reasoning associated with the *P* values reported in journal articles is applicable. When investigators compare two treatments, the question they ask is, "How likely is the observed difference due to chance alone?" If we accept the conventional boundary or threshold (*P* < .05), we will reject the null hypothesis and conclude that the treatment has some effect when the answer to this question is that repetitions of the experiment would yield differences as extreme as or more extreme than those we have observed less than 5% of the time.

Let us return to the example of the randomized trial in which investigators compared enalapril to the combination of hydralazine and nitrates in 804 men with heart failure. Results of this study illustrate hypothesis testing using a dichotomous (yes/no) outcome—in this case, mortality.[1] During the follow-up period, which ranged from 6 months to 5.7 years, 132 of 403 patients (33%) assigned to enalapril died, as did 153 of 401 (38%) of those assigned to hydralazine and nitrates. Application of a statistical test that compares proportions (the *chi-square test*) reveals that if there were actually no difference in mortality between the two groups, differences as large or larger than those actually seen would be expected 11 times per 100 (*P* = .11). Using the hypothesis-testing framework and the conventional threshold of *P* < .05, we would conclude that we cannot reject the null hypothesis and that the difference observed is compatible with chance.

THE RISK OF A FALSE-NEGATIVE RESULT

A clinician might comment on the results of the comparison of treatment with enalapril with that of a combination of hydralazine and nitrates as follows: "Although I accept the 5% threshold and therefore agree that we cannot reject the null hypothesis, I am nevertheless still suspicious that enalapril results in a lower mortality than does the combination of hydralazine and nitrates. The experiment still leaves me in a state of uncertainty." In making these statements, the clinician recognizes a second type of error that an investigator can make: falsely concluding that an effective treatment is useless. A *type II error* occurs when one erroneously dismisses an actual treatment effect—and a potentially useful treatment.

In the comparison of enalapril with hydralazine and nitrates, the possibility of erroneously concluding there is no difference between the two treatments looms large. The investigators found that 5% fewer patients receiving enalapril died than those receiving the alternative vasodilator regimen. If the true difference in mortality really were 5%, we would readily conclude that patients will receive an important benefit if we prescribe enalapril. Despite this, we were unable to reject the null hypothesis.

Why is it that the investigators observed an important difference between the mortality rates and yet were unable to conclude that enalapril is superior to hydralazine and nitrates? The answer is that their study did not enroll enough patients to warrant confidence that the important difference they observed is a real difference. The likelihood of missing an important difference (and, therefore, of making a type II error) decreases as the sample size gets larger. When a study is at high risk of making a type II error, we say it has inadequate power. The larger the sample size, the lower the risk of type II error and the greater the power. Although the 804 patients recruited by the investigators conducting the vasodilator trial may sound like a substantial number, for dichotomous outcomes such as mortality, very large sample sizes often are required to detect small treatment effects. For example, researchers conducting the trials that established the optimal treatment of acute myocardial infarction with thrombolytic agents both anticipated and found absolute differences between treatment and control mortality of less than 5%. Because of these small absolute differences between treatment and control they required—and recruited—thousands of patients to ensure adequate power.

Whenever a trial has failed to reject the null hypothesis (ie, when $P > .05$), the investigators may have missed a true treatment effect, and you should consider whether the power of the trial was adequate. In these negative studies, the stronger the nonsignificant trend in favor of the experimental treatment, the more likely it is that the investigators missed a true treatment effect.[2] Another section in this book describes how to decide if a study is large enough (see Part 2C, "Therapy and Understanding the Results, Confidence Intervals").

Some studies are not designed to determine whether a new treatment is better than the current one, but, rather, whether a treatment that is less expensive, easier to administer, or less toxic yields more or less the same treatment effect as standard therapy. Such studies are often referred to as *equivalence studies*.[3] In equivalence studies, considering whether investigators have recruited an adequate sample size to make sure they will not miss small but important treatment effects is even more important. If the sample size of an equivalence study is inadequate, the investigator runs the risk of concluding that the treatments are equivalent when, in fact, patients given standard therapy derive important benefits in comparison to the easier, less expensive, or less toxic alternative.

AN EXAMPLE USING A CONTINUOUS MEASURE OF OUTCOME

To this point, all of our examples have used outcomes such as yes/no, heads or tails, or dying or not dying, all of which we can express as a proportion. Often, investigators compare the effects of two or more treatments using a variable such as spirometric measurements, cardiac output, creatinine clearance, or score on a quality-of-life questionnaire. We call such variables, in which results can take a large number of values with small differences between those values, continuous variables.

The study of enalapril vs hydralazine and nitrates in patients with heart failure described above[1] provides an example of the use of a *continuous variable* as an outcome in a hypothesis test. The investigators compared the effect of the two regimens on exercise capacity. In contrast to the effect on mortality, which favored enalapril, exercise capacity improved with hydralazine and nitrates but not with enalapril. Using a test (the *t* test) appropriate for continuous variables, the investigators compared the changes in exercise capacity from baseline to 6 months in the patients receiving hydralazine and nitrates to those changes in the enalapril group over the same period of time. Exercise capacity in the hydralazine group improved more, and the differences between the two groups are unlikely to have occurred by chance ($P = .02$).

TAKING ACCOUNT OF BASELINE DIFFERENCES

Readers will often find that investigators have conducted their hypothesis tests taking account of baseline differences in the groups under study—an *adjusted analysis*. Randomization, a process whereby chance alone dictates to which group a patient is allocated, generally produces comparable groups. If, however, the investigator is unlucky, prognostic factors that determine outcome might have substantially different distributions in the two groups. For example, in a trial in which it is known that older patients have a poorer outcome, a larger proportion of the older patients may be randomly allocated to one of the two treatments being compared. Since older patients are at greater risk of adverse events, an imbalance in age could threaten the validity of an analysis that did not take age into account. The adjusted test yields a P value corrected for differences in the age distribution of the two groups. In this example, readers can consider that investigators are providing them with the probability that would have been generated had the age distribution in the two groups been the same. Investigators can make adjustments for several variables at once, and you can interpret the P value in the same way as we have already explained.

MULTIPLE TESTS

University students have long been popular subjects for all sorts of experiments. In keeping with this tradition, we have chosen medical students as the subjects for our next hypothetical experiment.

Picture a medical school in which two instructors teach an introductory course on medical statistics. One instructor is more popular than the other instructor. The dean of the medical school has no substitute for the less popular faculty member. She has a particular passion for fairness and decides that she will deal with the situation by assigning the 200 medical students in her first-year class to one instructor or the other by a process of random allocation through which each student has an equal chance (50%) of being allocated to one of the two instructors.

The instructors decide to take advantage of this decision and illustrate some important principles of medical statistics. They therefore ask the question: are there characteristics of the two groups of students that differ beyond a level that could be explained by the play of chance? The characteristics they choose include sex distribution, eye color, height, grade-point average in the last year of college before entering medical school, socioeconomic status, and favorite type of music. The instructors formulate null hypotheses for each of their tests. For instance, the null hypothesis associated with sex distribution is as follows: the students are drawn from the same group of people and, therefore, the true proportion of females in the two groups is identical. You will note that, in fact, the students were drawn from the same underlying population and were assigned to the two groups by random allocation. The null hypothesis in each case is true; therefore, any time in this experiment in which the hypothesis is rejected will represent a false-positive result.

The instructors survey their students to determine their status on each of the six variables of interest. For five of these variables they find that the distributions are similar in the two groups, and all of the P values associated with formal tests of the differences between groups are >.10. The instructors find that for eye color, however, 25 of 100 students in one group have blue eyes, whereas 38 of 100 in the other group have blue eyes. A formal statistical analysis reveals that if the null hypothesis were true (which it is), then differences in the proportion of people with blue eyes in the two groups as large or larger than the difference observed would occur slightly less than five times per 100 repetitions of the experiment. Using the conventional boundary, the instructors would reject the null hypothesis.

How likely is it that in testing six independent hypotheses on the same two groups of students, the instructors would have found at least one that crossed the threshold of 0.05 by chance alone? By *independent* we mean that the result of a test of one hypothesis does not depend in any way on the results of tests of any of the other hypotheses. Since our likelihood of crossing the significance threshold for any one characteristic is 0.05, the likelihood of not crossing the threshold for that same characteristic is $1.0 - 0.05$, or 0.95. When two hypotheses are tested, the probability that neither one would cross the threshold would be 0.95 multiplied by 0.95 (or the square of 0.95); when six hypotheses are tested, the probability that not a single one would cross the 5% threshold is 0.95 to the sixth power, or 74%. When six independent hypotheses are tested, the probability that at least one result is statistically significant is therefore 26% (100% – 74%)—or approximately one in four, rather than one in 20. If we wished to maintain our overall standard of 0.05, we would have to divide the threshold P value by six so each of the six tests would use a boundary value of 0.008.

The message here is twofold. First, rare findings do occasionally happen by chance. Even with a single test, a finding with a P value of .01 will happen 1% of the time. Second, one should beware of multiple hypothesis testing that may yield misleading results. Examples of this phenomenon abound in the clinical literature. For example, in a survey of 45 trials from three leading medical journals, Pocock et al found that the median number of endpoints mentioned was six, and most were tested for statistical significance.[2]

We find a specific example of the dangers of use of multiple endpoints in a randomized trial of the effect of rehabilitation on quality of life after myocardial infarction. In this study, investigators randomized patients to receive standard care, an exercise program, or a counseling program, and they obtained patient reports on work, leisure, sexual activity, satisfaction with outcome, compliance with advice, quality of leisure and work, psychiatric symptoms, cardiac symptoms, and general health.[4] For almost all of these variables, there was no difference among the three groups. However, at follow-up after 18 months, patients were more satisfied with the exercise regimen than with the other two regimens, families in the counseling group were less protective than in the other groups, and patients participating in the counseling group worked more hours and had sexual intercourse more frequently. Does this mean that both exercise and rehabilitation programs should be implemented because of the small number of outcomes that changed in their favor, or that they should be rejected because most of the outcomes showed no difference? The authors themselves concluded that their results did not support the effectiveness of rehabilitation in improving quality of life. However, a program's advocate might argue that if even some of the ratings favored treatment, the intervention is worthwhile. The use of multiple instruments opens the door to such potential controversy.

A number of statistical strategies exist for dealing with the issue of testing multiple hypotheses on the same data set. We have illustrated one of these in a previous example: dividing the P value by the number of tests. One can also specify, before the study is undertaken, a single primary outcome on which the major conclusions of the study will hinge. A third approach is to derive a single global test statistic (a pooled effect size, for instance) that effectively combines the multiple outcomes into a single measure. Full discussion of these strategies for dealing with multiple outcomes is beyond the scope of this book, but the interested reader can find a cogent discussion elsewhere.[5]

LIMITATIONS OF HYPOTHESIS TESTING

At this point, some clinicians may be entertaining a number of questions that leave them uneasy. Why, for example, use a single cutpoint when the choice of a cutpoint is so arbitrary? Why dichotomize the question of whether a treatment is effective into a yes/no issue, when it may be viewed more appropriately as a continuum (eg, from, for instance, very unlikely to be effective to almost certainly effective)?

We believe that clinicians asking these questions are on the right track. They can look to another part of this book (see Part 2C, "Therapy and Understanding the Results, Confidence Intervals") for an explanation of why we consider an alternative to hypothesis testing a superior approach.

References

1. Cohn JN, Johnson G, Ziesche S, et al. A comparison of enalapril with hydralazine-isosorbide dinitrate in the treatment of chronic congestive heart failure. *N Engl J Med*. 1991;325:303-310.

2. Detsky AS, Sackett DL. When was a "negative" trial big enough? How many patients you needed depends on what you found. *Arch Intern Med*. 1985;145:709-715.

3. Kirshner B. Methodological standards for assessing therapeutic equivalence. *J Clin Epidemiol*. 1991;44:839-849.

4. Mayou R, MacMahon D, Sleight P, Florencio MJ. Early rehabilitation after myocardial infarction. *Lancet*. 1981;2:1399-1401.

5. Pocock SJ, Geller NL, Tsiatis AA. The analysis of multiple endpoints in clinical trials. *Biometrics*. 1987;43:487-498.

THERAPY AND UNDERSTANDING THE RESULTS
Confidence Intervals

Gordon Guyatt, Stephen Walter, Deborah Cook, and Roman Jaeschke

The following EBM Working Group members also made substantive contributions to this section: Mark Wilson and Martin Stockler

IN THIS SECTION

Hypothesis testing involves estimating the probability that observed results would have occurred by chance if a *null hypothesis*, which most commonly states that there is no difference between a treatment condition and a control condition, were true (see Part 2B, "Therapy and Understanding the Results, Hypothesis Testing"). Health researchers and medical educators have increasingly recognized the limitations of hypothesis testing; consequently, an alternative approach, estimation, is becoming more popular. A number of authors[1-5] have outlined the concepts that we will introduce here, and you can use the full expanse of their discussions to supplement our presentation. We will illustrate the concepts with an example introduced earlier in this book (see Part 2B, "Therapy and Understanding the Results, Hypothesis Testing").

HOW SHOULD WE TREAT PATIENTS WITH HEART FAILURE? A PROBLEM IN INTERPRETING STUDY RESULTS

In a double-blind randomized controlled trial of 804 men with heart failure, investigators compared treatment with enalapril to that with a combination of hydralazine and nitrates.[6] In the follow-up period, which ranged from 6 months to 5.7 years, 132 of 403 patients (33%) assigned to receive enalapril died, as did 153 of 401 patients (38%) assigned to receive hydralazine and nitrates. The *P* value associated with the difference in mortality is .11.

Looking at this study as an exercise in hypothesis testing (see Part 2B, "Therapy and Understanding the Results, Hypothesis Testing") and adopting the usual 5% risk of obtaining a false-positive result, we would conclude that chance cannot be excluded as an explanation of the study results. We would classify this as a negative study (ie, we would conclude that no important difference existed between the treatment and control groups). The investigators also conducted an analysis that compared not only the proportion of patients surviving at the end of the study, but also the time pattern of the deaths occurring in both groups. This survival analysis, which generally is more sensitive than the test of the difference in proportions (see Part 2D, "Therapy and Understanding the Results, Measures of Association"), showed a nonsignificant P value of .08, a result that leads to the same conclusion as the simpler analysis that focused on results at the end of the study. However, the authors also tell us that the P value associated with differences in mortality at 2 years ("a point predetermined to be a major endpoint of the trial") was significant at .016.

At this point, clinicians could be excused for being a little confused. Ask yourself: is this a positive study dictating use of an angiotensin-converting enzyme (ACE) inhibitor instead of the combination of hydralazine and nitrates, or is it a negative study, showing no difference between the two regimens and leaving the choice of drugs open?

SOLVING THE PROBLEM: WHAT ARE CONFIDENCE INTERVALS?

How can clinicians deal with the limitations of hypothesis testing and resolve the confusion? The solution comes from an alternative approach that does not ask about how compatible the results are with the null hypothesis, or whether the P values differ significantly. By contrast, this approach poses two questions: (1) what is the single value most likely to represent the true difference between treatment and control?

and (2) given the observed difference between treatment and control, what is the plausible range of differences between them within which the true difference might actually lie? This second question can be answered using *confidence intervals*. Before applying them to resolve the issue of enalapril vs hydralazine and nitrates in patients with heart failure, we will illustrate the use of confidence intervals with a coin-toss experiment.

Suppose that we have a coin that may or may not be balanced. That is, although it may be that the true probability of heads on any individual coin toss is 0.5, it may also be that the true probability is as high as 1.0 in favor of heads (every toss will yield heads) or 1.0 in favor of tails (every toss will yield tails). We now decide to conduct an experiment to determine the true nature of the coin.

We begin by tossing the coin twice, observing one head and one tail. At this point, what is our best estimate of the probability of heads on any given coin toss? Is it the value we have obtained (otherwise known as the *point estimate*), which is 0.5? What is the plausible range within which the true probability of finding a head on any individual coin toss might lie? This range is very wide, and most people would think that the probability might still be as high or higher than 0.9—or as low as or lower than 0.1. In other words, if the true probability of heads on any given coin toss is 0.9, it would still not be terribly surprising if, in any sample of two coin tosses, one were heads and one were tails. Hence, after our two coin tosses we are not much further ahead in determining the true nature of the coin.

We proceed with eight additional coin tosses; after a total of 10 tosses, we have observed five heads and five tails. Our best estimate of the true probability of heads on any given coin toss remains 0.5, the point estimate. The range within which the true probability of heads might plausibly lie has narrowed, however. It is no longer plausible that the true probability of heads is as great as 0.9. That is, if the true probability were 0.9, it would be very unlikely that in a sample of 10 coin tosses, one would observe five tails. People's sense of the range of probabilities that might still be plausible may differ, but most would agree that a probability greater than 0.8 or less than 0.2 is very unlikely.

After 10 coin tosses, values between 0.2 and 0.8 are not all equally plausible. The most likely value for the probability is the point estimate, 0.5, but probabilities close to that point estimate (0.4 or 0.6, for instance) are also quite likely. The further the probability from the point estimate, the less likely it is that the value represents the truth.

Ten coin tosses have still left us with considerable uncertainty about our coin, so we conduct another 40 repetitions. After 50 coin tosses, we have observed 25 heads and 25 tails and our point estimate remains 0.5. We are now beginning to believe that the coin is very unlikely to be extremely biased, and our estimate of the range of probabilities, which is still reasonably consistent with 25 heads in 50 coin tosses, might be 0.35 to 0.65. This range still is quite wide and we may persist with another 50 repetitions. If after 100 tosses we observed 50 heads, we might guess that the true probability is unlikely to be more extreme than 0.40 or 0.60. If we were willing to endure the tedium of 1000 coin tosses and if we observed 500 heads, we would be very confident (but still not certain) that our coin is minimally, if at all, biased.

What we have done through this experiment is to use common sense to generate confidence intervals around an observed proportion, 0.5. In each case, the confidence interval represents the range within which the truth plausibly lies. The smaller the sample size, the wider the confidence interval. As the sample size gets very large, we become increasingly certain that the truth is not far from the point estimate we have calculated from our experiment and the confidence interval is smaller.

It is fortunate that, since people's common sense differs considerably, we can turn to statistical techniques for precise estimation of confidence intervals. To use these techniques, we must first be a little more specific about what we mean by "plausible." In our coin-toss example, we might ask "what is the range of probabilities within which, 95% of the time, the truth would lie?" Table 2C-1 presents the actual 95% confidence intervals around the observed proportion of 0.5 for our experiment. If we need not be quite so certain, we could ask about the range within which the true value would lie 90% of the time. This 90% confidence interval, also presented in Table 2C-1, is somewhat narrower.

TABLE 2C-1

Confidence Intervals Around a Proportion of 0.5 in a Coin-Toss Experiment

Number of Coin Tosses	Observed Result	95% Confidence Interval	90% Confidence Interval
2	1 head, 1 tail	0.01–0.99	0.03–0.98
10	5 heads, 5 tails	0.19–0.81	0.22–0.78
50	25 heads, 25 tails	0.36–0.65	0.38–0.62
100	50 heads, 50 tails	0.40–0.60	0.41–0.59
1000	500 heads, 500 tails	0.47–0.53	0.47–0.53

The coin-toss example also illustrates how the confidence interval tells you whether the study is large enough to answer the research question. If you wanted to be reasonably sure that the bias was no greater than 10% (that is, the ends of the confidence interval are within 10% of the point estimate), you would need approximately 100 coin tosses. If you needed greater precision—with 3% in either direction—

1000 coin tosses would be required. All you have to do to obtain greater precision is to make more measurements. In clinical research, this involves enrolling more patients or increasing the number of measurements in each patient who is enrolled.

USING CONFIDENCE INTERVALS TO INTERPRET THE RESULTS OF CLINICAL TRIALS

How do confidence intervals help us interpret the results of the trial of vasodilators in patients with heart failure? The mortality in the ACE inhibitor arm was 33% and in the hydralazine plus nitrate group it was 38%, an absolute difference of 5%. The difference of 5% is the point estimate, our best single estimate of the mortality benefit from using an ACE inhibitor. The 95% confidence interval around this difference works out to −1.2% to 12%.

How can we now interpret the study results? The most likely value for the mortality difference between the two vasodilator regimens is 5%, but the true difference may be as high as 1.2% in favor of the combination of hydralazine and nitrates or as high as 12% in favor of the ACE inhibitor. Values progressively farther from 5% will be less and less probable. We can conclude that patients offered ACE inhibitors will most likely (but not certainly) die later than patients offered hydralazine and nitrates—but the magnitude of the difference may be either trivial or quite large. This way of understanding the results avoids the yes/no dichotomy of hypothesis testing and the possible consequences of spending time and energy deciding about the legitimacy of the authors' focus on mortality at 2 years. It also obviates the need to argue whether the study should be considered positive or negative. One can conclude that, all else being equal, an ACE inhibitor is the appropriate choice for patients with heart failure, but the strength of this inference is weak. Toxicity, expense, and evidence from other studies would all bear on the final treatment decision (see Part 1F, "Moving From Evidence to Action"). Since a number of large randomized trials have now shown a mortality benefit from ACE inhibitors in patients with heart failure,[7] one can confidently recommend this class of agents as the treatment of choice.

INTERPRETING APPARENTLY "NEGATIVE" TRIALS

Another example of the use of confidence intervals in interpreting study results comes from the results of the Swedish Co-operative Stroke Study, a randomized trial that was designed to determine whether patients with cerebral infarction might have fewer subsequent strokes if they took aspirin.[8,9] The investigators gave placebos to 252 patients, of whom 18 (7%) subsequently had nonfatal stroke. They also gave aspirin to 253 patients, of whom 23 (9%) had recurrent nonfatal stroke. The point estimate from these results is a 2% increase in the incidence of strokes among those patients in the aspirin group.

This trial of more than 500 patients might appear to exclude any possible benefit from aspirin. The 95% confidence interval on the absolute difference of 2% in favor of placebo, however, is from 7% in favor of placebo to 3% in favor of aspirin. Were the truth that 3% of the patients who would otherwise have strokes been spared had they taken aspirin, many patients would want to receive that drug.

This would represent a 43% relative risk reduction, suggesting that we would need to treat only 33 patients to prevent a stroke. One can thus conclude that the trial has not excluded a patient-important benefit and, in that sense, was not large enough.

This example emphasizes that many patients must participate if trials are to generate precise estimates of treatment effects. In addition, it illustrates why we recommend that, whenever possible, clinicians turn to systematic reviews that pool data from the most valid studies.[10] In this case, such an overview shows that administration of antiplatelet agents in patients with transient ischemic attack or stroke reduces the relative risk of subsequent events by approximately 25% (with confidence intervals ranging from approximately 19% to 31%).[11] Given these data, many patients whose event rates without treatment would be over 10% (a number needed to treat of 50 or less) or even 5% (a number needed to treat of 100 or less) would be enthusiastic about taking aspirin.

This example also illustrates that when you see an apparently negative trial (one that, in our previous hypothesis-testing framework, fails to exclude the null hypothesis), you can focus on the upper end of the confidence interval (that is, the end that suggests the largest benefit from treatment). If the upper boundary of the confidence interval excludes any important benefit of treatment, you can conclude the trial is definitively negative. If, on the other hand, the confidence interval includes an important benefit, the possibility has not been ruled out that the treatment still might be worthwhile.

This logic of the negative trial is crucial in the interpretation of studies designed to help determine whether we should substitute a treatment that is less expensive, easier to administer, or less toxic for an existing treatment. In such an *equivalence study,* we will be ready to make the substitution only if we are sure that the standard treatment does not have important additional benefit beyond the less expensive or more convenient substitute. We will be confident that we have excluded the possibility of important additional benefit of the standard treatment if the upper boundary of the confidence interval around the difference is below our threshold.

INTERPRETING APPARENTLY "POSITIVE" TRIALS

How can confidence intervals be informative in a positive trial (one that, in the previous hypothesis-testing framework, makes chance an unlikely explanation for observed differences between treatments)? In another double-blind randomized controlled trial of patients with heart failure, treatment with enalapril was compared to that with placebo.[12] Of 1285 patients randomized to the ACE inhibitor, 613 (48%) died or were hospitalized for accelerated heart failure, whereas 736 (57%) of 1284 patients in the placebo group experienced one of these adverse outcomes. The point estimate of the difference in death or hospitalization for heart failure is 10%, and the 95% confidence interval is 6% to 14%. Thus, the smallest effect of the ACE inhibitor that is compatible with the data is a 6% reduction in the number of patients with the adverse outcomes. If you consider it worthwhile to treat 17 patients to prevent one patient from dying or developing heart failure (6% is equivalent to about one in 17), then this represents a definitive trial. If, before treating, you would require a greater reduction than 6% in the proportion of patients who are spared an adverse advent, a larger trial (with a correspondingly narrower confidence interval) would be required.

WAS THE TRIAL LARGE ENOUGH?

As implied in our discussion to this point, confidence intervals provide a way of answering the question: "Was the trial large enough?" We illustrate the approach in Figure 2C-1. In this figure, we present the distribution of randomized trial results you would expect from two treatments—one that results in an absolute reduction in mortality of 5% and one that results in an absolute increase in mortality of 1%. The vertical line in the center of the figure represents an absolute risk reduction of zero, when the experimental and control groups have exactly the same mortality. Values to the right of the vertical line represent results in which the treated group had a lower mortality than the control group. Values to the left of the vertical line represent results in which the treated group fared worse and had a higher mortality rate than the control group.

FIGURE 2C-1

Deciding Whether a Trial Is Definitive: Distributions of the Results of Trials of Two Therapies

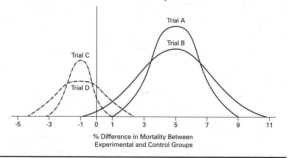

A represents the results of large trials of a therapy with an absolute mortality reduction of 5%; **B** represents the results of smaller trials of a therapy with an absolute reduction in mortality of 5%; **C** represents the results of large trials of a therapy with an absolute mortality increase of 1%; **D** represents the results of smaller trials of a therapy with an absolute reduction in mortality increase of 1%.

Reproduced with permission from the Canadian Medical Association.

For each of the two treatments, we present two distributions of results: one for a set of trials with a relatively small sample size, and one for a set of trials with a relatively large sample size. For each of the four distributions, the highest point of the distribution represents the underlying truth, the actual change in mortality. Distributions A and B come from the trials of the therapy that reduced mortality by 5%, and distributions C and D come from trials of the therapy that increased mortality by 1%.

Now, suppose we assume that absolute reductions in mortality greater than 1% warrant treatment. That is, the benefits outweigh the risks and costs whenever the absolute reduction in risk is 1% or greater (see Part 1F, "Moving From Evidence to Action"), whereas reductions less than 1% do not warrant treatment (that is, the risks outweigh the benefits). For instance, if experimental treatment results in a true reduction in mortality from 5% to less than 4%, we would want to use the treatment. If, on the other hand, the true reduction in mortality was 5% to 4.5%, we would consider that the experimental treatment was not worth the associated toxicity and expense. What implications does this have for the way we will interpret the results of studies of this treatment?

In distribution A, more than 95% of the distribution lies above an absolute risk reduction of 1% (distribution A, like the others, depicts a simplified presentation of the situation—probabilities never actually sink to zero). Based on trials of this therapy and on this sample size, 95% confidence intervals would, in most instances, exclude an absolute risk reduction as small as 1%. In such trials, we could be confident that the true treatment effect is above our threshold, 1%, and we have a definitive positive trial. That is, we would be very confident that the true reduction in risk is greater than 1% (and, most likely, is appreciably greater), suggesting that many patients would be interested in receiving the treatment. The sample size in such trials would be adequate to demonstrate that the treatment provides a clinically important benefit.

Distribution B also comes from trials of a therapy that reduces mortality by 5%, but these trials include fewer patients. Whereas some of these trials would exclude the null hypothesis (that is, no difference is assumed between the treatment and control groups), many of the 95% confidence intervals would include mortality reductions less than 1%. When the 95% confidence interval includes values less than 1%, the data are consistent with an absolute risk reduction less than 1%. For such trials, we are left in doubt that the treatment effect is really greater than our threshold. Such trials would still be perceived as positive, but their results would not be definitive. The sample size of these trials would be inadequate to definitively establish the appropriateness of administering the experimental treatment.

Distribution C shows the results of a set of trials, all of which would be negative in that they would not exclude the null hypothesis of "no treatment effect." On average, investigators conducting these trials would observe a mortality rate that was 1% higher in the treatment group than in the control group. Most such trials would generate a narrow 95% confidence interval, all of which would lie to the left of our 1% threshold. The fact that the upper limit of the confidence interval is less than 1% would mean that we can be very confident that, if there is a benefit, it is very small and is unlikely to be appreciably greater than the risks, costs, and inconvenience of therapy. These trials would therefore exclude any patient-important benefit of treatment and they could be considered definitive. We would therefore dismiss the experimental treatment—at least for this type of population.

Distribution D comes from the same therapy as is reflected in distribution C, in which the mortality is 1% higher in the experimental group than in the control group. Distribution D, however, depicts trials with smaller sample size and, consequently, a much wider distribution of results. Because the confidence interval of most of these trials would include an appreciable portion that lies above our 1% threshold, we would conclude that it remains plausible (though unlikely) that the true effect of the experimental treatment is a reduction in mortality greater than 1%. Although we would still refrain from using this treatment (indeed, we would conclude it most likely kills people), we would not totally dismiss it. Most trials from distribution D, therefore, would not be definitive, and we would require larger trials enrolling more patients to exclude a clinically important treatment effect.

CONCLUSION

We can restate our message as follows: in a positive trial establishing that the effect of treatment is greater than zero, look to the lower boundary of the confidence interval to determine whether sample size has been adequate. If this lower boundary—the smallest plausible treatment effect compatible with the data—is greater than the smallest difference that you consider important, the sample size is adequate and the trial is definitive. If the lower boundary is less than this smallest important difference, the trial is nondefinitive and further trials are required.

In a negative trial, look to the upper boundary of the confidence interval to determine whether sample size has been adequate. If this upper boundary, the largest treatment effect compatible with the data, is less than the smallest difference that you consider important, the sample size is adequate and the trial is definitively negative. If the upper boundary exceeds the smallest important difference, there may still be an important positive treatment effect, the trial is nondefinitive, and further trials are required.

References

1. Simon R. Confidence intervals for reporting results of clinical trials. *Ann Intern Med.* 1986;105:429-435.

2. Gardner MJ, Altman DG, eds. *Statistics With Confidence: Confidence Intervals and Statistical Guidelines*. London: BMJ Publishing Group; 1989.

3. Bulpitt CJ. Confidence intervals. *Lancet.* 1987;1:494-497.

4. Pocock SJ, Hughes MD. Estimation issues in clinical trials and overviews. *Stat Med.* 1990;9:657-671.

5. Braitman LE. Confidence intervals assess both clinical significance and statistical significance. *Ann Intern Med.* 1991;114:515-517.

6. Cohn JN, Johnson G, Ziesche S, et al. A comparison of enalapril with hydralazine-isosorbide dinitrate in the treatment of chronic congestive heart failure. *N Engl J Med.* 1991;325:303-310.

7. Garg R, Yusuf S. Overview of randomized trials of angiotensin-converting enzyme inhibitors on mortality and morbidity in patients with heart failure. Collaborative Group on ACE Inhibitor Trials. *JAMA.* 1995;273:1450-1456.

8. Britton M, Helmers C, Samuelsson K. High-dose salicylic acid after cerebral infarction: a Swedish co-operative study. *Stroke.* 1997;18:325.

9. Sackett DL, Haynes RB, Guyatt GH, Tugwell P. *Clinical Epidemiology; A Basic Science for Clinical Medicine*. Boston: Little, Brown and Company; 1991:218-220.

10. Oxman AD, Guyatt GH. Guidelines for reading literature reviews. *CMAJ.* 1988;138:697-703.

11. Antiplatelet Trialists' Collaboration. Secondary prevention of vascular disease by prolonged antiplatelet treatment. *BMJ.* 1988;296:320-331.

12. The SOLVD Investigators. Effect of enalapril on survival in patients with reduced left ventricular ejection fractions and congestive heart failure. *N Engl J Med.* 1991;325:293-302.

THERAPY AND UNDERSTANDING THE RESULTS
Measures of Association

Roman Jaeschke, Gordon Guyatt, Alexandra Barratt, Stephen Walter, Deborah Cook, Finlay McAlister, and John Attia

Sharon Straus also made substantive contributions to this section

IN THIS SECTION

When clinicians consider the results of clinical trials, they are interested in the association between a treatment and an outcome. The study under consideration may or may not demonstrate an association between treatment and outcome; for example, it may or may not demonstrate a decrease in the risk of adverse events in patients receiving experimental treatment.

The focus of this section is on yes/no or dichotomous outcomes like death, stroke, or myocardial infarction. In their presentation of the results of studies addressing intervention effects on dichotomous outcomes, authors generally include the proportion of patients in each group who suffered an adverse event. As depicted in Figure 2D-1, consider three different treatments that reduce mortality administered to three different populations. The first treatment, administered to a population with a 30% risk of dying, reduces the risk to 20%. The second treatment, administered to a population with a 10% risk of dying, reduces the risk to 6.7%. The third treatment reduces the risk of dying from 1% to 0.67%.

FIGURE 2D-1

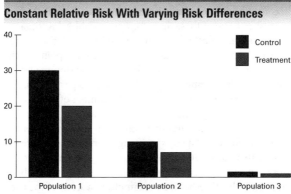

Constant Relative Risk With Varying Risk Differences

Although all three treatments reduce the risk of dying by a third, this piece of information is not adequate to fully capture the impact of treatment. Expressing the strength of the association as a *relative risk (RR)*, a *relative risk reduction (RRR)*, an *absolute risk reduction (ARR)* or *risk difference (RD)*, an *odds ratio (OR)*, or a *number needed to treat (NNT)* or *number need to harm (NNH)* conveys a variety of different information.

DICHOTOMOUS AND CONTINUOUS OUTCOMES

A study's primary analysis often is concerned with the proportion of patients who suffer a particular target outcome, endpoint, or event in the treatment and control groups. This is true whenever the outcome captures the presence or absence of negative events like stroke, myocardial infarction, cancer recurrence, or death. It is also true for positive events like ulcer healing or resolution of symptoms. Even if the outcome is not one of these dichotomous variables, investigators sometimes elect to present the results as if this were the case. For example, investigators may present endpoints such as the duration of exercise time before the development of chest pain, the number of episodes of angina per month, the change in pulmonary function, or the number of visits to the emergency department as the mean values in the two groups. Alternatively, they may transform these variables into dichotomous data by specifying a threshold or degree of change that constitutes an important improvement or deterioration and then examine the proportion of patients above and below this threshold. For example, in a study of the use of forced expiratory volume in 1 second (FEV_1) in the assessment of the efficacy of oral corticosteroids in patients with chronic stable airflow limitation, investigators defined an event as an improvement in FEV_1 over baseline of more than 20%.[1] In another study in patients with chronic lung disease, investigators examined the difference in the proportion of patients who achieved an important improvement in health-related quality of life.[2] The investigators' choice of the magnitude of change required to designate an improvement as "important" can affect the apparent effectiveness of the treatment (although less so for odds ratios, discussed later in this section, than for the other measures of association).

THE 2 X 2 TABLE

Table 2D-1 depicts a 2 x 2 table that captures the information for a dichotomous outcome of a clinical trial. For instance, in a randomized trial, investigators compared mortality rates in patients with bleeding esophageal varices controlled either by endoscopic ligation or endoscopic sclerotherapy.[3] After a mean follow-up of 10 months, 18 of 64 participants assigned to ligation died, as did 29 of 65 patients assigned to sclerotherapy (Table 2D-2).

TABLE 2D-1

The 2 x 2 Table

		Outcome	
		Yes	No
Exposure	Yes	a	b
	No	c	d

Relative Risk (RR) $\quad = \quad \dfrac{a/(a + b)}{c/(c + d)}$

Relative Risk Reduction (RRR) $\quad = \quad \dfrac{c/(c + d) - a/(a + b)}{c/(c + d)}$

Absolute Risk Reduction (ARR) $\quad = \quad \dfrac{c}{c + d} - \dfrac{a}{a + b}$

Number Needed to Treat (NNT) $\quad = \quad \dfrac{1}{ARR}$

Odds Ratio (OR) $\quad = \quad \dfrac{a/b}{c/d} = \dfrac{ad}{cb}$

TABLE 2D-2

Results From a Randomized Trial of Endoscopic Sclerotherapy as Compared With Endoscopic Ligation for Bleeding Esophageal Varices*

		Outcome		
		Death	**Survival**	**Total**
Exposure	Ligation	18	46	64
	Sclerotherapy	29	36	65

Relative Risk (RR) = 0.63

Relative Risk Reduction (RRR) = 0.37

Absolute Risk Reduction (ARR) = 0.165

Number Needed to Treat (NNT) = 6

Odds Ratio (OR) = 0.49

* Data from reference 3.

THE ABSOLUTE RISK

The simplest measure of association to understand is the *absolute risk*. The absolute risk of dying in the ligation group is 28% (18/64, or $a/a+b$), and the absolute risk of dying in the sclerotherapy group is 45% (29/65, or $c/c+d$). We often refer to the risk of the adverse outcome in the control group as the *baseline risk* or *control event rate*.

THE ABSOLUTE RISK REDUCTION

One can relate these two absolute risks by calculating the difference between them. We refer to this difference as the *absolute risk reduction* (ARR) or the risk difference (RD). Algebraically, the formula for calculating the ARR or RD is $[a/(a+c)]-[b/(b+d)]$ (see Table 2D-1). This measure of effect tells us what proportion of patients are spared the adverse outcome if they receive the experimental therapy, rather than the control therapy. In our example, the ARR is 0.446 − 0.281, or 0.165 (ie, an ARR of 16.5%).

THE RELATIVE RISK

Another way to relate the absolute risks in the two groups is to take the ratio of the two; this is called the *relative risk* or *risk ratio (RR)*. The RR tells us the proportion of the original risk (in this case, the risk of death with sclerotherapy) that is still present when patients receive the experimental treatment (in this case, ligation). Looking at our 2 x 2 tables, the formula for this calculation is $[a/(a+c)]/[b/(b+d)]$ (see Table 2D-1). In our example, the RR of dying after receiving initial ligation versus sclerotherapy is 18/64 (the risk in the ligation group) divided by 29/65 (the risk in the sclerotherapy group), or 63%. In other words, we would say the risk of death with ligation is about two thirds of that with sclerotherapy.

THE RELATIVE RISK REDUCTION

Another measure used when assessing effectiveness of treatment is the *relative risk reduction (RRR)*. An estimate of the proportion of baseline risk that is removed by the therapy, it is calculated by dividing the absolute risk reduction by the absolute risk in the control group (see Table 2D-1). In our bleeding varices example, the RRR is 16.5% (the ARR) divided by 44.6% (the risk in the sclerotherapy group), or 0.37. One may also derive the RRR as (1.0 − RR). In the example, we have RRR = 1.0 − 0.63 = 0.37, or 37%. Using nontechnical language, we would say that ligation decreases the relative risk of death by 37% compared to sclerotherapy.

THE ODDS RATIO

Instead of looking at the risk of an event, we could estimate the odds of having vs not having an event. You might be most familiar with odds in the context of sporting events, when bookies or newspaper commentators quote the chances for and against a horse, a boxer, or a tennis player winning a particular event. When used in medicine, the *odds ratio (OR)* represents the proportion of patients with the target event divided by the proportion without the target event. In most instances in medical investigation, odds and risks are approximately equal—so much so that many authors calculate relative odds and then report the results as if they had calculated relative risks. The following discussion will inform clinicians who wish to understand what an odds ratio is and who wish to be alert to those circumstances when treating an odds ratio as a relative risk will be misleading.

To provide a numerical example: If 1/5 of the patients in a study suffer a stroke, the odds of their having a stroke is (1/5)/(4/5) or 0.20/0.80, or 0.25. It is easy to see that because the denominator is the same in both the top and bottom expressions, it is canceled out, leaving the number of patients with the event (1) divided by the number of patients without the event (4). To convert from odds to risk, divide the odds by 1 plus the odds. For instance, if the odds of a poor surgical outcome is 0.5, the risk is 0.5/1 + 0.5, or 0.33. Table 2D-3 presents the relationship between risk and odds. Note that the greater the magnitude of the risk, the greater is the divergence between the risk and odds.

TABLE 2D-3

Risks and Odds*

Risk	Odds
80%	4
60%	1.5
50%	1.0
40%	0.67
33%	0.50
25%	0.33
20%	0.25
10%	0.11
5%	0.053

* Risks are equal to odds / 1 + odds. Odds are equal to risk / 1 – risk.

In our example, the odds of dying in the ligation group are 18 (death) vs 46 (survival), or 18 to 46 or 18/46 (*a/b*), and the odds of dying in the sclerotherapy group are 29 to 36 (*c/d*). The formula for the ratio of these odds is (*a/c*)/(*b/d*) (see Table 2D-1); in our example, this yields (18/46)/(29/36), or 0.49. If one were formulating a terminology parallel to risk (where we call a ratio of risks a relative risk), one would call the ratio of odds a *relative odds*. Epidemiologists, who have been averse to simplifying parallel terminology, have chosen *relative risk* as the preferred term for a ratio of risks and *odds ratio* for a ratio of odds.

Clinicians have a good intuitive understanding of risk and even of a ratio of risks. Gamblers have a good intuitive understanding of odds. No one (with the possible exception of certain statisticians) intuitively understands a ratio of odds.[4,5] Nevertheless, until recently the OR has been the predominant measure of association.[6] The reason is that the OR has a statistical advantage in that it is essentially independent of the arbitrary choice between a comparison of the risks of an event (such as death) or the corresponding nonevent (such as survival), which is not true of the RR.[7]

As clinicians, we would like to be able to substitute the RR—which we intuitively understand—for the OR—which we do not understand. Looking back at our 2 x 2 table (see Table 2D-1), we see that the validity of this substitution requires that $[a/(a+b)]/[c/(c+d)]$—the RR—be more or less equal to $(a/b)/(c/d)$—the OR. For this to be the case, a must be much less than b, and c much less than d; in other words, the outcome must occur infrequently in both the treatment and the control groups. As we have noted, Table 2D-3 demonstrates that as the risk falls, the odds and risk come closer together. For low event rates, common in most randomized trials, the OR and RR are very close. The RR and OR will also be closer together when the magnitude of the treatment effect is small (that is, OR and RR are close to 1.0) than when the treatment effect is large.

When event rates are high and effect sizes are large, there are ways of converting the OR to RR.[8,9] Fortunately, clinicians will rarely need to consult such tables. To see why, consider a meta-analysis of ligation vs sclerotherapy for esophageal varices,[10] which demonstrated a rebleeding rate of 47% with sclerotherapy—as high an event rate as one is likely to find in most trials. The OR associated with treatment with ligation was 0.52—a large effect. Despite the high event rate and large effect, the RR is 0.60, which is not very different from the OR. The two are close enough—and this is the crucial point— that choosing one measure or the other is unlikely to have an important influence on treatment decisions.

RELATIVE RISK AND ODDS RATIO VS ABSOLUTE RELATIVE RISK: WHY THE FUSS?

Having decided that distinguishing between OR and RR will seldom have major importance, introducing hypothetical changes to the 2 x 2 table (see Table 2D-2) shows us why we must pay much more attention to distinguishing between the OR and RR vs the ARR. Let us assume that the number of patients dying decreased by approximately 50% in both groups. We now have nine deaths among 64 patients in liga- tion group and 14 deaths among 65 patients in the scle- rotherapy group. The risk of death in the ligation group decreases from 28% to 14%, and in the sclerotherapy group, it decreases from 44.6% to 22.3%. The RR becomes 14/22.3 or 0.63, the same as before. The OR becomes (9/55)/(14/51) or 0.60, moderately different from 0.49 and closer to the RR. The absolute risk reduction decreases quite dramati- cally from 16.5% to approximately 8%. Thus, the decrease in the proportion of those dying in both groups by a factor of two leaves the RR unchanged, results in a moderate increase in the OR, and reduces the ARR by a factor of 2. This (see Figure 2D-1) shows how the same RR can be asso- ciated with quite different ARRs—and that although the RR does not reflect changes in the risk of an adverse event without treatment (or, as in this case, with the inferior treatment), the ARR can change markedly with changes in this baseline risk.

Thus, a RR of 0.67 may represent both a situation in which a treatment reduces the risk of dying from 1% to 0.67%, or from 30% to 20% (see Figure 2D-1). Assume that the frequency of severe side effects associated with such a treatment were 10%—we might encounter this situation in offering chemotherapy to a patient with cancer, for instance. Under these circumstances we would probably not recommend the treatment to most patients if it reduced the probability of dying by 0.33% (from 1% to 0.67%), but we may well be willing to recommend this treatment if the probability of an adverse outcome drops from 30% to 20%. In the latter situation, 10 patients per 100 would benefit, whereas one would suffer adverse effects—a tradeoff that most would consider worthwhile.

The RRR behaves the same way as the RR and does not reflect the change in the underlying risk in the control population. In our example, the RRR will be of the same magnitude if the frequency of events decreases by approximately half in both groups: $(22.3 - 14)/22.3$, or 0.37.

THE NUMBER NEEDED TO TREAT

One can also express the impact of treatment by the number of patients one would need to treat to prevent an adverse event, the *number needed to treat (NNT)*.[11] Table 2D-2 shows that the risk of dying in the ligation group is 28.1%, and in the sclerotherapy group, it is 44.6%. If these estimates are accurate, treating 100 patients with ligation rather than sclerotherapy will result in between 15 and 16 patients avoiding death (the ARR, the control event rate minus the intervention event rate). If treating 100 patients results in avoiding 16 events, how many patients do we need to treat to avoid one event? The answer, 100 divided by 16, or approximately 6 (that is, 100 divided by the risk difference expressed as a percentage), is the NNT. One can also arrive at this number by taking the reciprocal of the ARR expressed as a proportion; that is, one can calculate the NNT by the formula 1/ARR (see Table 2D-1). You may see that both the NNT and the ARR change with the difference in the underlying risk—which is not surprising, because the NNT is the reciprocal of the ARR. Given knowledge of the baseline risk and relative risk reduction, a nomogram presents a third way of arriving at the NNT (see Figure 2D-2).[12]

The NNT is inversely related to the proportion of patients in the control group who suffer an adverse event. If the risk of an adverse event doubles, we need treat only half as many patients to prevent an adverse event. If the risk decreases by a factor of 4, we will have to treat four times as many people. In our example, if the frequency of events (the baseline risk) decreases by a factor of 2 while the RRR remains constant, treating 100 patients with ligation would then result in avoiding eight events (22 – 14) and the NNT would double to 12.

The NNT is also inversely related to the RRR. A more effective treatment with twice the RRR will reduce the NNT by half. If the relative risk reduction with one treatment is only a quarter of that achieved by an alternative strategy, the NNT will be four times greater. Table 2D-4 presents hypothetical data that illustrate these relationships.

FIGURE 2D-2

Nomogram for Calculating the Number Needed to Treat

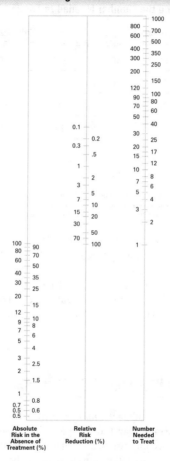

TABLE 2D-4

Relationship Between the Baseline Risk, the Relative Risk Reduction, and the Number Needed to Treat*

Control Event Rate	Intervention Event Rate	Relative Risk	Relative Risk Reduction	Risk Difference	NNT
0.02	0.01	50%	50%	0.01	100
0.4	0.2	50%	50%	0.2	5
0.04	0.02	50%	50%	0.02	50
0.04	0.03	75%	25%	0.01	100
0.4	0.3	75%	25%	0.1	10
0.01	0.005	50%	50%	0.005	200

* Relative risk is equal to the intervention event rate/control event rate; the relative risk reduction is equal to 1– relative risk; the risk difference is equal to control event rate – intervention event rate; the NNT is equal to 1 / risk difference.

Using ARR and its reciprocal, the NNT, incorporates the influence of the changing baseline risk. If all we know is the ARR or the NNT, however, we remain ignorant of the size of the baseline risk. For example, an ARR of 5% (and a corresponding NNT of 20) may represent reduction of the risk of death from 10% to 5% (a RRR of 50%) or from 50% to 45% (a RRR of 10%).

THE NUMBER NEEDED TO HARM

Clinicians can calculate the *number needed to harm* (NNH) in exactly the same way. If one expects that five of 100 patients will become fatigued when given a beta blocker, one will have to treat 20 patients to cause one to become tired, and the NNH is 20.

In this discussion we have not mentioned the problem that investigators may report odds ratios instead of relative risks. As we have mentioned, the best way of dealing with this situation when event rates are low is to assume the RR will be very close to the OR. The higher the risk, the less secure is the assumption. Tables 2D-5 and 2D-6 provide a guide for making an accurate estimate of the NNT and NNH when you know the patient's baseline risk and the investigator has provided only an odds ratio.

TABLE 2D-5

Deriving the NNT From the Odds Ratio*

Control Event Rate	Therapeutic Intervention (OR)								
	0.5	0.55	0.6	0.65	0.7	0.75	0.8	0.85	0.9
0.05	41	46	52	59	69	83	104	139	209
0.1	21	24	27	31	36	43	54	73	110
0.2	11	13	14	17	20	24	30	40	61
0.3	8	9	10	12	14	18	22	30	46
0.4	7	8	9	10	12	15	19	26	40
0.5	6	7	8	9	11	14	18	25	38
0.7	6	7	9	10	13	16	20	28	44
0.9	12	15	18	22	27	34	46	64	101

* Adapted from reference 18.

The formula for determining the NNT is:

$$NNT = \frac{1 - CER(1 - OR)}{CER(1 - CER)(1 - OR)}$$

(CER = control event rate, OR = odds ratio)

TABLE 2D-6

Deriving the NNH From the Odds Ratio*

Control Event Rate	Therapeutic Intervention (OR)								
	1.1	1.2	1.3	1.4	1.5	2	2.5	3	3.5
0.05	212	106	71	54	43	22	15	12	9
0.1	112	57	38	29	23	12	9	7	6
0.2	64	33	22	17	14	8	5	4	4
0.3	49	25	17	13	11	6	5	4	3
0.4	43	23	16	12	10	6	4	4	3
0.5	42	22	15	12	10	6	5	4	4
0.7	51	27	19	15	13	8	7	6	5
0.9	121	66	47	38	32	21	17	16	14

* Adapted from reference 18.

The formula for determining the NNH is:

$$NNH = \frac{CER(OR - 1) + 1}{CER(OR - 1)(1 - CER)}$$

(CER=control event rate, OR=odds ratio)

BACK TO THE 2 X 2 TABLE

Whichever way of expressing the magnitude of the treatment effect we choose, the 2 x 2 table reflects results at a given point in time. Therefore, our comments on RR, ARR, RRR, OR, and NNT or NNH must be qualified by imposing a time frame on them. For example, we have to say that using ligation rather than sclerotherapy resulted in absolute risk reduction of death of 17% and an NNT of 6 over a mean time of 10 months. The results could be different if the duration of observation was very short (if there was no time to develop an event) or very long (after all, if an outcome is death, after 100 years of follow-up, everybody will die).

CONFIDENCE INTERVALS

We have presented all of the measures of association of the treatment with ligation vs sclerotherapy as if they represented the true effect. The results of any experiment, however, represent only an estimate of the truth. The true effect of treatment may actually be somewhat greater—or less—than what we observed. The confidence interval tells us, within the bounds of plausibility, how much greater or smaller the true effect is likely to be (see Part 2C, "Therapy and Understanding the Results, Confidence Intervals"). Statistical programs permit computation of confidence intervals for each of the measures of association we have discussed.

SURVIVAL DATA

As we pointed out, the analysis of a 2 x 2 table implies an examination of the data at a specific point in time. This analysis is satisfactory if we are looking for events that occur within relatively short periods of time and if all patients have the same duration of follow-up. In longer-term studies, however, we are interested not only in the total number of events, but in their timing as well. For instance, we may focus on whether therapy for patients with a uniformly fatal condition (severe congestive heart failure or unresectable lung cancer, for example) delays death.

When the timing of events is important, investigators could present the results in the form of several 2 x 2 tables constructed at different points of time after the study began. For example, Table 2D-2 represented the situation after a mean of 10 months of follow-up. Similar tables could be constructed describing the fate of all patients available for analysis after their enrollment in the trial for 1 week, 1 month, 3 months, or whatever time frame we choose to examine. The analysis of accumulated data that takes into account the timing of events is called *survival analysis*. Do not infer from the name, however, that the analysis is restricted to deaths; in fact, any dichotomous outcome will qualify.

The survival curve of a group of patients describes the status of patients at different time points after a defined starting point.[13] In Figure 2D-3, we show the survival curve from the bleeding varices trial. Because the investigators followed approximately half of the patients for a longer time, the survival curve extends beyond the mean follow-up of 286 days. At some point, prediction becomes very imprecise because there are few patients available to estimate the probability of survival. Confidence intervals around the survival curves capture the precision of the estimate.

Even if the true relative risk, or relative risk reduction, is the same for each duration of follow-up, the play of chance will ensure that the point estimates differ. Ideally then, we would estimate the overall relative risk reduction by applying an average, weighted for the number of patients available, for the entire survival experience. Statistical methods allow just such an estimate. The weighted relative risk over the entire study is known as the *hazard ratio*.

FIGURE 2D-3

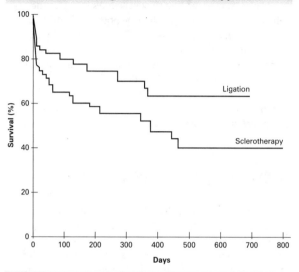

Survival Curves for Ligation and Sclerotherapy

Reproduced with permission from the Massachusetts Medical Society.

Assuming the null hypothesis (ie, that there is no difference between two survival curves), we can generate a *P* value that informs us about the likelihood that chance explains the differences in results. Statistical techniques (most commonly, the *Cox regression model*) allow the results to be adjusted or corrected for differences in the two groups at baseline (see "Part 2C, Therapy and Understanding the Results, Confidence Intervals"). If one group was older (and, thus, was at higher risk) or had less severe disease (and, thus, was at lower risk), the investigators might focus on an analysis that takes these differences into account. This, in effect, tells us what would have happened had the two groups had comparable risk factors for adverse outcome at the start of the trial.

Another way of reading survival curves is to plot the points at which a chosen percentage of the patients in each group have reached an endpoint. The difference between these points is a reflection of the delay in outcomes in the treatment group. For example, although ACE inhibitors may be associated with an up to 25% decrease in mortality in patients with postmyocardial infarction, this translates into an extra few months of life for patients in the treatment group, a result that may not appear as impressive.[14]

CASE-CONTROL STUDIES

Up to now, our examples have come from prospective randomized controlled trials. In these trials, we start with a group of patients who are exposed to an intervention and a group of patients who are not exposed to the intervention. The investigators follow the patients over time and record the frequency of events. The process is similar in observational studies termed *prospective cohort studies*, although in this study design the exposure or treatment is not controlled by the investigators. For randomized trials and prospective cohort studies we can calculate risks, absolute risk reductions, and relative risks.

In case-control studies, investigators choose or sample participants not according to whether they have been exposed to the treatment or risk factor, but on the basis of whether they have experienced a target outcome. Participants start the study with or without the event, rather than with or without the exposure or intervention. Investigators compare patients with the adverse outcome—be it stroke, myocardial infarction, or cancer—to controls who have not suffered the outcome. The usual question asked is if there are any factors that seem to be more commonly present in one of these groups than in the other group.

In one case-control study, investigators examined the question of whether sunbeds or sunlamps increase the risk of skin melanoma.[15] They identified 583 patients with melanoma and 608 controls. The control patients and the cases had similar distributions of age, sex, and residence. Table 2D-7 presents the findings for the men who participated in this study.

TABLE 2D-7

Results From a Case-Control Study Examining the Association of Cutaneous Melanoma and the Use of Sunbeds and Sunlamps*

	Exposure	Cases	Controls
Sunbeds or sunlamps	Yes	67	41
	No	210	242

* Data from reference 11.

If the information in Table 2D-7 came from a prospective cohort study or randomized controlled trial, we could begin by calculating the risk of an event in the exposed and control groups. This would not make sense in the case-control study because the number of patients who did not have melanoma was chosen by the investigators. For calculation of relative risk, we need to know the population at risk, and a case-control study does not provide this information.

The OR provides the only sensible measure of association in a case-control study. One can ask whether the odds of having been exposed to sunbeds or sunlamps among people with melanoma were the same as the odds of exposure among the control patients. In the study, the odds of exposure were

67/210 in the melanoma patients and 41/242 in the control patients. The OR is therefore (67/210)/(41/242), or 1.88 (95% CI, 1.20-2.98), suggesting an association between using sunbeds or sunlamps and developing melanoma. The fact that the confidence interval does not overlap or include 1.0 suggests that the association is unlikely to have resulted from chance.

Even if the association were not chance related, it does not necessarily mean that the sunbeds or sunlamps were the cause of melanoma. Potential explanations could include greater recollection of using these devices among people with melanoma (recall bias), longer sun exposure among these people, and different skin color; of these explanations, the investigators addressed many. To be confident that exposure to sunbeds or sunlamps was the cause of melanoma would require additional confirmatory studies.

WHICH MEASURE OF ASSOCIATION IS BEST?

As evidence-based practitioners, we must decide which measure of association deserves our focus. Does it matter? The answer is "yes." The same results, when presented in different ways, may lead to different treatment decisions.[16-20] For example, Forrow and colleagues[16] demonstrated that clinicians were less inclined to treat patients after presentation of trial results as the absolute change in the outcome compared with the relative change in the outcome. In a similar study, Naylor and colleagues[17] found that clinicians rated the effectiveness of an intervention lower when events were presented in absolute terms rather than using relative risk reduction. Moreover, effectiveness was rated lower when results were expressed in terms of NNT than when the same data were presented as relative or absolute risk reductions. The pharmaceutical industry's awareness of this phenomenon may be responsible for their propensity to present physicians with treatment-associated relative risk reductions.

Patients turn out to be as susceptible as clinicians to the mode in which results are communicated.[12, 21-23] In one study, when researchers presented patients with a hypothetical life-threatening illness, those patients were more likely to choose a treatment described in terms of relative risk reduction than in terms of the equivalent absolute risk reduction.[12]

Aware that they will perceive results differently depending on how they are presented, what are clinicians to do? We believe that the best option is to consider all of the data (either as a 2 x 2 table or as a survival analysis) and then consider both the relative and the absolute figures. As you examine the results, you will find that if you can calculate the ARR and its reciprocal, the NNT, in an individual patient, these will be most useful in deciding whether to institute treatment. The conscientious evidence-based practitioner will use all available information to formulate the likely risks and benefits for the individual patient.

References

1. Callahan CM, Dittus RS, Katz BP. Oral corticosteroid therapy for patients with stable chronic obstructive pulmonary disease: a meta-analysis. *Ann Intern Med.* 1991;114:216-223.

2. Guyatt GH, Juniper EF, Walter SD, Griffith LE, Goldstein RS. Interpreting treatment effects in randomised trials. *BMJ.* 1998;316:690-693.

3. Stiegmann GV, Goff JS, Michaletz-Onody PA, et al. Endoscopic sclerotherapy as compared with endoscopic ligation for bleeding esophageal varices. *N Engl J Med.* 1992;326:1527-1532.

4. Sinclair JC, Bracken MB. Clinically useful measures of effect in binary analyses of randomized trials. *J Clin Epidemiol*. 1994;47:881-889.

5. Sackett DL. Down with odds ratios! *Evid Based Med*. 1996; 1:164-166.

6. Laird NM, Mosteller F. Some statistical methods for combining experimental results. *Int J Technol Assess Health Care*. 1990; 6:5-30.

7. Walter SD. Choice of effect measure for epidemiological data. *J Clin Epidemiol*. 2000;53:931-939.

8. Davies HT, Crombie IK, Tavakoli M. When can odds ratios mislead? *BMJ*. 1998;316:989-991.

9. Zhang J, Yu KF. What's the relative risk? A method of correcting the odds ratio in cohort studies of common outcomes. *JAMA*. 1998;280:1690-1691.

10. Laine L, Cook D. Endoscopic ligation compared with sclerotherapy for treatment of esophageal variceal bleeding: a meta-analysis. *Ann Intern Med*. 1995;123:280-287.

11. Laupacis A, Sackett DL, Roberts RS. An assessment of clinically useful measures of the consequences of treatment. *N Engl J Med*. 1988;318:1728-1733.

12. Chatellier G, Zapletal E, Lemaitre D, Menard J, Degoulet P. The number needed to treat: a clinically useful nomogram in its proper context. *BMJ*. 1996;312:426-429.

13. Coldman AJ, Elwood JM. Examining survival data. *CMAJ*. 1979;121:1065-1068, 1071.

14. Tan LB, Murphy R. Shifts in mortality curves: saving or extending lives? *Lancet*. 1999;354:1378-1381.

15. Walter SD, Marrett LD, From L, Hertzman C, Shannon HS, Roy P. The association of cutaneous malignant melanoma with the use of sunbeds and sunlamps. *Am J Epidemiol*. 1990;131:232-243.

16. Forrow L, Taylor WC, Arnold RM. Absolutely relative: how research results are summarized can affect treatment decisions. *Am J Med*. 1992;92:121-124.

17. Naylor CD, Chen E, Strauss B. Measured enthusiasm: does the method of reporting trial results alter perceptions of therapeutic effectiveness? *Ann Intern Med*. 1992;117:916-921.

18. Hux JE, Levinton CM, Naylor CD. Prescribing propensity: influence of life-expectancy gains and drug costs. *J Gen Intern Med*. 1994;9:195-201.

19. Redelmeier DA, Tversky A. Discrepancy between medical decisions for individual patients and for groups. *N Engl J Med*. 1990;322:1162-1164.

20. Bobbio M, Demichelis B, Giustetto G. Completeness of reporting trial results: effect on physicians' willingness to prescribe. *Lancet*. 1994;343:1209-1211.

21. Malenka DJ, Baron JA, Johansen S, Wahrenberger JW, Ross JM. The framing effect of relative and absolute risk. *J Gen Intern Med*. 1993;8:543-548.

22. McNeil BJ, Pauker SG, Sox HC Jr, Tversky A. On the elicitation of preferences for alternative therapies. *N Engl J Med*. 1982;306:1259-1262.

23. Hux JE, Naylor CD. Communicating the benefits of chronic preventive therapy: does the format of efficacy data determine patients' acceptance of treatment? *Med Decis Making*. 1995;15:152-157.

APPENDIX
Calculations

Raymond Leung

IN THIS SECTION

TREATMENT AND HARM

(see *Part 1B1, "Therapy"; Part 1B2, "Harm"; Part 2B2, "Therapy and Understanding the Results, Measures of Association"*)

		Outcome	
		Present	**Absent**
Exposure/Treatment	Present	a	b
	Absent	c	d

$$\text{Controlled Event Rate (CER)} = \frac{c}{(c + d)}$$

$$\text{Experimental Event Rate (EER)} = \frac{a}{(a + b)}$$

$$\text{Relative Risk (RR)} = \frac{a/(a + b)}{c/(c + d)}$$

$$\text{Relative Risk Reduction (RRR)} = 1 - RR$$

$$= \frac{c/(c + d) - a/(a + b)}{c/(c + d)}$$

$$\text{Absolute Risk Reduction (ARR)} = \frac{c}{c + d} - \frac{a}{a + b}$$

$$\text{Number Needed to Treat (NNT)} = \frac{1}{ARR}$$

$$\text{Odds Ratio (OR)} = \frac{a/b}{c/d} = \frac{ad}{cb}$$

Deriving number needed to treat from controlled event rate and odds ratio

$$NNT = \frac{1 - CER(1 - OR)}{CER(1 - CER)(1 - OR)}$$

Deriving number needed to harm from controlled event rate and odds ratio

$$NNH = \frac{1 + CER(1 - OR)}{CER(1 - CER)(1 - OR)}$$

DIAGNOSIS

(see *Part 1C2, "Diagnostic Tests"*)

		Reference Standard	
		Positive	**Negative**
Test Result	Positive	a	b
	Negative	c	d

$$\text{True Positive} = a$$

$$\text{True Negative} = d$$

$$\text{False Positive} = b$$

$$\text{False Negative} = c$$

$$\text{Sensitivity} = \frac{a}{a + c}$$

$$\text{Specificity} = \frac{d}{b + d}$$

$$\text{Likelihood Ratio for Positive Test (LR+)} = \frac{a/(a + c)}{b/(b + d)}$$

$$\text{Likelihood Ratio for Negative Test (LR--)} = \frac{c/(a + c)}{d/(b + d)}$$

$$\text{Positive Predictive Value (PPV)} = \frac{a}{a + b}$$

$$\text{Negative Predictive Value (NPV)} = \frac{d}{c + d}$$

$$\text{Diagnostic Accuracy} = \frac{a + d}{a + b + c + d}$$

$$\text{Pretest Probability (prevalence)} = \frac{a + c}{a + b + c + d}$$

$$\text{Pretest Odds} = \frac{prevalence}{1 - prevalence} = \frac{a + c}{b + d}$$

$$\text{Posttest Odds} = \text{pretest odds} \times \text{likelihood ratio}$$

$$\text{Posttest Probability} = \text{posttest odds} / (1 + \text{posttest odds})$$

CHANCE-CORRECTED AGREEMENT: KAPPA

(see *Part 2C, "Diagnosis, Measuring Agreement Beyond Chance"*)

		Rater B's Observation	
		Present	**Absent**
Rater A's Observation	Present	a	b
	Absent	c	d

$$\text{Raw agreement} = \frac{a + d}{a + b + c + d}$$

$$\text{Kappa } (\kappa) = \frac{\dfrac{observed}{agreement} - \dfrac{expected}{agreement}}{1 - expected\ agreement}$$

$$\text{where observed agreement} = \frac{a + d}{a + b + c + d}$$

$$\text{and expected agreement} = \frac{(a + b)(a + c)}{a + b + c + d} + \frac{(c + d)(b + d)}{a + b + c + d}$$

$$\text{Odds Ratio (OR)} = \frac{ad}{bc}$$

$$\text{Phi } (\Phi) = \frac{\sqrt{OR} - 1}{\sqrt{OR} + 1} + \frac{\sqrt{ab} - \sqrt{bc}}{\sqrt{ad} + \sqrt{bc}}$$

THRESHOLD NUMBER NEEDED TO TREAT (NNT)

(see *Part 2F, "Moving From Evidence to Action, Grading Recommendations—A Quantitative Approach"*)

$$NNT_T = \frac{Cost_{target} + value_{target}}{Cost_{treatment} + \Sigma(Cost_{AE})(Rate_{AE}) + \Sigma(Value_{AE})(Rate_{AE})}$$

Where

NNT_T = the threshold number needed to treat

$Cost_{treatment}$ = the cost of treating one patient

$Cost_{target}$ = the cost of treating one target event

$Cost_{AE}$ = the cost of treating one adverse event

$Rate_{AE}$ = the proportion of treated patients who suffer an adverse event

$Value_{target}$ = the dollar value we assign to preventing one target event

$Value_{AE}$ = the dollar value we assign to preventing one adverse event

CONFIDENCE INTERVALS

(see *Part 2B2, "Therapy and Understanding the Results, Confidence Intervals"*)

For the 2 x 2 sample set:

	Column 1	Column 2	Total
Row 1	a	b	c
Row 2	c	d	m

the following confidence intervals can be calculated[1]:

	Point Estimate	Confidence Intervals	Examples
Binomial proportion	$\dfrac{a}{n}$	$\dfrac{a}{n} \pm z\sqrt{\dfrac{a(n-a)}{n^3}}$	CER, EER, Sensitivity, Specificity, PPV, NPV
Difference between 2 proportions	$\dfrac{a}{n} - \dfrac{c}{m}$	$\left(\dfrac{a}{n} - \dfrac{c}{m}\right) \pm z\sqrt{\dfrac{a(n-a)}{n^3} + \dfrac{c(m-c)}{m^3}}$	ARR
Ratio between 2 proportions	$\dfrac{a/n}{c/m}$	$\dfrac{a/n}{c/m} e^{\pm z\sqrt{\frac{1}{a} - \frac{1}{n} + \frac{1}{c} - \frac{1}{m}}}$	RR, LR+, LR−
Ratio between 2 ratios	$\dfrac{a/b}{c/d}$	$\dfrac{a/b}{c/d} e^{\pm z\sqrt{\frac{1}{a} + \frac{1}{b} + \frac{1}{c} + \frac{1}{d}}}$	OR

where $z = 1.96$ for 95% confidence intervals.

Reference

1. SAS Institute Inc. SAS OnlineDoc, Version 8. Cary, NC: SAS Institute Inc; 1999. Availiable at: http://v8doc.sas.com/sashtml/. Accessed February 21, 2001.

Glossary

Legend:

Used for indicates an alternative to the preferred term

See indicates the preferred term

See also indicates related terms

Term	Definition	See Also
Absolute Risk Increase (ARI)	Difference in the absolute risk (percentage or proportion of patients with an outcome) in the exposed vs the unexposed. Typically used with a harmful exposure.	Absolute Risk Reduction (ARR); Number Needed to Harm (NNH)
Absolute Risk Reduction (ARR)	Difference in the absolute risk (percentage or proportion of patients with an outcome) in the exposed (experimental event rate [EER]) vs the unexposed (control event rate [CER]). Use restricted to a beneficial exposure or intervention.	Absolute Risk Increase (ARI); Number Needed to Treat (NNT); Risk
Active Alternatives	See *Differential Diagnosis*	
Adjusted Analysis	An adjusted analysis takes into account differences in prognostic factors between groups that may influence the outcome. For instance, in comparison between an experimental treatment and control, if the experimental group is on average older, and thus at higher risk of an adverse outcome, than the control group, the adjusted analysis will show a larger treatment effect than the unadjusted analysis.	Cox Regression Model

Term	Definition	See Also
Alerting Systems	Alerting systems monitor a continuous signal or stream of data and generate a message (an alert) in response to items or patterns that might require action on the part of the clinician.	Reminder Systems
Algorithm	An explicit description of an ordered sequence of steps to be taken in patient care under specified circumstances.	
Allocation Concealment	Randomization is concealed if the person who is making the decision about enrolling a patient is unaware of whether the next patient enrolled will be entered in the treatment or control group. If randomization was not concealed, patients with better prognoses may tend to be preferentially enrolled in the active treatment arm resulting in exaggeration of the apparent benefit of therapy (or even falsely concluding that treatment is efficacious). Used for *Concealment*	Blind
Alpha Level	The probability of erroneously concluding there is a difference between two treatments when there is in fact no difference. Typically, investigators decide on the chance of a false positive result they are willing to accept when they plan the sample size for a study.	
Autocorrelation	Autocorrelation occurs when the likelihood of an observation is not independent of its relationship with other observations. For example, autocorrelation occurs when a "good day" for a patient with chronic disease is more likely to follow a "good day" than a "bad day."	
Baseline Risk	The risk of an adverse outcome in the control group of an experiment. Synonymous with control event rate (CER).	
Bayesian Analysis	An analysis that starts with a particular probability of an event (the prior probability) and incorporates new information to generate a revised probability (a posterior probability).	
Before-After Trial	Investigation of an intervention in which the investigators compare the status of patients before and after the intervention.	Crossover Trial

Term	Definition	See Also
Bias	A sytematic tendency to produce an outcome that differs from the underlying truth	

a) **Channeling effect or Channeling bias:** The tendency of clinicians to prescribe treatment based on a patient's prognosis. As a result of the behavior, comparisons between treated and untreated patients will yield a biased estimate of treatment effect.

b) **Data completeness bias:** Using the information system to log episodes in the treatment group and using a manual system in the non-CDSS (computer decision support system) group can create a data completeness bias.

c) **Detection bias:** The tendency to look more carefully for an outcome in one of two groups being compared.

d) **Incorporation bias:** When investigators study a diagnostic test that incorporates features of the target outcome.

e) **Interviewer bias:** Greater probing by an interviewer in one of two groups being compared.

f) **Publication bias:** Publication bias occurs when the publication of research depends on the direction of the study results and whether they are statistically significant.

g) **Recall bias:** Recall bias occurs when patients who experience an adverse outcome have a different likelihood of recalling an exposure than the patients who do not have an adverse outcome, independent of the true extent of exposure.

h) **Surveillance bias:** Synonymous with detection bias; the tendency to look more carefully for an outcome in one of two groups being compared.

i) **Verification Bias:** Results of a diagnostic test influence whether patients are assigned to a treatment group.

Used for *Work-up Bias*

Term	Definition	See Also
Blind (or Blinded or Masked)	The participant of interest is unaware of whether patients have been assigned to the experimental or control group. Patients, clinicians, those monitoring outcomes, judicial assessors of outcomes, data analysts, and those writing the paper can all be blinded or masked. To avoid confusion the term *masked* is preferred in studies in which vision loss of patients is an outcome of interest.	Allocation Concealment
Bootstrap Technique	A statistical technique for estimating parameters such as standard errors and confidence intervals based on resampling from an observed data set with replacement.	
Case Reports	Descriptions of individual patients.	
Case Series	A study reporting on a consecutive collection of patients treated in a similar manner, without a control group. For example, a surgeon might describe the characteristics of an outcome for 100 consecutive patients with cerebral ischemia who received a revascularization procedure.	Consecutive Sample
Case-Control Study	A study designed to determine the association between an exposure and outcome in which patients are sampled by outcome (that is, some patients with the outcome of interest are selected and compared to a group of patients who have not had the outcome), and the investigator examines the proportion of patients with the exposure in the two groups.	
Chance-Corrected Agreement	Of the possible agreement beyond what one would expect by chance alone, the proportion achieved.	
Channeling Effect (or Channeling Bias)	See *Bias*	
Checklist Effect	The effect on clinicians' behavior of having them record information, or their orders, using a structured data collection form.	

Term	Definition	See Also
Chi-square Test	A statistical test that examines the distribution of categorical outcomes in two groups, the null hypothesis of which is that the underlying distributions are identical.	
Clinical Prediction Rules (or Clinical Decision Rules)	A clinical prediction rule is generated by initially examining, and ultimately combining, a number of variables to predict the likelihood of a current diagnosis or a future event. Sometimes, if the likelihood is sufficiently high or low, the rule generates a suggested course of action.	
Cointerventions	Interventions other than treatment under study that may be differentially applied to experimental and control groups and, thus, potentially bias the results of a study.	
Comorbidity	Disease(s) that coexist(s) in a study participant in addition to the index condition that is the subject of the study.	
Cohort	A group of persons with a common characteristic or set of characteristics. Typically, the group is followed for a specified period of time to determine the incidence of a disorder or complications of an established disorder (prognosis).	Cohort Study
Cohort Study (or Cohort Analytic Study)	Prospective investigation of the factors that might cause a disorder in which a cohort of individuals who do not have evidence of an outcome of interest but who are exposed to the putative cause are compared with a concurrent cohort who are also free of the outcome but not exposed to the putative cause. Both cohorts are then followed to compare the incidence of the outcome of interest. Used for *Prospective Study*	Cohort; Inception Cohort
Complete Follow-up	See *Follow-up*	
Computer Decision Support Systems (CDSS)	Computer software designed to aid directly in clinical decision-making about individual patients.	

Term	Definition	See Also
Concealment	See *Allocation Concealment*	
Concepts	Concepts are the basic building blocks of theory.	
Conceptual Framework	An organization of ideas that provides a system of relationships between those ideas.	
Conditional Probabilities	The probability of a particular state, given another state. That is, the probability of A, given B – $P(A/B)$.	
Confidence Interval (CI)	Range of two values within which it is probable that the true value lies for the whole population of patients from whom the study patients were selected.	
Confounder	A factor that distorts the true relationship of the study variable of interest by virtue of also being related to the outcome of interest. Confounders are often unequally distributed among the groups being compared. Randomized studies are less likely to have their results distorted by confounders than are observational studies. Used for *Confounding Variable*	
Confounding Variable	See *Confounder*	
Consecutive Sample	A sample in which all potentially eligible patients seen over a period of time are enrolled. Used for *Sequential Sample* Case Series	
Consequentialist (or Utilitarian)	A consequentialist or utilitarian view of distributive justice would contend that even in individual decision-making, the clinician should take a broad social view in which the action that would provide the greatest good to the greatest number is favored. In this broader view, the effect on others of allocating resources to a particular patient's care would bear on the decision. An alternative to the deontological view.	

Term	Definition	See Also
Construct Validity	A construct is a theoretically derived notion of the domain(s) we wish to measure. An understanding of the construct will lead to expectations about how an instrument should behave if it is valid. Construct validity therefore involves comparisons between measures, and examination of the logical relationships, which should exist between a measure and characteristics of patients and patient groups.	
Contamination	Contamination occurs when participants in either the experimental or control group receive the intervention intended for the other arm of the study.	
Continuous Variables	A variable that can theoretically take any value and in practice can take a large number of values with small differences between them.	
Control Event Rate (CER)	See *Event Rate, Baseline Risk*	
Control Group	A group that does not receive the experimental intervention. In many studies, the control group receives either the standard of care currently delivered in the community or the best care that is available on the basis of the current evidence.	
Controlled Trial	See *Randomized Controlled Trial*	
Convenience Sample	Individuals or groups selected at the convenience of the investigator or primarily because they were available at a convenient time or place.	
Corollary Orders	Orders that are needed to detect or ameliorate adverse reactions (also called response orders).	
Correlation	The magnitude of the relationship between different variables or phenomena.	
Correlation Coefficient	A numerical expression of the strength of the relationship between two variables, which can take values from –1.0 to 1.0	

Term	Definition	See Also
Cost Analysis	If two strategies are analyzed but only costs are compared, this comparison would inform only the resource-use half of the decision (the other half being the expected outcomes) and is termed a cost analysis.	
Cost Benefit Analysis	A form of economic analysis in which both the costs and the consequences (including increases in the length and quality of life) are expressed in monetary terms.	
Cost-Effectiveness Analysis	An economic analysis in which the consequences are expressed in natural units. Some examples would include cost per life saved or cost per unit of blood pressure lowered.	
Cost Minimization Analysis	An economic analysis conducted in situations where the consequences of the alternatives are identical, and so the only issue is their relative costs.	
Cost-to-Charge Ratio	Where there is a systematic deviation between costs and charges, an economic analysis may adjust charges using a cost-to-charge ratio. The goal is to approximate real costs.	
Cost-Utility Analysis	A type of cost-effectiveness analysis in which the consequences are expressed in terms of life-years adjusted by peoples' preferences. Typically, one considers the incremental cost per incremental gain in quality adjusted life-years (QALYs).	Quality-Adjusted Life-Year (QALY)
Cox Regression Model	A regression technique that allows adjustment for known differences in baseline characteristics between experimental and control groups applied to survival data.	Adjusted Analysis
Criterion Standard	A method having established or widely accepted accuracy for determining a diagnosis, providing a standard with which a new screening or diagnostic test can be compared. The method need not be a single or simple procedure but could include follow-up of patients to observe the evolution of their conditions or the consensus of an expert panel of clinicians, as is frequently used in the study of psychiatric conditions. Used for *Gold Standard, Reference Standard*	

Term	Definition	See Also
Critiquing	When the computer evaluates a clinician's decision and generates an appropriateness rating or an alternative suggestion, the decision support approach is called critiquing.	
Crossover Trial	A study design in which all patients receive both experimental and control treatments in sequence.	Before-After Trial
Cross-Sectional Survey	The observation of a defined population at a single point in time or during a specific time interval. Exposure and outcome are determined simultaneously.	
Data Completeness Bias	See *Bias*	
Data-dredging	Searching a data set for differences between groups on particular outcomes, or in subgroups of patients, without explicit a priori hypotheses.	
Decision Aid	A tool that endeavors to present patients with the benefits and risks of alternative courses of action in a manner that is quantitative, comprehensive, and understandable.	
Decision Analysis	A systematic approach to decision making under conditions of uncertainty. It involves identifying all available alternatives and estimating the probabilities of potential outcomes associated with each alternative, valuing each outcome, and, on the basis of the probabilities and values, arriving at a quantitative estimate of the relative merit of the alternatives.	
Decision Tree	Most clinical decision analyses are built as decision trees. Articles about clinical decision analyses usually will include one or more diagrams showing the structure of the decision tree used for the analysis.	
Degrees of Freedom	A technical term in a statistical analysis that has to do with the power of the analysis. The more degrees of freedom, the more powerful the analysis.	

Term	Definition	See Also
Deontological	A deontological approach to distributive justice holds that the clinician's only responsibility should be to best meet the needs of the individual under her care. An alternative to the consequentialist or utilitarian view.	
Dependent Variable	In a regression analysis we identify predictor or independent variables and the target or dependent variable.	
Detection Bias	See *Bias*	
Determinants of Outcome	The causal factors that determine whether or not a target event will occur.	
Dichotomous Outcomes	"Yes" or "no" outcomes that either happen or do not happen, such as cancer recurrence, myocardial infarction, and death.	
Dichotomous Variable	A variable that can take one of two values, such as pregnant or not pregnant, dead or alive, having suffered a stroke or not having suffered a stroke.	
Differential Diagnosis	The set of diagnoses that can plausibly explain a patient's presentation.	
Disability-Adjusted Life-Years (DALY)	The number of years of life after downward adjustment for disabilities that patients experience.	Quality-Adjusted Life-Year (QALY)
Discriminant Analysis	A statistical technique, similar to logisitic regression analysis, that identifies variables that are associated with the presence or absence of a particular outcome.	
Dose-Dependence	Risk of an outcome increases as the quantity or the duration of exposure to the putative harmful agent increases. Used for *Dose-Response Gradient*	
Dose-Response Gradient	See *Dose-Dependence*	

Term	Definition	See Also
Downstream Costs	Costs due to resources consumed in the future and associated with clinical events that are attributable to the therapy.	
Drug Class Effects (or Class Effects)	Similar effects produced by most or all members of a class of drugs (such as beta blockers, calcium antagonists, or angiotensin converting enzyme inhibitors)	
Economic Analysis	A set of formal, quantitative methods used to compare two or more treatments, programs, or strategies with respect to their resource use and their expected outcomes.	
Economic Evaluation	Comparative analysis of alternative courses of action in terms of both their costs and consequences.	
Effect Size	The effect size is the difference in outcomes between the intervention and control groups divided by some measure of variability, typically the standard deviation.	
Efficiency	Technical efficiency is the relationship between inputs (costs) and outputs (in health, quality-adjusted life-years [QALYs]). Treatments that provide more QALYs for the same or fewer resources are more efficient. Technical efficiency is assessed using cost minimization, cost-effectiveness, and cost-utility analysis. Allocative efficiency recognizes that health is not the only goal that society wishes to pursue, so competing goals must be weighted and then related to costs. This is typically done through cost-benefit analysis.	
Endpoint	Endpoints refer to health events or outcomes that lead to completion or termination of follow-up of an individual in a trial or cohort study, for example, death or major morbidity.	Outcomes; Treatment Targets
Equivalence Studies (or Equivalence Trials)	Studies designed to determine if an intervention that has a cost (cheaper), toxicity (less toxic), or administrative (simpler to administer) advantage is equivalent in terms of its benefit to the current standard.	

Term	Definition	See Also
Event Rate	Proportion of patients in a group in whom an event is observed. Control event rate (CER) and experimental event rate (EER) are used to refer to this in control and experimental groups of patients, respectively. Used for *Experimental Event Rate (EER)*	Treatment Effects; Baseline Risk
Evidence-Based Medicine (EBM)	The conscientious, explicit, and judicious use of current best evidence in making decisions about the care of individual patients. The practice of evidence-based medicine requires integration of individual clinical expertise and patient preferences with the best available external clinical evidence from systematic research.	
Evidence-Based Practice (EBP)	See *Evidence Based Medicine*	
Evidence-Based Health Care (EBHC)	See *Evidence-Based Medicine*	
Exclusion Criteria	Criteria that render potential subjects ineligible to participate in a particular study.	
Experimental Event Rate (EER)	See *Event Rate*	
Experimental Therapy	A therapeutic alternative, often new or innovative, to standard or control therapy.	
Explode	When searching Medline, the "explode" command identifies all articles that have been indexed using a given Medical Subjects Heading (MeSH) term as well as articles indexed using more specific terms.	
Exposure	A condition to which patients are exposed (either a potentially harmful agent or a potentially beneficial one) that may impact on their health.	
Face Validity	A measurement instrument has face validity if it appears to be measuring what it is intended to measure.	

Term	Definition	See Also
False-Negative	In a treatment study, treatment is considered ineffective when it actually is effective. In a diagnosis study, the patient suffers from the target condition, but the test suggests the patient does not.	
False-Positive	In a treatment study, the treatment is deemed effective when it actually is ineffective. In a diagnosis study, the patient does not suffer from the target condition, but the test suggests the patient does.	
Feedback Effect	The impact of performance evaluations on clinicians' behavior.	
Focus Groups	Investigators use focus groups, typically gatherings of 4 to 8 people with similar background or experience, to understand their attitudes or their response to a particular situation or experience.	
Follow-up	The investigators are aware of the outcome in every patient who participated in a study.	
Generalizibility	The ability to generalize the findings of a study to a larger group of similar people.	
Gold Standard	See *Criterion Standard*	
Harm	Adverse consequences of exposure to a stimulus.	
Hawthorne Effect	Human performance that is improved when participants are aware that their behavior is being observed.	
Hazard Ratio	Investigators may compute the relative risk over a period of time, as in a survival analysis, and call it a hazard ratio, the weighted relative risk over the entire study.	
Health	A state of optimal physical, mental, and social well-being; not merely the absence of disease and infirmity (World Health Organization definition).	
Health Care Personnel	Such persons include physicians, internists and medical doctors, nurses, nurse practitioners, physician assistants, and other allied health personnel.	Health Care Professionals

Term	Definition	See Also
Health Condition	A broad term for a health state that may include diseases, disorders, syndromes, and symptoms.	Health State
Health Costs	These concern the use of health care resources (direct and indirect) and the inability to use the same resources for other worthwhile purposes (opportunity costs). Used for *Health Care Costs*	
Health Outcome	All possible changes in health status that may occur for a defined population or that may be associated with exposure to an intervention. These include changes in the length and quality of life as a result of detecting or treating disease when it is present, the false security associated with failing to detect disease when it is present, and the mislabeling associated with detecting disease when it is really absent.	
Health Professionals	All persons with health-based certification: physicians, nurses, medical doctors, physiotherapists, pharmacists, occupational therapists, respiratory technicians, and counselors.	Health Care Personnel
Health Profile	Health profiles are instruments, intended for use in the entire population (including the health, the very sick, and patients with any sort of health problem), that attempt to measure all-important aspects of Health-Related Quality of Life (HRQL).	Health-Related Quality of Life
Health State	The health condition of an individual or group over a specified interval of time (commonly assessed at a particular point in time).	
Health-Related Quality of Life	Measurements of how people are feeling or the value they place on their health state.	Health Profile
Heterogeneity	Differences between patients or differences in the results of different studies.	
Inception Cohort	A designated group of persons assembled at a common time early in the development of a specific clinical disorder (eg, at the time of first exposure to the putative cause or the time of initial diagnosis) and who are followed thereafter.	Cohort; Cohort Study

Term	Definition	See Also
Incidence	Number of new cases of disease occurring during a specified period of time; expressed as a percentage of the number of people at risk.	Prevalence
Inclusion criteria	Investigators specify the inclusion criteria to define the population who will be eligible for a study.	
Incorporation Bias	See *Bias*	
Independent Association	When a variable is associated with an outcome after adjusting for multiple other potential prognostic factors, the association is an independent association.	
Independent Variables	Explanatory or predictor variables that may be associated with a particular outcome. The term is usually used in the context of a regression analysis.	
Index Date	The date of an important event that marks the beginning of monitoring patients for the occurrence of the outcome of interest.	
Indirect Costs and Benefits	The impact of alternative patient management strategies on the productivity of the patient and others involved in the patient's care.	
Informed Consent	A potential participant's expression of willingness, after full disclosure of the implications, to participate in a study.	
Intention-to-Treat (ITT) Principle (or Intention-to-Treat Analysis)	Analyzing patient outcomes based on which group into which they were randomized regardless of whether they actually received the planned intervention. This analysis preserves the power of randomization, thus maintaining that important unknown factors that influence outcome are likely equally distributed in each comparison group.	
Interviewer Bias	See *Bias*	
Inverse Rule of 3s	A rough rule of thumb, called the inverse rule of 3s, tells us the following: If an event occurs, on average, once every "x" days, we need to observe 3x days to be 95% confident of observing at least one event.	

Term	Definition	See Also
Investigator Triangulation	Investigator triangulation requires more than one investigator to collect and analyze the raw data, such that the findings emerge through consensus between or among investigators.	
Kaplan-Meier Curve	See *Survival Curve*	
Kappa Statistic (or Weighted Kappa)	A measure of the extent to which observers achieve the possible agreement beyond any agreement expected to occur by chance alone. Kappa can take values from –1.0 to 1.0.	
Law of Multiplicative Probabilities	The law of multiplicative probabilities for independent events (where one event in no way influences the other) tells us that the probability of 10 consecutive heads can be found by multiplying the probability of a single head (1/2) 10 times over; that is, 1/2 × 1/2 × 1/2, and so on.	
Leading Hypothesis (or Working Diagnosis)	The clinician's single best explanation for the patient's clinical problem(s).	
Likelihood	See *Likelihood Ratio*	
Likelihood Functions	Functions constructed from a statistical model and a set of observed data that give the probability of that data for various values of the unknown model parameters. Those parameter values that maximize the probability are the maximum likelihood estimates of the parameters.	
Likelihood Ratio	For a screening or diagnostic test (including clinical signs or symptoms), expresses the relative likelihood that a given test would be expected in a patient with (as opposed to one without) a disorder of interest.	Used for *Likelihood*
Likert-Type Scales	Scales, typically with from 3 to 9 possible values, that include extremes of attitudes or feelings (such as from totally disagree to totally agree) and that investigators present to respondents to obtain their ratings of their responses.	Visual Analogue Scale

Term	Definition	See Also
Linear Regression	The term used for a regression analysis when the dependent or target variable is a continuous variable and the relationship between the dependent and independent variables is thought to be linear.	
Logical Operator (or Boolean Ope rators)	Words used by a search engine to perform specific tasks such as combining terms (AND/OR) or excluding terms (NOT) from the search strategy.	
Logistic Regression	A term used for a regression analysis in which the dependent or target variable is dichotomous and which uses a model that relies on logarithms.	
Longitudinal Study	See *Cohort Study*	
Lost to Follow-up	Patients whose status on the outcome or endpoint of interest is unknown.	
Marginal Utility	The change in a person's utility (preference or relative value) for an outcome as the outcome increases in magnitude.	
Masked	See *Blind*	
Matching	A deliberate process to make the study group and comparison group comparable with respect to factors (or confounders) that are extraneous to the purpose of the investigation but that might interfere with the interpretation of the studies' findings. For example, in case control studies, individual cases may be matched with specific controls on the basis of comparable age, gender, and/or other clinical features.	
Median Survival	Length of time that one half of the study population survives.	
Member Checking	Member checking involves sharing draft study findings with the participants to inquire whether their viewpoints were faithfully interpreted, to determine whether there are gross errors of fact, and to ascertain whether the account makes sense to participants with different perspectives.	

Term	Definition	See Also
Meta-Analysis	An overview that incorporates a quantitative strategy for combining the results of several studies into a single pooled or summary estimate.	
Mortality	Measure of rate of death.	
Multivariable Regression Equation	A type of regression that provides a mathematical model that explains or predicts the dependent or target variable by simultaneously considering all of the independent or predictor variables.	Multivariate Analysis
Multivariate Analysis	An analysis that simultaneously considers a number of predictor variables.	Multivariable Regression Equation
Negative Studies	Studies in which the authors have concluded that the experimental treatment is no better than control therapy.	
No Test Threshold (or Test Threshold)	The probability below which the clinician decides a diagnosis warrants no further consideration.	
N of 1 RCT	An experiment in which there is only a single participant, designed to determine the effect of an intervention or exposure on that individual.	
Nomogram	Graphical scale facilitating calculation of a probability.	
Non randomized Trial	Experiment in which assignment of patients to the intervention groups is at the convenience of the investigator or according to a preset plan that does not conform to the definition of random.	Randomized Control Trial (RCT)
Null Hypothesis	In the hypothesis-testing framework, the starting hypothesis the statistical test is designed to consider and, possibly, reject.	
Number Needed to Harm (NNH)	The number of patients who would need to be treated over a specific period of time before one adverse side effect of the treatment will occur. It is the inverse of the absolute risk increase.	Absolute Risk Increase (ARI)

Term	Definition	See Also
Number Needed to Treat (NNT)	The number of patients who need to be treated over a specific period of time to prevent one bad outcome. When discussing NNT, it is important to specify the treatment, its duration, and the bad outcome being prevented. It is the inverse of the absolute risk reduction (ARR).	Absolute Risk Reduction (AAR)
Observational Studies (or Observational Study Design)	Studies in which patient or physician preference determines whether a patient receives treatment or control.	
Odds	A ratio of probability of occurrence to nonoccurrence of an event.	
Odds Ratio (OR)	A ratio of the odds of an event in an exposed group to the odds of the same event in a group that is not exposed. Used for *Cross-Product Ratio*	Used for *Relative Odds*
Open-ended, Semi-structured, and Contrast Questions	Open-ended questions offer no specific structure for the respondent's answer. Semi-structured questions offer a limited structure for the respondent's answer.	
Opportunity Costs	The value of (health or other) benefits forgone in alternative uses when a resource is used.	
Outcomes	Changes in health status that may occur in following subjects or that may stem from exposure to a causal factor or to a therapeutic intervention.	Treatment targets; Endpoints
Overview	A type of review in which primary research relevant to a question is examined and summarized, and an effort is made to identify all available literature (published or unpublished) that pertains to that question.	Systematic Review
Palliate	Palliative care or treatment is a set of actions taken for patients in whom cure is unlikely. *Stedman's Medical Dictionary*, 27th edition, defines palliative as mitigating or reducing the severity of symptoms without reducing the underlying disease. These actions are often multiple and can include family members and significant others.	

Term	Definition	See Also
Patient Expected Event Rate	The probability of the occurrence of the endpoint or outcome of interest.	
Patient Preferences	The relative value that patients place on varying health states.	
Performance Criteria	Concerns how interventions are performed without regard to whether they should be performed. An example would be the acceptable range of results reported for reference cholesterol samples sent to clinical laboratories.	
Phase I Studies	See *Studies*	
Phase II Studies	See *Studies*	
Phase III Studies	See *Studies*	
Phase IV Studies	See *Studies*	
Phi (or Phi Statistic)	A measure of chance-independent agreement calculated by the following formula (where OR indicates odds ratio): $$\frac{\sqrt{OR}-1}{\sqrt{OR}+1}$$	
Placebo Effect	The impact of a treatment independent of its biological effect.	
Placebos	Interventions (typically a pill or capsule) without biologically active ingredients.	
Point Estimate	The results of a study which represent the best estimates of the treatment.	
Positive Study or Positive Trial	A study in which the effect of experimental intervention differs from that of the control.	
Postmarketing Surveillance Studies	See *Studies*	

Term	Definition	See Also
Posttest Odds	The odds of the target condition being present after the results of a diagnostic test are available.	
Posttest Probability	The probability of the target condition being present after the results of a diagnostic test are available.	
Power	In a comparison of two interventions, the ability to detect a difference between the two experimental if one in fact exists.	
Practice Guidelines	Guidelines are systematically developed statements to assist practitioner and patient decisions about appropriate health care for specific clinical circumstances. They are a set of statements, directions, or principles presenting current or future clinical rules or policy concerning the proper indications for performing a procedure or treatment or the proper management for specific clinical problems. Guidelines may be developed by government agencies, institutions, organizations such as professional societies or governing boards, or by the convening of expert panels.	
Predictive Value (PPV or NPV)	Two categories: Positive Predictive Value—the proportion of people with a positive test who have the disease; Negative Predictive Value—proportion of people with a negative test and who are free of disease.	
Prefiltered	By prefiltered, we mean that someone has reviewed the literature and chosen only the methodologically strongest studies.	
Pretest Odds	The odds of the target condition being present before the results of a diagnostic test are available.	
Pretest Probability	The probability of the target condition being present before the results of a diagnostic test are available.	
Prevalence	Proportion of persons affected with a particular disease at a specified time. Prevalence rates obtained from high- quality studies can inform clinicians' efforts to set anchoring pretest probabilities for their patients.	Incidence

Term	Definition	See Also
Prevent	A preventative maneuver is an action that arrests the threatened onset of disease. Primary prevention is done to stop a condition from starting. Secondary prevention stops progression of a disease or disorder when patients have a disease and are at risk for developing something related to their current disease. Very often secondary prevention is indistinguishable from treatment. An example of primary prevention is vaccination for pertussis; an example of secondary prevention is administration of an antiosteoporosis intervention to women with low bone density and evidence of a vertebral fracture to prevent	subsequent fractures.
Primary Care	Medical care provided by the clinician of first contact for the patient. Typically, the primary care physician is a general practitioner, family practitioner, primary care internist, or primary care pediatrician. Primary care may also be administered by health professionals other than physicians, notably specially trained nurses (nurse practitioners) and paramedics. Usually, a general practitioner, family practitioner, nurse practitioner, or paramedic provides only primary care services, but an individual with specialty qualifications may provide primary care, alone or in combination with referral services. Thus, it is the nature of the contact (first vs referred) that determines the care designation rather than the qualifications of the practitioner.	Referred Care
Primary Care Setting	Medical care facility that offers first contact health care only. Patients requiring specialized medical care are referred elsewhere. Some primary care centers provide a mixture of primary and referred care. Thus, it is the nature of the service provided (first contact) rather than the setting per se that distinguishes primary from more advanced levels of care.	Primary Care; Referred Care; Tertiary Care Center
Primary studies	Studies that collect original data. Primary studies are differentiated from systematic reviews that summarize the results of primary studies.	

Term	Definition	See Also
Probability	Quantitative estimate of the likelihood of a condition existing (as in diagnosis) or of subsequent events (such as in a treatment study).	P-value
Prognosis	The possible outcomes of a disease and the frequency with which they can be expected to occur.	
Prognostic Factors	Patient or study participant characteristics that confer increased or decreased risk of a positive or adverse outcome.	
Prognostic Study	A study that enrolls patients at a point in time and follows them forward to determine the frequency and timing of subsequent events.	
Prospective Study	See *Cohort Study*	
Provider Adherence or Compliance	Provider adherence or compliance refers to the extent that health care providers (physicians, nurses, etc) carry out the host of diagnostic tests, monitoring equipment, interventional requirements, and other technical specifications that define optimal patient management.	
Publication Bias	See *Bias*	
Purposive Sampling	In qualitative research, the consecutive or random selection of participants, common in quantitative research, is replaced by a conscious selection of a small number of individuals meeting particular criteria—a process called purposive sampling.	
P-value	The probability that results as or more extreme than those observed would occur if the null hypothesis were true and the experiment were repeated over and over.	Probability
Qualitative Research	Qualitative research offers insight into social, emotional, and experiential phenomena in health care.	Quantitative Research

Term	Definition	See Also
Quality Assurance	Any procedure, method, or philosophy for collecting, processing, or analyzing data that is aimed at maintaining or improving the appropriateness of health care services.	
Quality of Care	The extent to which health care meets technical and humanistic standards of optimal care.	
Quality-Adjusted Life-Expectancy	The number of years of expected life corrected for the quality of life that patients are expected to experience in those years.	
Quality-Adjusted Life-Year (QALY)	A unit of measure for survival that accounts for the effects of suboptimal health status and the resulting limitations in quality of life. For example, if a patient lives for 10 years and her quality of life is decreased by 50% because of chronic lung disease, her survival would be equivalent to 5 quality-adjusted life years.	Cost-Utility Analysis
Quantitative Research	Aims to test well-specified hypotheses concerning predetermined variables that yield numbers suitable for statistical analysis.	Qualitative Research
Random	Governed by a formal chance process in which the occurrence of previous events is of no value in predicting future events. The probability of assignment of, for example, a given participant to a specified treatment group is fixed and constant (typically 0.5), but the participant's actual assignment cannot be known until it occurs.	Randomization; Random Error
Random Error	We can never know with certainty the true value of a treatment effect because of random error. It is inherent in all measurement. The observations that are made in a study are only a sample of all possible observations that could be made from the population of relevant patients. Thus, the average value of any sample observations is subject to some variation from the true value for that entire population. When the level of random error associated with a measurement is high, the measurement is less precise and we are less certain about the value of that measurement.	Random; Random Sample

Term	Definition	See Also
Random Sample	A sample derived by selecting sampling units (eg, individual patients) such that each unit has an independent and fixed (generally equal) chance of selection. Whether or not a given unit is selected is determined by chance, for example, by a table of randomly ordered numbers.	Random; Random Error
Randomization or Random Allocation	Allocation of individuals to groups by chance, usually done with the aid of table of random numbers. Not to be confused with systematic allocation (eg, on even and odd days of the month) or allocation at the convenience or discretion of the investigator.	Random; Random Sample; Random Error
Randomized Controlled Trial	See *Randomized Trial*	
Randomized Trial	Experiment in which individuals are randomly allocated to receive or not receive an experimental preventative, therapeutic, or diagnostic procedure and then followed to determine the effect of the intervention. Used for *Controlled Trial* Used for *Randomized Controlled Trial*	Non randomized Trial
Recall Bias	See *Bias*	
Receiver Operating Characteristic (ROC) Curve	A figure depicting the power of a diagnostic test. The ROC curve presents the test's true positive rate (ie, sensitivity) on the horizontal axis and the false positive rate (ie, 1-specificity) on the vertical axis for different cut-points dividing a positive from a negative test. An ROC curve for a perfect test has an area under the curve equal to 1.0 while a test that performs no better than by chance has an area under the curve of only .5.	
Recursive Partitioning Analysis	A technique for determining the optimal way of using a set of predictor variables to estimate the likelihood of an individual experiencing a particular outcome. The technique repeatedly divides the population (eg, old vs young; among young and old, the men and the women) according to their status on variables that discriminate between those who will have the outcome of interest and those who will not.	

Term	Definition	See Also
Reference Standard	See *Criterion Standard*	
Referred Care	Medical care provided to a patient when referred by one health professional to another with more specialized qualifications or interests. There are two levels of referred care: secondary and tertiary. Secondary care is usually provided by a broadly skilled specialist such as a general surgeon, general internist, or obstetrician. Used for *Secondary Care*	Primary Care
Regression	A technique that uses predictor or independent variables to build a statistical model that predicts an individual patient's status with respect to a dependent or target variable.	
Rehabilitation	A set of actions designed to restore, following disease or injury, the ability to function in a normal or near-normal manner.	
Relative Odds	A synonym for odds ratio: a ratio of the odds of an event in an exposed group to the odds of the same event in a group that is not exposed.	
Relative Risk (RR)	Ratio of the risk of an event among an exposed population to the risk among the unexposed.	Relative Risk Reduction (RRR); Risk; Risk Ratio
Relative Risk Reduction (RRR)	An estimate of the proportion of baseline risk that is removed by the therapy, it is calculated by dividing the absolute risk reduction by the absolute risk in the control group.	Relative Risk (RR); Risk; Treatment Effect
Reliability	Refers to consistency or reproducibility of data.	Reproducibility
Reminder Systems	Reminder systems notify clinicians of important tasks that need to be done before an event occurs.	Alerting Systems
Reproducibility	Ability of a measure to yield the same result when reapplied to stable patients.	Reliability

Term	Definition	See Also
Review	A general term for all attempts to obtain and synthesize the results and conclusions of two or more publications on a given topic.	
Risk	Measure of the association between exposure and outcome (including incidence, side effects, toxicity).	Absolute Risk (AR); Absolute Risk Reduction (ARR); Relative Risk (RR); Relative Risk Reduction (RRR)
Risk Aversion	People are said to be risk averse if they would accept a fixed outcome with certainty rather than a lottery with a higher expected value. For example, they would choose $10 for sure rather than a 50/50 chance of $0 or $30.	
Risk Factors	Authors often distinguish between prognostic factors and risk factors, which are those patient characteristics associated with the development of the disease in the first place.	
Risk Ratio	A synonym for relative risk: ratio of the risk of an event among an exposed population to the risk among the unexposed.	
Screening	Services, designed to detect people at high risk of suffering from a condition associated with a modifiable adverse outcome, to be offered to persons who have neither symptoms of, nor risk factors (other than age or gender) for a target condition.	Selective Screening
Secondary Care	See *Referred Care*	
Secular Trends	Changes in the probability of events with time, independent of known predictors of outcome.	

Term	Definition	See Also
Selective Screening	Services to be offered to asymptomatic persons with one or more risk factors for a target condition, such as family history of the disease, certain personal behaviors, or membership in a population with increased prevalence of the disease.	Screening
Sensitivity	The proportion of people who truly have a designated disorder who are so identified by the test. The test may consist of, or include, clinical observations.	Sensitivity Analysis; Specificity; SnNout
Sensitivity Analysis	Any test of the stability of the conclusions of a health care evaluation over a range of probability estimates, value judgments, and assumptions about the structure of the decisions to be made. This may involve the repeated evaluation of a decision model in which one or more of the parameters of interest are varied.	
Sentinal Effect	Human performance may improve when participants are aware that their behavior is being evaluated.	
Sequential Sample	See *Consecutive Sample*	
Sequential Tests	Tests conducted in sequence, rather than simultaneously.	
Sign	Any abnormality indicative of disease, discoverable by the clinician at an examination of the patient. It is an objective aspect of a disease.	
Sign Test	A statistical hypothesis test used when an outcome is dichotomous and in which the null hypothesis is that there is an equal likelihood of either outcome occurring.	
Silo Effect	One of the main reasons for considering narrower viewpoints in conducting an economic analysis is to assess the impact of change on the main budget holders, as budgets may need to be adjusted before a new therapy can be adopted (often termed the silo effect).	

Term	Definition	See Also
SnNout	When a test with a high sensitivity is negative, it effectively rules out the diagnosis of disease.	Sensitivity
Snowball Sampling	Purposive sampling might aim to represent any of the following: typical cases, unusual cases, critical cases, cases that reflect important political issues, or cases with connections to other cases (ie, snowball sampling).	
Specificity	The proportion of people who are truly free of a designated disorder who are so identified by the test. The test may consist of, or include, clinical observations.	Sensitivity; SpPin
SpPin	When a test is highly specific, a positive result can rule in the diagnosis.	Specificity
Standard Error	The standard deviation of an estimate of a population parameter (thus, the standard error of the mean is the standard deviation of the estimate of the population mean value).	
Standard Gamble	A direct preference or utility measure that effectively asks the respondent to rate their quality of life on a scale from 0 to 1.0, where 0 is death and 1.0 is full health. The respondent chooses between a specified time x in their current health state and a gamble in which they have probability p (anywhere from 0 to .99) of full health for time x, and a probability $1 - P$ of immediate death.	
Standards	Authoritative statements of minimal levels of acceptable performance or results, excellent levels of performance or results, or the range of acceptable performance or results.	
Statistical Inference	Statistical methodologies to make deductions about underlying truth. There are two principle functions: (1) to predict or estimate a population parameter from a sample statistic, and (2) to test statistically based hypotheses.	
Statistical Significance	A result is statistically significant if the null hypothesis is rejected. That is, the probability of the observed results, given the null hypothesis, falls below an arbitrary threshold (most often .05).	

Term	Definition	See Also
Studies or Study Design	The way a drug study is organized or constructed. a) Phase I Studies: Studies that investigate a drug's physiological effect or ensure that it does not manifest unacceptable early toxicity, often conducted in normal volunteers. b) Phase II Studies: Initial studies on patients, which provide preliminary evidence of possible drug effectiveness. c) Phase III Studies: Randomized control trials designed to definitively establish the magnitude of drug benefit. d) Phase IV Studies or Postmarketing Surveillance Studies: Studies conducted after the effectiveness of a drug has been established and the drug marketed, typically to establish the frequency of unusual toxic effects.	
Surrogate Outcomes (or Substitute Endpoints or Surrogate Endpoints)	Outcomes that are not in themselves important to patients, but are associated with outcomes that are important to patients (eg, bone density for fracture, cholesterol for myocardial infarction, and blood pressure for stroke).	
Surveillance Bias	See *Bias*	
Survey	Observational or descriptive non-experimental study in which individuals are systematically examined for the absence or presence (or degree of presence) of characteristics of interest.	
Survival Analysis	An analysis that considers not only the proportion of patients who experience an outcome or endpoint, but also the time pattern of the occurrence of outcomes or endpoints.	
Survival Curve	A curve that starts at 100% of the study population and shows the percentage of the population still surviving (or free of disease or some other outcome) at successive times for as long as information is available. Used for *Kaplan Meier Curve*	

Term	Definition	See Also
Symptom	Any morbid phenomenon or departure from the normal in function, appearance, or sensation reported by the patient and indicative of disease. Symptoms are considered subjective.	
Syndrome	A collection of signs and/or symptoms and/or physiological abnormalities.	
Syndrome Diagnosis	When no reference standards exist, investigators' degree of diagnostic certainty is much lower. In these situations, known sometimes as syndrome diagnosis, diagnostic criteria usually rely on a list of clinical features required for the diagnosis.	Syndrome
Systematic Review	A critical assessment and evaluation of research (not simply a summary) that attempts to address a focused clinical question using methods designed to reduce the likelihood of bias.	Overview
Target Condition	In diagnostic test studies, the condition the investigators or clinicians are particularly interested in identifying (eg, tuberculosis, lung cancer, or iron-deficiency anemia).	
Target Outcomes (or Target Events or Target Endpoints)	In treatment studies, the condition the investigators or clinicians are particularly interested in identifying and which it is anticipated the intervention will decrease (eg, myocardial infarction, stroke, or death) or increase (eg, ulcer healing).	Cohort Study
Target-Negative	In diagnostic test studies, patients who do not have the target condition.	
Target-Positive	In diagnostic test studies, patients who do have the target condition.	
Tertiary Care	See *Referred Care*	

Term	Definition	See Also
Tertiary Care Center	A medical facility that receives referrals from both primary and secondary care levels and usually offers tests, treatments, and procedures that are not available elsewhere. Most tertiary care centers offer a mixture of primary, secondary, and tertiary care services so that it is the specific level of service rendered rather than the facility that determines the designation of care in a given study.	Referred Care; Primary Care
Test Threshold	Probability below which a clinician dismisses a diagnosis and orders no further tests.	Treatment Threshold
Theoretical Saturation (or Informational Redundancy)	The point at which iterations among data collection, analysis, and theory development yield a well-developed conceptual framework and further observations yield minimal or no new information to further challenge or elaborate the framework.	
Theory	Theory consists of concepts and their relationships.	
Theory Triangulation	Theory triangulation is a process whereby emergent findings are corroborated with existing social science theories.	
Time Series	Typically used in observational studies, time series design monitors the occurrence of outcomes or endpoints over a number of cycles and determines if the pattern changes coincident with an intervention or event.	
Treatment Effect	The results of comparative clinical studies can be expressed using various treatment effect measures. Examples are absolute risk reduction (ARR), relative risk reduction (RRR), odds ratio (OR), number needed to treat (NNT), and effect size. The appropriateness of using these to express a treatment effect and whether probabilities, means, or medians are used to calculate them depends upon the type of outcome variable used to measure health outcomes. For example, ARR, RRR, and NNT are used for dichotomous variables, and effect sizes are normally used for continuous variables.	Absolute Risk Reduction (ARR); Relative Risk Reduction (RRR); Odds Ratio (OR); Number Needed to Treat (NNT)

Term	Definition	See Also
Treatment Target	The manifestation of illness (a symptom, sign, or physiological abnormality) toward which a treatment is directed.	Endpoints; Outcomes
Treatment Threshold	Probability above which a clinician would consider a diagnosis confirmed and would stop testing and initiate treatment.	Test Threshold
Trial of Therapy	In a trial of therapy, the physician offers the patient an intervention, reviews the impact of the intervention on that patient at some subsequent time, and, depending on the impact, recommends either continuation or discontinuation of the intervention.	
Triangulation	In the course of qualitative analysis, key findings are also corroborated using multiple sources of information, a process called triangulation.	
Trigger orders	Orders in response to which the computer decision support system (CDSS) would initiate action.	Corollary Orders
Univariable Regression (or Simple Regression)	Regression where there is only one independent variable.	Regression
Up-Front Costs	Costs incurred to "produce" the treatment, such as the physician's time, nurse's time, materials, and so on.	
Utility	Patient preferences that are measured with techniques consistent with modern utility theory. Patient preferences refer to the degrees of subjective satisfaction, distress, or desirability that patients or potential patients associate with a particular health outcome. Utility theory is based on specific axioms that describe how a rational decision-maker ought to make a decision when the outcomes of that decision are uncertain. Commonly used measures of utility include the "standard gamble" or "time trade-off" techniques.	

Term	Definition	See Also
Utility Measures	Measures that provide a single number that summarizes all of Health-Related Quality of Life (HRQL) are preference- or value-weighted; these have the preferences or values anchored to death and full health and are called utility measures.	Health-Related Quality of Life (HRQL)
Utilization Review	An organized procedure carried out through committees to review admissions, duration of stay, and professional services furnished, and to evaluate the medical necessity of those services and promote their most efficient use.	
Validity	In relation to studies of diagnosis or therapy, a study is valid insofar as the results represent an unbiased estimate of the underlying truth. In relation to health-related quality of life measures, validity represents the extent to which an instrument is measuring what is intended to measure.	
Values	The basis for individual personal preferences.	
Variance	The technical term for the statistical estimate of the variability in results.	
Verification Bias	See *Bias*	
Washout Period	In a trial, the period required for the treatment to cease to act once it has been discontinued.	
Work-up Bias	See *Bias*	

CD-ROM
Installation Instructions

INSTALLATION INSTRUCTIONS FOR MICROSOFT WINDOWS

To run the hypertext *Users' Guides* on a PC, you must have a PC-compatible computer running Windows 95, 98, ME, NT, or 2000; a CD-ROM drive; and Microsoft Internet Explorer 4 or later installed. To run the program, follow these steps:

1. Insert the CD-ROM into your CD-ROM drive. The setup program will run automatically. If it does not, continue to Step 2.

2. Click START, select RUN, select BROWSE, and select your CD-ROM drive.

3. Select the setup.exe file form the CD-ROM and click OK or RUN.

4. Follow the instructions provided by the *Users' Guides* setup program.

A hypertext version of the *Users' Guides*, with links to an Adobe Acrobat navigable version, will appear on your computer hard drive, and a shortcut to the *Users' Guides* will be placed on your Windows desktop.

INSTALLATION INSTRUCTIONS FOR MACINTOSH COMPUTERS

To run the read-only, PDF navigable version of the *Users' Guides* on a Macintosh, you must have a CD-ROM drive and Adobe Acrobat Reader software, version 4 or more recent, installed. If you do not have Adobe Acrobat Reader, a current version can be obtained from the Adobe Web site at www.adobe.com. Once you have Adobe Acrobat Reader installed, follow these steps:

1. Insert the CD-ROM into your CD-ROM drive.

2. Click the CD icon that appears on your desktop to open the CD-ROM.

3. Open the Mac folder.

4. Click start.pdf to open the read-only, PDF navigable version of the *Users' Guides*.

Index